Assessing and Treating Behavioral Addictions

Rommel Johnson
University of Texas Rio Grande Valley, USA

Reuben Mwangi
Central Michigan University, USA

IGI Global
Scientific Publishing
Publishing Tomorrow's Research Today

Vice President of Editorial Melissa Wagner
Director of Acquisitions Mikaela Felty
Director of Book Development Jocelynn Hessler
Production Manager Mike Brehm
Cover Design Jose Rosado

Published in the United States of America by
IGI Global Scientific Publishing
701 East Chocolate Avenue
Hershey, PA, 17033, USA
Tel: 717-533-8845
Fax: 717-533-7115
Website: https://www.igi-global.com E-mail: cust@igi-global.com

Library of Congress Cataloging-in-Publication Data

Names: Johnson, Rommel, 1979- editor | Mwangi, Reuben, 1963- editor
Title: Assessing and treating behavioral addictions / edited by Rommel Johnson, Reuben Mwangi.
Description: Hershey, PA : IGI Global Scientific Publishing, [2026] | Includes bibliographical references and index. | Summary: "This book delves into the multifaceted world of behavioral addictions, exploring their significance, symptoms, and treatment options. It provides a comprehensive overview of various forms of behavioral addiction, including gambling, gaming, shopping, love and romance, sex and pornography and social media use, examining how these behaviors can become compulsive and interfere with daily life creating distress for individuals, relationships and families"-- Provided by publisher.
Identifiers: LCCN 2025007602 (print) | LCCN 2025007603 (ebook) | ISBN 9798337305189 hardcover | ISBN 9798337305196 paperback | ISBN 9798337305202 ebook
Subjects: LCSH: Compulsive behavior--Diagnosis | Compulsive behavior--Treatment
Classification: LCC RC533 .A857 2025 (print) | LCC RC533 (ebook)
LC record available at https://lccn.loc.gov/2025007602
LC ebook record available at https://lccn.loc.gov/2025007603

British Cataloguing in Publication Data
A Cataloguing in Publication record for this book is available from the British Library.

Table of Contents

Detailed Table of Contents

Internet addiction (IA) is a growing public health concern, particularly among adolescents and those with psychological vulnerabilities. As digital connectivity expands, excessive internet use is linked to social isolation, mental health issues, and cognitive impairment. This chapter explores the demographic, psychological, and environmental factors contributing to IA, emphasizing impulsivity, emotional distress, and social influences. It examines IA's neurobiological basis, drawing parallels with substance use disorders, focusing on dopamine dysregulation and reward processing. Cultural perspectives show how societal norms and technology access shape IA prevalence. Peer pressure, family dynamics, and socioeconomic disparities are analyzed as risk factors. Effective treatments are reviewed, including cognitive-behavioral therapy (CBT), motivational interviewing (MI), family therapy, and exercise-based interventions. The chapter highlights relapse prevention, advocacy, and policy recommendations to promote responsible technology use and support affected individuals.

This chapter explores the impact of problematic social media use on mental wellbeing, examining its diverse effects across various age groups and demographics, including individuals with disabilities. It synthesizes empirical research and practical insights and intends to create awareness regarding the detriments of excessive social media engagement, while also offering effective strategies for treatment and intervention. The chapter delves into the symptoms of social media addiction, like excessive use and withdrawal, and outlines treatment options, including Cognitive Behavioral Therapy (CBT), group therapy, and the promotion of digital literacy. By integrating robust case studies, empirical research, and relevant statistical analyses, this chapter aims to clarify the underlying issues surrounding problematic social media use, highlight its varied implications, and propose effective strategies for treatment and intervention.

This chapter explores Gaming Disorder (GD) and its impact on adolescents. GD is defined as a condition in which excessive gaming negatively affects various life aspects (American Psychiatric Association, 2023). The chapter identifies key sources for recognizing GD symptoms, which can aid practitioners (American Psychiatric Association, 2023). It examines the prevalence of GD among adolescents, highlighting contributing factors like stress, family dynamics, and mental health conditions such as depression and ADHD (Gao et al., 2022). Emphasizing the importance of therapists understanding the gaming world of adolescents, it discusses how gaming practices can lead to addiction, thus guiding effective treatment (Van der Schyff et al., 2023). The chapter outlines strategies for parents to prevent GD (Young, 2009) and highlights effective counseling techniques for practitioners (Kim & Chun, 2022). Lastly, it promotes healthy gaming practices, helping adolescents engage in gaming more balanced and healthfully (Educational Advancement, 2022).

Addiction is not having control over doing something to the extent that it is harmful to an individual. Recent studies show pornographic addiction can also lead to such compulsivity in behavior. The technological advancements and long quarantine period of the COVID-19 pandemic have caused a significant increase in the user base of pornographic materials. It is estimated that about 74% of men and 41% of women watch porn. The purpose of this study is to examine the consequences of pornographic addiction on the life of an individual. This is a systematic review paper and it is based on data collected from Research Papers Existing literature on pornographic addictions shows that it can lead to impairments in the psychological well-being (Feelings of loneliness, frustration, guilt,t, etc.) of an individual. Additionally, it can lead to depression, stress disorders, mood disorders, etc. Pornographic addiction also hampers one's ability to sustain good social relationships. Moreover, it was also reported by previous studies that pornography hurts the sexual life of an individual.

use, and other psychiatric issues. The chapter also highlights cultural considerations and concludes with advocacy goals, and proposals for further research.

Preface

OVERVIEW

Behavioral addictions encompass a wide range of maladaptive behaviors that are both phenomenologically and neurobiologically distinct from substance-related disorders, necessitating greater attention and a nuanced understanding in the field of behavioral health care. Despite the long-standing acknowledgment of substance use disorders, the increasing prevalence of behavioral addictions poses unique clinical challenges, particularly in accurately identifying, differentiating, and effectively intervening in these compulsive patterns. Given their significant incidence and frequent comorbidity with various psychiatric conditions, it is likely that mental health practitioners will encounter clients whose functional impairments are primarily due to behavioral addiction phenomena.

Authored by an international consortium of thirty researchers, clinicians, and scholars—both within and outside the traditional boundaries of addiction and behavioral health fields—this book explores the multifactorial landscape of behavioral addictions. The text provides a detailed examination of several prominent forms, including internet addiction, problematic social media engagement, gaming disorder, pornography addiction, compulsive purchasing, and exercise dependency, analyzing how these behaviors can evolve into compulsive, maladaptive patterns that profoundly disrupt individual functioning and destabilize relational and familial dynamics.

Through an integrative approach that includes critical literature reviews, case studies, expert testimonies, and cutting-edge empirical research, this volume outlines the psychological, social, and neurobiological factors underlying these disorders. Each chapter emphasizes not only the psychosocial and neurofunctional effects on individuals and their networks but also suggests practical, evidence-based strategies for early detection, preventive actions, and therapeutic interventions. By promoting a thorough understanding of the complexities of behavioral addiction, this work aims to provide behavioral health professionals with the crucial knowledge and teaching tools needed to improve clinical awareness, enable targeted support, and advocate for innovative, community-level treatment models.

Fit In Today's World

In the contemporary landscape, behavioral addictions have become increasingly prominent, reflecting broader societal shifts driven by digital technology, the proliferation of social media, and changing cultural norms around consumption and fitness. Despite a longstanding recognition of substance use disorders, the rising prevalence and complexity of behavioral addictions—such as internet use, social media engagement, gaming, pornography, compulsive shopping, and exercise—highlight critical challenges in diagnosis, differentiation, and treatment within behavioral health care. As these maladaptive behaviors frequently co-occur with other psychiatric conditions and significantly impair individual functioning and social relationships, understanding their multifaceted neurobiological, psychological, and social foundations is essential. This evolving phenomenon underscores the importance of a nuanced, multidisciplinary approach to training and intervention strategies for mental health practitioners, emphasizing early detection, prevention, and community-based treatment to effectively address these pervasive issues in today's interconnected, digitally driven society.

Target Audience

By integrating empirical research with practical applications, this volume aims to enhance the skills of a wide variety of professionals in the behavioral health field. The intended audience for this introductory and intermediate-level resource includes behavioral health professionals, addiction counselors, addiction medicine physicians, nurse practitioners, physician assistants, clinicians, researchers, residents, fellows, students, parents, and policymakers. Its primary objective is to provide a comprehensive understanding of behavioral addictions while fostering a more profound commitment to developing essential competencies in this vital area of behavioral health practice.

CHAPTER DESCRIPTION AND SUMMARY

Chapter 1: Neurobiological Mechanisms and Therapeutic Interventions in Behavioral Addictions

This introductory chapter examines the neurobiological mechanisms underlying behavioral addictions, including gambling, internet/gaming, and food addiction. It highlights the role of dopaminergic pathways, neurotransmitter imbalances, and neural circuits involved in reward processing and impulse control. The chapter discusses diagnostic methods, psychometric tools, and neuroimaging techniques used to understand these addictions. It also reviews treatment options, including Cognitive Behavioral Therapy (CBT), mindfulness practices, and pharmacological interventions. In addition, the chapter addresses associated challenges like stigma, co-occurring mental health conditions, and high relapse rates. Furthermore, it emphasizes prevention strategies, including education, community support, and industry regulation, to mitigate the societal impact of behavioral addictions. Lastly, the chapter explores future directions in personalized medicine, genetic research, and digital tools for intervention. By integrating neuroscience, clinical practice, and public health perspectives, it aims to provide a comprehensive foundation for understanding and managing these complex conditions.

Chapter 2: Unraveling Internet Addiction: Clinical Perspectives, Implications, and Interventions

This chapter examines internet addiction (IA) as a growing concern driven by technological advancements and the internet's deep integration into daily life. It defines IA as compulsive behavior leading to negative impacts on personal, social, educational, and occupational functioning. The chapter highlights symptoms such as withdrawal, increased tolerance, and continued use despite adverse consequences. It notes that while IA is not formally recognized in the DSM-5 (though internet gaming disorder is), it is acknowledged as a public health issue in some countries, with the COVID-19 pandemic worsening the problem. Understanding IA's impact is crucial for interventions, policymaking, and promoting healthier lifestyles. Furthermore, the chapter delves into cognitive and behavioral indicators of IA, including compulsive internet use, withdrawal symptoms, and the tendency to prioritize online engagement over real-life responsibilities. Cultural and societal influences significantly shape IA's perception and prevalence, as differing cultural norms and attitudes play a role. Specific vulnerable populations, such as adolescents and those with pre-existing psychological conditions, are examined. The chapter further explores the neurobiological aspects of IA, focusing on dopamine dysregulation and altered brain activity, and highlights various treatment approaches, including CBT, Motivational Interviewing (MI), family-centered therapy, and exercise-based interventions.

Chapter 3: Exploring the Digital Abyss: The Consequences of Problematic Social Media Use on Mental Wellbeing

This chapter explores the pervasive impact of problematic social media use on mental well-being across diverse populations. It examines the phenomenon of social media addiction and its symptoms, including excessive use, withdrawal, cravings, and emotional sensitivity, along with associated risks such as social isolation, body image problems, sleep disturbances, and cyberbullying. The chapter examines how various age groups—adolescents, adults, and older adults—experience these challenges, using case studies to illustrate the distinct difficulties they encounter. It emphasizes that social media's design can be inherently addictive, stimulating reward systems in the brain and perpetuating a cycle of validation-seeking and negative emotions. The chapter then discusses various treatment options.

These include self-help strategies such as setting time limits and practicing mindfulness, CBT to address distorted thinking, group therapy to combat isolation, and digital literacy training to enhance critical thinking and evaluation skills. It highlights the importance of preventive measures, such as educational initiatives in schools and formal guidelines in the workplace, to promote responsible social media use. The chapter calls for continued research to understand the long-term effects of problematic social media use, particularly within rapidly evolving technologies. It emphasizes the need for targeted interventions for marginalized communities. Ultimately, the chapter advocates for a balanced approach to online engagement, prioritizing mental well-being and fostering an online environment that promotes mental health and encourages positive human connections.

Chapter 4: Gaming Disorder and Its Impact on Adolescents' Mental Health

This chapter provides an overview of Gaming Disorder (GD), also known as Internet Gaming Disorder (IGD), highlighting its definition, controversies, and recognition by the WHO as a mental health condition. It discusses the prevalence among adolescents, noting both potential benefits and negative impacts such as sleep issues, bullying, and academic decline, while emphasizing the importance for therapists to understand gaming behaviors, mechanics, and psychological factors driving addiction. It also examines the neurological effects of GD, which are comparable to substance use disorders, and explores long-term consequences on sleep, nutrition, social interactions, and academic performance. Risk factors, including stress, psychological issues, and family challenges, are underscored, along with societal stigmas. The chapter reviews global regulations, especially China's restrictions, and the pandemic's role in increasing gaming. Finally, it presents assessment approaches and practical interventions, including counseling techniques and parental strategies to promote healthy gaming habits.

Chapter 5: Intra-Interpersonal Consequences of Pornographic Addiction in Youth

This chapter delivers a comprehensive exploration of pornographic addiction, focusing on its increasing prevalence and detrimental impacts, especially on vulnerable youth and adolescents. Beginning with definitions and historical context, it outlines how technological advancements have fueled accessibility, contributing to its transformation from a discreet commodity to a pervasive online phenomenon. The chapter emphasizes that easy accessibility, affordability, and anonymity (AAA) contribute to the compulsive consumption patterns, turning casual engagement into problematic addiction. The core of the chapter explores the specific consequences of pornographic addiction, detailing both intrapersonal and interpersonal effects such as psychological distress, including guilt, irritability, stress, and depression, as well as cognitive changes impairing focus, memory, and emotional regulation. The chapter discusses the neurological underpinnings of addiction, explaining how pornography affects the brain's reward system, leading to increased impulsivity and decreased executive control. It also notes that exposure to pornography distorts expectations about consent, gender roles, and sexual performance. The role of society is touched upon, which then leads to limited treatment options, including the importance of CBT. The chapter concludes by advocating for further research to understand better and address pornographic addiction and by providing recommendations for supporting individuals, including promoting awareness among parents, teachers, and policymakers.

Chapter 6: Unraveling Compulsive Buying Disorder- A Comprehensive Review of the Causes, Impact, and Treatment of Compulsive Buying Disorder

This chapter provides an overview of Compulsive Buying Disorder (CBD), a behavioral addiction affecting 2-8% of the population, especially women and youth. Characterized by uncontrollable shopping despite adverse consequences, CBD involves psychological factors like impulsivity, low self-esteem, and stress, as well as neurobiological mechanisms similar to substance addiction, involving brain regions linked to dopamine pathways. Sociocultural influences, including materialism, gender roles, digital marketing, and easy credit, contribute to its development. Treatment strategies discussed include CBT, Motivational Interviewing, and Acceptance and Commitment Therapy (ACT), with CBT being the most supported by research. Pharmacological options and support groups are also considered, but relapse remains a challenge. The chapter emphasizes the need for standardized diagnosis, integrated treatment approaches, and further research into neurological and behavioral factors, as well as financial literacy to reduce compulsive buying behaviors.

Chapter 7: Exercise Addiction

This chapter examines exercise addiction (EA) and tracks its evolution from a beneficial activity to a recognized behavioral disorder. It defines EA as a compulsive pattern characterized by a loss of control, dependence, and negative consequences while highlighting the absence of formal diagnostic criteria. Prevalence varies by demographics: men are more prone to experience primary EA related to performance, while women often develop secondary EA associated with body dissatisfaction and eating disorders. The neurobiological basis includes brain reward systems, tolerance, cravings, and withdrawal, with psychological factors such as impulsivity and distorted thoughts also playing a role. Comorbidities like anxiety and depression can exacerbate EA. Social and environmental influences comprise family dynamics, media exposure, societal pressures, and the increasing presence of fitness apps that reinforce certain ideals. Treatment approaches, including CBT, rational-emotive behavior therapy (REBT), and mindfulness, are discussed along with limited pharmacological options. The chapter emphasizes the importance of assessment, awareness campaigns, and further research to develop standardized diagnostic criteria and interdisciplinary interventions, especially given EA's connection to other conditions like eating disorders.

CONCLUSION AND IMPACT

This comprehensive volume significantly advances the field of behavioral health by systematically clarifying the complex and multifaceted nature of behavioral addictions. By integrating empirical research, neurobiological insights, and practical intervention strategies, the book provides a strong framework for understanding a diverse range of behavioral disorders—from internet and social media addiction to gaming, pornography, compulsive buying, and exercise dependence. Its multidisciplinary approach addresses the biological, psychological, and social dimensions of these conditions, offering clinicians, researchers, and policymakers essential tools for early detection, prevention, and customized treatment.

By highlighting the prevalence, neurobiological mechanisms, societal influences, and therapeutic options for behavioral addictions, this work fills vital gaps in the current literature, particularly the need for standardized diagnostic criteria and integrated intervention models. Moreover, its international perspective and inclusion of cutting-edge research foster a global understanding of these pervasive issues. Ultimately, this book catalyzes ongoing research, informed clinical practice, and policy development, shaping a more nuanced and practical approach to behavioral addictions. In doing so, it significantly enriches the academic discourse and practical strategies within the evolving landscape of behavioral health.

Chapter 1

Neurobiological Mechanisms and Therapeutic Interventions in Behavioral Addictions

Jawad Laadraoui
https://orcid.org/0000-0002-9784-1265
Faculty of Sciences, Hassan II University, Casablanca, Morocco

Mehdi Aitlarradia
Ministry of Health and Social Protection, Beni Mellal, Morocco

Khadija Oubella
https://orcid.org/0000-0003-1943-9454
Faculty of Sciences, University Cadi Ayyad, Marrakech, Morocco

Fatimzahra Agouram
https://orcid.org/0000-0002-8073-2126
Faculty of Sciences, University Cadi Ayyad, Marrakech, Morocco

Sara Oufquir
Faculty of Sciences, University Cadi Ayyad, Marrakech, Morocco

Abdelfatah Ait Baba
https://orcid.org/0000-0002-5650-3868
Independent Researcher, Morocco

Hamid Kabdy
https://orcid.org/0009-0004-7438-3638
Faculty of Sciences, University Cadi Ayyad, Marrakech, Morocco

Bilal El-Mansoury
https://orcid.org/0000-0002-2583-7515
Royal College of Surgeons in Ireland, Ireland & University of Medicine and Health Sciences, Dublin, Ireland

ABSTRACT

Behavioral addictions, including gambling, internet/gaming, and food addiction, profoundly affect individuals and society. This chapter examines their neurobiological underpinnings, highlighting dopaminergic pathways, neurotransmitter imbalances, and the neural circuits involved in reward processing and impulse control.

DOI: 10.4018/979-8-3373-0518-9.ch001

It covers diagnostic methods, psychometric tools, and neuroimaging, and reviews treatments such as Cognitive Behavioral Therapy, mindfulness, and pharmacological interventions. Stigma, comorbidities, and relapse risks are addressed, alongside prevention strategies emphasizing education, community support, and regulation. Future directions focus on personalized medicine, genetic and epigenetic research, and digital tools for intervention. By integrating neuroscience, clinical practice, and public health, this chapter offers a comprehensive foundation for understanding and managing behavioral addictions.

1. INTRODUCTION

Behavioral addictions, also known as non-substance addictions, refer to compulsive engagement in certain behaviors that can lead to significant impairment or distress. These behaviors activate the brain's reward system in ways similar to substance-based addictions, resulting in a cycle of craving, reinforcement, and loss of control (Jawad et al., 2019; Grant et al., 2010). The distinction between behavioral and substance-based addictions is a topic of ongoing research and debate. While both share core characteristics, including impaired control, continued engagement despite adverse effects, and withdrawal symptoms, the primary difference lies in the consumption of psychoactive substances, such as alcohol or drugs in substance-based addictions (American Psychiatric Association, 2013). In contrast, behavioral addictions revolve around activities that can be engaging and rewarding, such as gambling, internet use, gaming, or excessive shopping (Potenza, 2014; Ricciutti et al., 2024).

The scope of behavioral addictions is broad and multifaceted, raising important questions regarding diagnosis, treatment, and societal impact. As technology evolves and digital behaviors proliferate, concerns over conditions such as internet gaming disorder and social media addiction have come to the forefront of clinical and public health discussions (Lemmens et al., 2023). Understanding the definition and scope of behavioral addictions is crucial for developing effective therapeutic approaches and for promoting awareness among individuals, families, and professionals. Recent research has begun to explore the neurobiological underpinnings common to both substance abuse and behavioral addictions, revealing similar pathways in the brain that reinforce compulsive behavior (Uhl et al., 2019; İzci et al., 2022; Su et al., 2024). While both types of addictions share common features, including neurobiological pathways and psychological triggers, their assessment, progression, and recovery processes may differ significantly (Chen et al., 2017).

Research suggests that behavioral addictions affect millions of people worldwide, with a recent study estimating that approximately 1.5 billion individuals engage in addictive behaviors (Kuss & Griffiths, 2017). Behavioral addictions, such as internet addiction disorder (IAD), online gaming disorder, and social media addiction, are particularly prevalent among young people and adolescents. One study revealed a 24% increase in adolescents meeting IAD criteria between 2008 and 2018 (Kuss & Griffiths, 2017).

The societal impact of behavioral addictions is far-reaching, with individuals experiencing significant consequences, including mental and physical health problems, impaired social relationships, and reduced productivity (Billieux et al., 2015; Kuss & Griffiths, 2017). Internet addiction is linked to negative mental health outcomes, some argue that moderate internet use can foster social connections and provide support, potentially alleviating feelings of depression in certain contexts. Meta-analyses reveal a strong correlation between internet addiction and depression among adolescents, indicating a significant relationship between problematic internet use and depressive symptoms (Soriano-Molina et al., 2024; Zhang et al., 2024). Additionally, it is associated with suicidal ideation and attempts, particularly when depression is not controlled (He et al., 2024). Furthermore, behavioral addictions impose significant economic and social costs, affecting not only the individuals but also their families, friends, and community (Su et al., 2024).

2. NEUROBIOLOGICAL BASIS OF BEHAVIORAL ADDICTIONS

2.1. Role of the reward system (dopaminergic pathways).

The reward system plays a crucial role in regulating behaviors driven by pleasure and reinforcement. It enables the brain to associate certain stimuli or actions with pleasurable sensations, thereby encouraging the repetition of rewarding behaviors (Sayin, 2019). This mechanism is fundamental for vital activities such as feeding, reproduction, and learning, contributing to survival and adaptation (Schultz, 2015).

Dopamine (DA), the main neurotransmitter of this system, acts as a chemical signal that marks reward or its anticipation. When a pleasurable stimulus is perceived, neurons in the ventral tegmental area (VTA) release DA to key regions such as the nucleus accumbens (NAc) and the prefrontal cortex (PFC) (Chakravarthy et al., 2018). This process reinforces rewarding behaviors, influences decision-making, and motivates individuals to actively seek similar experiences (Panksepp and Wilson, 2016). Additionally, DA plays a role in reinforcement learning by strengthening neural connections between behaviors and outcomes, contributing to the formation of habits and social behaviors (Subramanian et al., 2022).

Figure 1. Primary dopaminergic pathways governing the brain's reward system. The mesolimbic pathway (highlighted in red) and mesocortical pathway (depicted in blue) are central to mediating reward processing and motivational behaviors (Ferrer-Pérez et al., 2024).

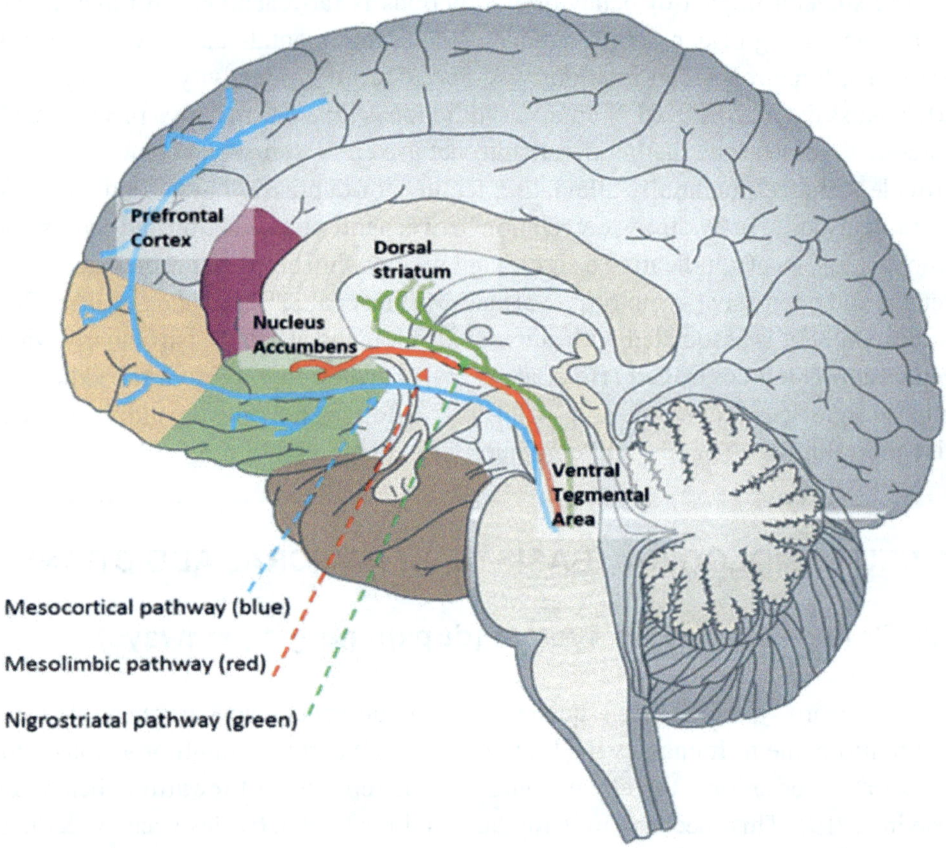

2.2. Neurotransmitter imbalances and their impact.

Neurotransmitter imbalances play a central role in influencing motivation, emotion regulation, and impulse control (Ghallab and Elassal, 2024). These alterations particularly affect the reward system, cognitive control circuits, and decision-making processes, promoting maladaptive behaviors such as behavioral addictions (Peng et al., 2025).

2.2.1. Role of Dopamine in Behavioral Addictions

Dopamine, a key player in the reward system, is involved in responses to addictive stimuli. In cases of behavioral addictions, excessive DA release in the NAc reinforces behaviors associated with these stimuli, generating pleasurable sensations that motivate their repetition (Volkow et al., 2017). However, this chronic overactivation often leads to a reduction in dopaminergic responses to natural rewards, promoting compulsive reward-seeking through the addictive activity despite its negative consequences (Ferrer-Pérez et al., 2024).

Imbalances in the dopaminergic system are also at the core of numerous neuropsychiatric and neurodegenerative disorders (Chanda and Surepalli, 2019), such as Parkinson's disease, characterized by the progressive loss of dopaminergic neurons in the substantia nigra, leading to motor deficits such as bradykinesia, tremors, and rigidity (Lee, 2023); depression, often associated with reduced DA release in the mesolimbic system (Belujon and Grace, 2017); and schizophrenia, particularly negative symptoms like apathy and reduced social interactions, linked to altered dopaminergic receptor function in the PFC (Singh et al., 2020).

2.2.2. Impact of Glutamate/GABA Imbalances

In parallel, imbalances between glutamate (neuronal excitation) and GABA (neuronal inhibition) contribute to loss of control and impulsive behaviors (Sears and Hewett, 2021). Excessive glutamatergic activity can exaggerate reward system responses, reinforcing addictive habits, while a GABA deficit weakens inhibitory mechanisms necessary to suppress these behaviors (Volkow et al., 2019).

2.3. Neural circuits implicated in impulse control and decision-making.

Complex neural circuits that balance immediate gratification with long-term consequences, playing a key role in impulse control and decision-making, regulate human behavior (Bickel et al., 2018).

These processes are primarily governed by interactions between the PFC, limbic structures (such as the amygdala), and the striatum, forming a complex network that regulates emotional responses and motivated actions (Pessoa, 2017; Šimić et al., 2021).

The PFC, particularly the ventromedial and dorsolateral regions, is central to cognitive control and impulse regulation. It is responsible for evaluating available options, predicting consequences, and inhibiting inappropriate automatic responses (Firat, 2019). In decision-making situations, the PFC communicates with the striatum, which integrates reward signals to modulate behavior (Goulet-Kennedy et al., 2016). Dysfunction in this circuit, such as prefrontal hypoactivity, can lead to impaired impulse inhibition, promoting impulsive behaviors (Li et al., 2020).

Limbic structures, such as the amygdala and hippocampus, also play a key role in integrating emotional and contextual signals into the decision-making process (Rolls, 2019; Kumar and Jha, 2024). The amygdala is particularly involved in responses to emotional stimuli, influencing short-term decisions under the effect of emotions (Gongora et al., 2019).

When the connection between limbic circuits and the PFC is disrupted, as seen in impulsivity disorders or behavioral addictions, decisions become more influenced by immediate emotions rather than a rational evaluation of long-term consequences (Hultman et al., 2016). These dysfunctions illustrate how impairments in neural circuits governing impulse control and decision-making can lead to maladaptive or risky behaviors (Dalley and Ersche, 2019).

Dopaminergic neurons project to various brain regions, forming several major pathways involved in impulse control and decision-making (Chakravarthy et al., 2018). The Nigrostriatal Pathway consists of neurons from the A9 group, located in the substantia nigra pars compacta (SNc), which project to the dorsal striatum and play a central role in motor control and goal-directed behaviors such as reward-related learning and cognition (Collins and Saunders, 2020; Young, 2023). The Mesolimbic and Mesocortical Pathways originate from A10 neurons in the VTA, extending to the nucleus NAc, PFC, and other limbic regions (Renard et al., 2018; Baik, 2020), where they regulate positive and negative reinforcement, incentive salience, aversion-related behaviors, and decision-making (Baik, 2020). The Tuberoinfundibular Pathway, located in the hypothalamus (A12 and A14 neurons), projects to the pituitary gland and regulates hormone synthesis and release, particularly prolactin (Lechan and Toni, 2016; Qi-Lytle et al., 2023). Imbalances in these pathways contribute to various neuropsychiatric and neurodegenerative disorders. For example, Parkinson's disease results from dopaminergic neuron degeneration in the nigrostriatal pathway, leading to motor deficits such as bradykinesia, tremors, and rigidity (Lee, 2023). Depression is often associated with reduced DA release in the mesolimbic system (Belujon and Grace, 2017), while schizophrenia, particularly its negative symptoms like apathy and reduced social interactions, is linked to dopaminergic receptor dysfunction in the PFC (Singh et al., 2020). Across species, including rodents, primates, and humans, dopaminergic neurons are identifiable by their immunohistochemical reactivity to tyrosine hydroxylase (TH), a rate-limiting enzyme in DA synthesis (Vecchio, 2016; Johnson et al., 2018). Although the distribution of dopaminergic neurons varies, the A9 and A10 populations dominate, accounting for approximately 95% of dopaminergic neurons, with A9 neurons being more predominant in primates and humans (German and Manaye, 1993; Baik, 2020).

Trauma, particularly in early life, can dysregulate stress response systems and alter dopaminergic pathways, increasing vulnerability to addictive behaviors (Teicher et al., 2016). Social determinants of health, such as socioeconomic disadvantage and lack of social support, further exacerbate this risk by contributing to chronic stress and limiting access to coping resources (Galea et al., 2011). Environmental factors, including exposure to addictive behaviors and cultural norms, also play a critical role in shaping addictive tendencies (Potenza, 2017). Therapeutic interventions for behavioral addictions must therefore address both neurobiological and psychosocial factors.

3. TYPES OF BEHAVIORAL ADDICTIONS

3.1. Gambling addiction

Gambling addiction, or pathological gambling, is a prominent example of behavioral addiction, characterized by compulsive and repetitive behavior aimed at seeking immediate gratification through games of chance or betting (Trivedi and Teichert, 2018). Affected individuals experience intense excitement at the prospect of winning, which becomes a powerful driving force, even in the face of financial losses or severe social consequences (Vinberg et al., 2021).

This addiction is linked to dysfunction in the dopaminergic reward system. Wins or the anticipation of wins trigger DA release in the NAc, reinforcing gambling behaviors (Laskowski, 2022). Over time, neural circuits become hypersensitive to gambling-related stimuli, while natural rewards lose their appeal, leading to compulsive gambling at the expense of personal responsibilities (Arrigoni, 2019).

Gambling addiction is also associated with deficits in cognitive control circuits, particularly in the PFC (van Timmeren et al., 2017). This region, responsible for decision-making and impulse inhibition, is often hypoactive in pathological gamblers, making it difficult to resist the urge to gamble despite negative consequences (Pallanti et al., 2021).

Research has also shown that DA plays a central role in gambling addiction (Zack et al., 2020). For example, the administration of L-DOPA (a dopamine precursor) facilitates the learning of winning strategies, thereby reinforcing the tendency to seek rewards (Kroemer et al., 2019). This phenomenon may explain why some patients treated for Parkinson's disease develop compulsive gambling behaviors (Napier et al., 2020).

In addition to reinforcing reward-related behaviors, DA also appears to respond to the unpredictability of stimuli, challenging the notion that its role is solely linked to reward processing (Lerner et al., 2021).

3.2. Internet and gaming addiction

Internet and video game addiction, as forms of behavioral addiction, manifest through excessive and compulsive use, significantly disrupting daily functioning, social relationships, and mental health (Remon, 2024). These behaviors originate from the constant availability of digital platforms and their highly engaging design. Although distinct in their specific manifestations, these addictions share common neurobiological mechanisms, primarily linked to the brain's reward system.

At the core of Internet and video game addiction lies a dysregulation of the dopaminergic reward system. This dysregulation is triggered by repeated DA release in key brain regions, such as the NAc, during activities perceived as rewarding, such as winning a game or receiving notifications (Weinstein and Lejoyeux, 2020).

Over time, frequent activation of the reward system leads to a desensitization of dopaminergic receptors. This phenomenon results in a reduced response to usual stimuli, requiring increased exposure to achieve the same level of satisfaction a mechanism known as tolerance (Volkow et al., 2010). In other words, individuals gradually become unable to experience similar pleasure from ordinary activities, such as social interactions or non-digital hobbies.

Simultaneously, structural and functional changes occur in the PFC, the brain region crucial for decision-making, planning, and impulse control. Hypoactivity in this area, frequently observed in addicted individuals, impairs their ability to inhibit compulsive behaviors (Li et al., 2020). This explains why they struggle to limit their Internet or video game use, even when faced with clear negative consequences.

These neurobiological changes resemble those observed in substance addictions, where craving and reinforcement mechanisms play a central role. For instance, the NAc, along with other structures such as the amygdala and hippocampus, encodes memory associations between addiction-related stimuli and reward sensations, intensifying the urge to engage in these behaviors (Naassila, 2014).

Neurobiological disruptions directly contribute to the emergence of psychological symptoms, such as anxiety, depression, and withdrawal manifestations like irritability and agitation upon deprivation. These effects extend to daily life, promoting social isolation, neglect of responsibilities, sleep disturbances, and a deterioration of interpersonal relationships (Martini et al., 2022).

3.3. Food addiction and binge-eating disorder

The concepts of food addiction and binge-eating disorder (BED) share common mechanisms while exhibiting distinct neurobiological and behavioral differences. Both disorders are characterized by a loss of control over food consumption, leading to detrimental effects on physical and mental health (Kalon et al., 2016; Giel et al., 2022).

Food addiction, considered a form of behavioral dependence, involves neurobiological responses similar to those observed in substance addiction (Kalon et al., 2016). Specifically, the consumption of foods high in sugar, fat, or salt activates the mesolimbic dopaminergic system, particularly the NAc, triggering DA release associated with sensations of pleasure and satisfaction (Campana et al., 2019). Over time, neuroplastic alterations emerge, including a reduced sensitivity to natural rewards, leading to compulsive consumption to maintain the same level of gratification. This process is reinforced by uncontrollable impulses, often linked to negative emotional states, promoting cycles of compulsive eating (Pascoli et al., 2016).

BED, on the other hand, is defined by episodes of excessive and rapid food intake in the absence of hunger, without compensatory behaviors such as vomiting. These episodes are frequently triggered by emotional factors, including anxiety, depression, or stress, and are accompanied by a pronounced sense of loss of control and post-episode distress (Dingemans et al., 2017). Although both disorders involve alterations in the reward system, their distinct mechanisms reflect differences in triggers and consequences. In BED, binge episodes are often associated with an exaggerated emotional response, whereas food addiction is more centered on the hedonic properties of food, particularly those rich in sugar and fat, which activate mu-opioid circuits, enhancing sensory pleasure (Gearhardt et al., 2011; Ratković et al., 2023).

A central mechanism shared by both disorders is impulsivity, defined as the tendency to act rapidly without considering potential negative consequences. Impulsivity serves both as a risk factor for the development of these disorders and as a consequence of their chronicity, with deficits observed in brain regions involved in inhibitory control and decision-making, such as the PFC (Veit et al., 2021). In the context of food addiction, impulsivity manifests as heightened reactivity to food-related stimuli and an inability to resist highly palatable foods. Similarly, individuals with BED exhibit attentional deficits, risky decision-making, and difficulties in adjusting their behavior in response to negative feedback (Ferracci et al., 2024).

Although these two disorders share converging neurobiological mechanisms particularly the involvement of the dopaminergic reward system and opioid circuits their differences justify distinct therapeutic approaches. Food addiction is often conceptualized as dependence on the addictive properties of food, whereas BED is more strongly influenced by emotional and psychological factors (Breault, 2020). Distinguishing between these conditions is essential for guiding prevention and treatment strategies. A deeper understanding of their shared and specific mechanisms could contribute to more effective management while informing ongoing debates regarding the classification of food addiction as a genuine form of behavioral addiction.

3.4. Other emerging addictions (e.g., shopping, exercise)

Emerging addictions, such as shopping or exercise addiction, although independent of substance use, have significant impacts on both mental and physical health (Colledge et al., 2020; Ünübol et al., 2022). These disorders share similar neurobiological mechanisms, primarily characterized by dysfunctions in brain circuits involved in reward processing and impulse regulation (Lezhari, 2020; Ünübol et al., 2022).

3.4.1. Shopping Addiction

This disorder is characterized by compulsive purchasing behaviors often triggered by negative emotions such as anxiety, stress, or depression. Hyperactivation of the dopaminergic system reinforces the urge to buy, even in the presence of negative consequences, while reduced activity in the PFC impairs impulse control. Additionally, imbalances in the serotonergic and opioid systems affect emotional regulation and amplify compulsive behaviors (Lee et al., 2014; Koob and Volkow, 2016).

The consequences include financial problems, social isolation, and an inability to restrain these behaviors, highlighting the complexity of the underlying mechanisms.

3.4.2. Exercise Addiction

Although physical exercise is essential for overall health, excessive engagement can become problematic. Official guidelines recommend at least 2 hours and 30 minutes of moderate-intensity exercise per week or 1 hour and 15 minutes of vigorous-intensity exercise (UDHHS, 2008). While exceeding these thresholds may provide additional benefits, excessive increases can lead to negative consequences, transforming exercise into an overwhelming and sometimes addictive activity (Hausenblas and Giacobbi, 2004).

Neurobiologically, excessive DA release in the NAc reinforces the positive effects of exercise, such as stress reduction and mood improvement, while promoting compulsive engagement (Greenwood, 2019). Furthermore, an impaired PFC weakens impulse control. This mechanism can lead to injuries, hormonal imbalances, and psychological distress due to the uncontrollable need to continue exercising despite health risks (Lichtenstein et al., 2017).

Both forms of addiction share neurobiological similarities with other impulse control disorders, such as pathological gambling. They reflect an imbalance between brain circuits involved in reward processing and emotional regulation, illustrating the complexity of compulsive behaviors (Matar and Abdelfattah, 2023).

4. DIAGNOSTIC TOOLS AND ASSESSMENT METHODS

4.1. Clinical criteria and diagnostic manuals (DSM-V and ICD-11).

The concept of behavioral addictions refers to non-substance-related compulsions that result in impairment to functioning and significant levels of psychological distress. Examples of such addictions include gambling disorder, internet gaming disorder. The rise of technology and changes in societal habits have led to an increased prevalence of behavioral addictions, thereby rendering them a prominent issue in the fields of clinical psychology and psychiatry. The diagnostic criteria for these conditions can be found in both the Diagnostic and Statistical Manual of Mental Disorders, Fifth Edition (DSM-V) and the International Classification of Diseases 11th Edition (ICD-11) (First et al., 2021), though the conceptualization of these conditions differs between the two systems.

a- Comparative analysis of the DSM-V and the ICD-11 criteria for behavioral addictions

Diagnostic Approach and Criteria: The fifth edition of the Diagnostic and Statistical Manual of Mental Disorders (DSM-V) places significant emphasis on the identification of symptom clusters, with a particular focus on behavioral patterns that include preoccupation, loss of control, and continued engagement in spite of negative consequences (Wakefield, 2013). This edition adopts a more symptom-based and individual-focused approach, rendering it applicable in clinical settings where the primary focus is on the diagnosis of specific mental health conditions. ICD-11, on the other hands, adopts a more expansive and inclusive stance on behavioral addictions. It encompasses a more extensive range of conditions, including compulsive sexual behavior, and employs a global diagnostic approach that considers environmental, cultural, and societal influences (WHO, 2024).

Global Applicability and Use: The fifth edition of the Diagnostic and Statistical Manual of Mental Disorders is extensively utilized in the United States, with a primary focus on a clinical perspective. The criteria employed in this edition reflect a Western-centric approach to the diagnosis of mental health conditions (Gouveia, 2024). Conversely, the International Classification of Diseases, 11th Revision (ICD-11) is recognized and employed on an international level. The criteria for this edition have been designed to be applicable across diverse cultures and healthcare systems. The inclusion of behavioral addictions within a global health framework is a salient feature of the ICD-11, which helps address the rising global prevalence of these disorders (First et al., 2015).

Inclusion of Additional Behavioral Addictions: The most recent edition of the Diagnostic and Statistical Manual of Mental Disorders currently includes only gambling disorder as a recognized behavioral addiction, while other behaviors such as internet gaming remain under investigation (Pinna et al., 2015). The International Classification of Diseases, 11th Revision officially recognizes internet gaming disorder as behavioral addictions, acknowledging the growing concern of these issues in both clinical and societal contexts (Stein et al., 2020).

4.2. Psychometric tools for assessing behavioral addictions.

Psychometric tools represent a fundamental component in the assessment of behavioral addictions, serving as standardized instruments designed to evaluate psychological traits and behaviors (Albrecht et al., 2007). The aforementioned tools are specifically designed for the quantification of symptoms, behaviors, and patterns of addiction, consequently aiding clinicians and researchers in the assessment and diagnosis of addiction.

b- Psychometric Tools for Assessing Behavioral Addictions

Gambling Addiction: The most widely utilized measure for gambling addiction is the Gambling Disorder Screening Tool (PGSI), which was developed by Ferris and Wynne in 2001. The PGSI employs a series of questions designed to assess the severity of gambling problems. The questions relate to behavioral symptoms, including preoccupation, tolerance, and attempts to control gambling (Adu-Akoh, 2022). Its reliability and validity have been well documented across diverse populations. The South Oaks Gambling Screen (SOGS) is another prominent diagnostic instrument. It was developed for the specific purpose of diagnosing gambling addiction in clinical and community settings (Esparza-Reig et al., 2021). The SOGS has been the subject of critique regarding its tendency to overestimate the prevalence of gambling addiction in certain demographics (Lind et al., 2021). However, its notable sensitivity and specificity continue to render it a crucial instrument in the realm of gambling disorder research.

Internet Addiction: The Internet Addiction Test (IAT) was developed by Kimberly Young in 1998 and is considered one of the earliest tools to assess internet addiction (Young, 2009). The IAT is a tool designed to evaluate problematic internet use, with self-report items focusing on the emotional and behavioral aspects of internet usage. These aspects include preoccupation, tolerance, and withdrawal symptoms (Kuss and Lopez-Fernandez, 2016). Despite its widespread utilization, the IAT has been the subject of critique, with concerns regarding its reliance on self-reporting and the absence of a universally accepted definition of internet addiction.

The development of the Internet Addiction Test (IAT-20), a condensed version of the original IAT, has been undertaken to enhance efficiency while maintaining the validity of the assessment. Despite its ease of administration, the IAT-20 still relies on self-reports, which may introduce biases into the assessment process (Feleke et al., 2024).

4.3. Role of neuroimaging and biomarkers in diagnosis.

Recent years have seen significant advancements in the field of neuroimaging and biomarkers, which have yielded considerable insights into the brain systems implicated in behavioral addictions, particularly with regard to reward processing, decision-making, and impulsivity. Neuroimaging techniques, including functional magnetic resonance imaging (fMRI) and positron emission tomography (PET), have emerged as powerful tools for direct observation of brain activity in individuals with behavioral addictions (Ekhtiari et al., 2024). Moreover, the presence of biomarkers, defined as molecular indicators found in blood, urine, or cerebrospinal fluid, has demonstrated potential in the identification of neurobiological alterations associated with these conditions (Quinones and Kaddurah-Daouk, 2009).

4.3.1. Neuroimaging in the Diagnosis

Neuroimaging techniques have emerged as a means of visualizing the structure and activity of the human brain that is both non-invasive and readily available to researchers in the field. These tools have been instrumental in the recent identification of key brain regions and circuits implicated in the pathophysiology of behavioral addictions.

Functional Magnetic Resonance Imaging (FMRI) is a technique that enables the observation of real-time brain activity by measuring changes in blood oxygen levels. Research has repeatedly demonstrated altered brain activity in individuals with behavioral addictions, particularly in reward-related brain regions (Amemiya et al., 2024).

FMRIs have revealed that individuals with Gambling Disorder (GD) exhibit increased activation in the ventral striatum, a key region implicated in reward processing, as a response to gambling-related cues (Raimo et al., 2021). Concurrently, diminished activity has been observed in the PFC, a region responsible for executive function and impulse control, suggesting potential deficits in inhibitory control in individuals with GD (Ceceli et al., 2023). The concept of Internet Gaming Disorder (IGD) has been subject to rigorous investigation through the utilization of functional magnetic resonance imaging (fMRI) studies (Chen et al., 2021; Liu et al., 2023). These studies have demonstrated that individuals afflicted with IGD exhibit heightened activation within the mesolimbic dopaminergic system, particularly in response to cues related to gaming (Von Deneen et al., 2022). This phenomenon bears a striking resemblance to the brain activity observed in individuals with substance use disorders, thereby suggesting that IGD may indeed exhibit significant neurobiological similarities with such traditional addictions.

Positron Emission Tomography (PET): The utilization of PET imaging, particularly in conjunction with radiolabeled tracers for neurotransmitters, has yielded insights into the neurochemical underpinnings of behavioral addiction (Royse et al., 2023). PET studies have revealed alterations in DA receptor availability within the striatum of individuals afflicted with behavioral addictions, thereby suggesting a dysfunction within the reward system. In the context of gambling disorder and IGD, a reduction in DA receptor binding has been observed, which may contribute to the compulsive pursuit of reward (Xie et al., 2024).

Electroencephalography (EEG): EEG is a method of measuring electrical activity in the brain (Da Silva, (2023). It has been used to study the neural basis of impulse control and reward processing in cases of behavioral addiction (Kbah et al., 2025). In individuals diagnosed with gambling disorder, increased theta and decreased alpha power have been linked to impulsivity and heightened reward sensitivity (Yin, et al., 2024) Likewise, individuals diagnosed with IGD show an alteration in brain wave activity during tasks that require decision-making (Zeng et al., 2024).

4.3.2. Biomarkers in the Diagnosis:

Neurochemical Biomarkers: Biomarkers may be identified by observing changes in the levels of neurotransmitters or their metabolites. For example, changes in DA and serotonin levels have been detected in individuals diagnosed with gambling disorder and IGD, and these changes may be used to measure the severity of the addiction (García-Castro et al., 2023).

Genetic Biomarkers: Genetics have been demonstrated to play a role in the propensity for behavioral addictions (İzci et al., 2022). Variations in genes connected to the DA system, such as the DRD2 gene, have been linked to an elevated risk of developing gambling disorder and other behavioral addictions. Nevertheless, genetic research in this domain is still developing, and the necessity for large-scale studies is evident to identify specific genetic markers that can be utilized for diagnostic purposes (İzci et al., 2022).

Endocrine Biomarkers: Behavioral addictions have been demonstrated to be associated with alterations in the endocrine system, particularly in the regulation of cortisol and other stress hormones (Yılmazer, 2024). Research has indicated that dysregulated stress responses are observable in individuals with gambling disorder and IGD (Pallanti et al., 2021). Biomarkers related to the hypothalamic-pituitary-adrenal (HPA) axis may assist in the assessment of the impact of chronic stress on addiction-related brain changes (Sinha, 2024).

5. THERAPEUTIC APPROACHES TO BEHAVIORAL ADDICTIONS

Behavioral addictions, encompassing conditions such as gambling disorder, internet gaming disorder, and compulsive buying, present significant challenges in mental health treatment. Effective management often necessitates a multifaceted approach, integrating psychotherapeutic interventions, pharmacological treatments, or a combination of both, tailored to the individual's specific needs (Brand et al., 2025).

5.1. Psychotherapeutic Interventions

Psychotherapeutic interventions represent a fundamental approach in the management of behavioral addictions, with Cognitive Behavioral Therapy (CBT) and mindfulness-based interventions (MBIs) being the most extensively studied and empirically supported methods (Grant & Chamberlain, 2016). CBT aims to identify and restructure dysfunctional thought patterns and maladaptive behaviors that contribute to addictive behaviors. For instance, in gambling disorder, CBT helps patients challenge irrational beliefs such as the "gambler's fallacy" or the illusion of control, which reinforce addictive behaviors (Petry et al., 2017). A meta-analysis conducted by Stevens et al. (2019) demonstrated that CBT significantly reduces symptoms of gambling disorder and internet gaming disorder, with moderate to large effect sizes. Key techniques include cognitive restructuring, behavioral experiments, and relapse prevention strategies, providing patients with effective tools to manage triggers and high-risk situations.

MBIs, such as Mindfulness-Based Cognitive Therapy (MBCT) and Mindfulness-Based Relapse Prevention (MBRP), have also shown promise in the treatment of behavioral addictions (Bowen et al., 2021). These approaches emphasize present-moment awareness and non-judgmental acceptance of thoughts and emotions, helping individuals disengage from automatic behavioral responses (Oberoi, 2024). A study conducted by Zhang et al. (2021) demonstrated that mindfulness interventions significantly reduce cravings and enhance emotional regulation in individuals with behavioral addictions (Sancho et al., 2018; Schwebel et al., 2020). Techniques such as meditation, breathing exercises, and acceptance-based strategies are particularly effective in addressing addictions related to technology use, where triggers are pervasive and immediate (Baer & Huss, 2008).

5.2. Pharmacological Treatments

Pharmacological treatments for behavioral addictions are continuously advancing, with several medications targeting neurotransmitter systems demonstrating potential in alleviating symptoms and enhancing therapeutic outcomes (Peng et al., 2025). DA modulators, such as naltrexone, an opioid receptor antagonist, have proven effective in managing gambling disorder and compulsive sexual behavior by modulating the hyperactivity of the reward system (Camardese et al., 2015; Ginley et al., 2019). A randomized controlled trial conducted by Grant & Chamberlain (2020) reported that naltrexone significantly reduced symptoms of gambling disorder when compared to a placebo. Similarly, bupropion, a DA and norepinephrine reuptake inhibitor, has been utilized off-label to treat internet gaming disorder, with studies indicating reductions in both gaming time and cravings (Vasile & Vasiliu, 2021).

Serotonin modulators, particularly selective serotonin reuptake inhibitors (SSRIs) such as fluoxetine and escitalopram, have been investigated for conditions like compulsive shopping and kleptomania (Williams et al., 2008). However, the evidence regarding SSRIs remains inconsistent, with some studies demonstrating modest benefits while others report limited efficacy (Brewer & Potenza, 2008; Müller & Mitchell, 2011). Glutamate modulators, such as N-acetylcysteine (NAC), have also attracted attention for their potential in reducing impulsivity and cravings associated with gambling disorder and internet addiction (Grant et al., 2013). A review by Minarini et al. (2017) emphasized NAC's ability to restore glutamate homeostasis and mitigate compulsive behaviors, positioning it as a promising candidate for further investigation.

Emerging pharmacological treatments include off-label applications of medications such as Topiramate (an anticonvulsant) and Memantine (an NMDA receptor antagonist), which focus on modulating impulsivity and reward processing (Bautovich, 2017). Furthermore, novel compounds that act on the endocannabinoid system are currently being explored, raising prospects for more precise and effective treatments in the future (Pallanti et al., 2021).

Figure 2. Overview of Pharmacological Treatments for Behavioral Addictions, with Gambling Disorder as an Example

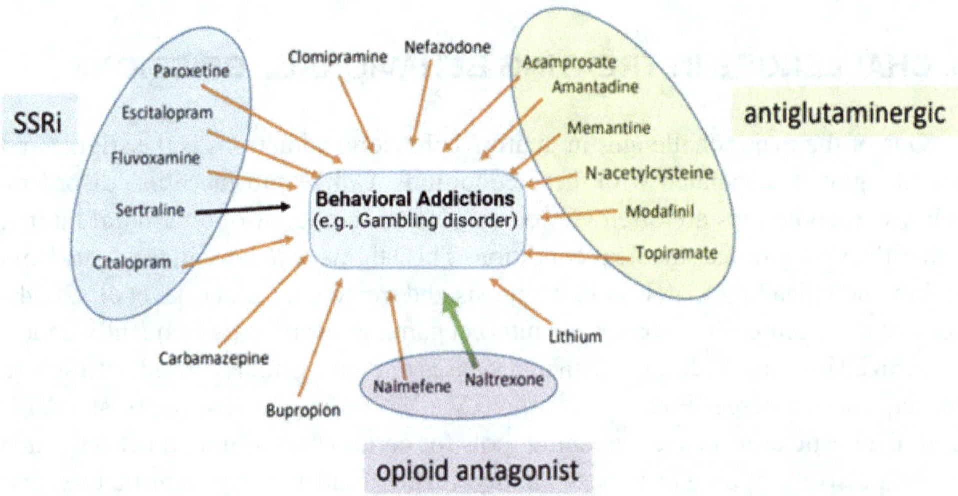

5.3. Combined Therapy Approaches and Their Efficacy

Combined therapeutic approaches, which integrate psychotherapeutic and pharmacological treatments, are gaining increasing recognition as an effective strategy for addressing the multifaceted nature of behavioral addictions. These approaches seek to target both the psychological and neurobiological mechanisms underlying addiction, offering a more holistic treatment framework(Brand et al., 2025). For instance, a randomized controlled trial demonstrated that the combination of CBT and naltrexone yielded significantly better outcomes in gambling disorder compared to either treatment alone (Ioannidis et al., 2024). The synergy between psychotherapy and pharmacotherapy enhances treatment efficacy by addressing cognitive distortions and maladaptive behaviors while concurrently reducing cravings and stabilizing mood (Sandua, 2024).

The advantages of combined therapy approaches include enhanced patient engagement, improved adherence, and better long-term maintenance of recovery. Psychotherapy equips patients with coping skills and relapse prevention strategies, while pharmacotherapy targets the neurochemical imbalances that underpin addictive behaviors (Singha, 2025). This integrated approach proves especially effective in cases of severe or treatment-resistant addictions, where single-modality interventions may be inadequate (de Oliveira, 2017). Future research should focus on optimizing combined therapy protocols and investigating their applicability across various types of behavioral addictions.

6. CHALLENGES IN TREATING BEHAVIORAL ADDICTIONS

One of the major challenges in treating behavioral addictions is the stigma and underdiagnosis associated with these conditions. Unlike substance use disorders, behavioral addictions are often viewed as a lack of self-control or a moral failing, rather than a legitimate medical condition. This stigma can deter individuals from seeking help, leading to delays in diagnosis and treatment (Gjoneska et al., 2024). For instance, gambling disorder and internet gaming disorder are frequently underrecognized in clinical settings, with many cases remaining undiagnosed until severe consequences emerge (Fineberg et al., 2022). Moreover, the absence of standardized diagnostic criteria and screening tools for certain behavioral addictions, such as compulsive shopping or hypersexuality, further hinders early identification and intervention.

Another significant challenge is the high prevalence of co-occurring mental health conditions, such as anxiety, depression, and personality disorders, among individuals with behavioral addictions. These comorbidities often exacerbate the severity of addictive behaviors and complicate treatment outcomes (Dom & Moggi, 2015). For example, studies have indicated that up to 60% of individuals with gambling disorder also meet the criteria for a mood or anxiety disorder (Dowling et al., 2015). Similarly, individuals with internet gaming disorder often report symptoms of depression and social anxiety, which can both contribute to and result from excessive gaming (M. W. Stevens et al., 2021). Effectively treating behavioral addictions in the context of these comorbidities requires integrated approaches that address both the addiction and the underlying mental health conditions. However, such comprehensive care is frequently lacking in clinical practice.

Finally, resistance to treatment and high relapse rates present significant challenges in the effective management of behavioral addictions. Many individuals with behavioral addictions exhibit ambivalence toward seeking help or may minimize the severity of their condition (Rosenberg, 2014). Even when treatment is initiated, the chronic and relapsing nature of these disorders makes sustained recovery particularly challenging. For instance, relapse rates for gambling disorder are estimated to be as high as 75% within the first year of treatment (Grant et al., 2024). Contributing factors to relapse include persistent triggers (e.g., gambling advertisements or easy access to technology), insufficient coping skills, and the lack of long-term support systems (Monaghan & Blaszczynski, 2009). Overcoming these challenges requires the implementation of innovative strategies, such as digital interventions, peer support programs, and continuous monitoring, to enhance treatment engagement and reduce the risk of relapse.

Figure 3. Challenges in treating behavioral addictions

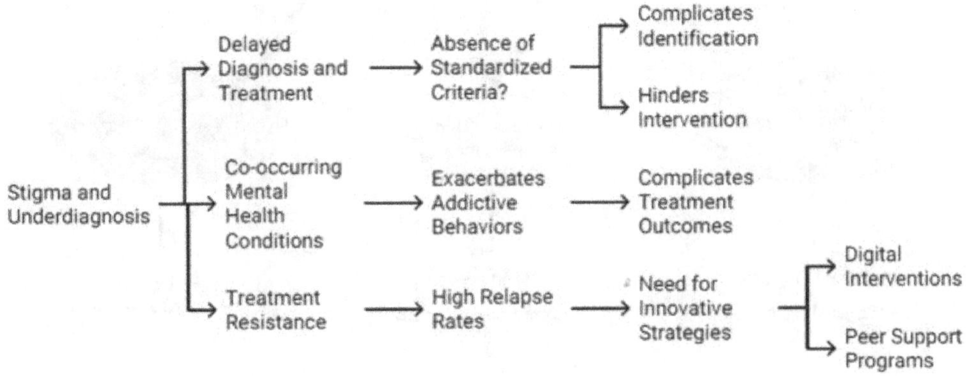

7. PREVENTION AND PUBLIC HEALTH STRATEGIES

Behavioral addictions pose significant challenges to public health, necessitating multifaceted prevention strategies that address individual, community, and systemic levels. Effective prevention requires a combination of education, community engagement, and regulatory measures to mitigate risk factors and promote healthier behaviors. This section explores these strategies, emphasizing their interconnected roles in reducing the societal burden of behavioral addictions (Figure 3).

Figure 4. Prevention and Public Health Strategies for Reducing Behavioral Addictions.

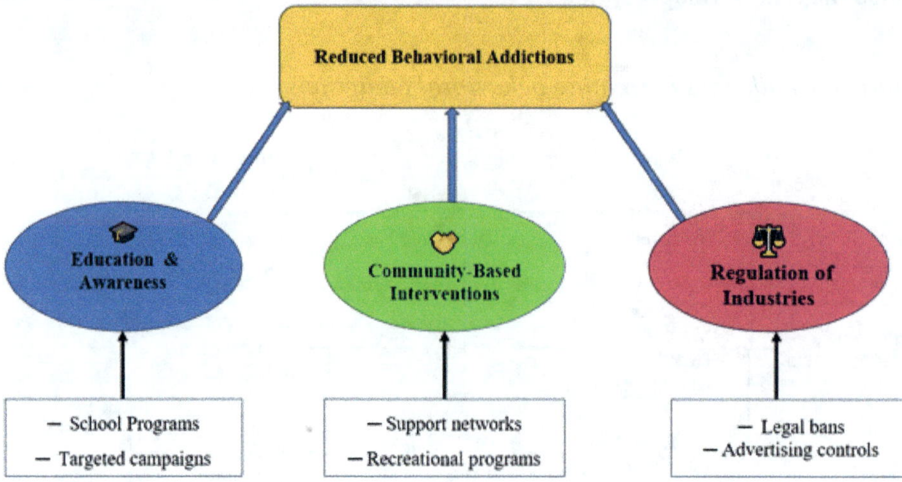

7.1. Role of Education and Awareness Campaigns

Education and awareness campaigns are foundational in preventing behavioral addictions by addressing misinformation and reducing stigma. Public knowledge about the neurobiological basis of these conditions such as DA dysregulation in gaming or gambling addictions can foster empathy and encourage early intervention (Rueda 2020). School-based programs that teach digital literacy and impulse control have shown promise in reducing adolescent susceptibility to internet addiction (Throuvala et al., 2019). For example, the ScreenSmart initiative in Australia integrates mindfulness exercises and critical thinking modules to help students recognize compulsive technology use (Dunlop et al., 2016).

Targeted campaigns are equally critical for high-risk populations. Problem gambling rates, for instance, are disproportionately higher among low-income individuals exposed to aggressive advertising by betting companies (Tran et al., 2024). Campaigns like the UK's Bet Regret, which uses social media to highlight the consequences of impulsive gambling, have demonstrated a 15% reduction in at-risk behaviors among young adults (Gambling Commission, 2020). Similarly, National Eating Disorders Awareness Week in the U.S. has expanded to address food addiction, emphasizing the distinction between disordered eating and substance-based addictions (NEDA, 2022).

7.2. Community-Based Interventions and Support Networks

Community-driven initiatives play a pivotal role in fostering environments that discourage addictive behaviors. Peer support groups, such as Gamblers Anonymous (GA) and Internet and Technology Addicts Anonymous (ITAA), provide safe spaces for individuals to share experiences and coping strategies. A meta-analysis by Tracy et al., (2016) found that participation in such groups correlates with a 30% reduction in relapse rates for gambling addiction.

Local governments and nonprofits can also implement alternative recreational programs to reduce isolation, a key risk factor for behavioral addictions. For instance, South Korea's *Jump Up Internet Rescue School* offers outdoor activities and counseling for adolescents with gaming addiction, resulting in improved social skills and reduced screen time (Koo et al., 2011). Similarly, community centers in urban areas have introduced gambling-free zones partnered with job training programs to address socioeconomic drivers of addiction (Matheson et al. 2022). Healthcare providers are essential in bridging clinical and community efforts. Integrating screening tools for behavioral addictions into primary care settings—such as the Problematic Media Use Measure (PMUM) for adolescents—ensures early detection and referrals to local resources (Domoff et al., 2019).

7.3. Regulation of Industries Associated with Addictive Behaviors

Structural interventions are critical to curbing the commercial determinants of behavioral addictions. The gaming and gambling industries, for example, employ manipulative design elements (e.g., loot boxes, variable rewards) that exploit psychological vulnerabilities (King & Delfabbro, 2019). Belgium and the Netherlands have banned loot boxes in video games, classifying them as gambling mechanisms under national law (Spicer et al., 2022). Similarly, the UK's prohibition of credit card uses for online gambling in 2021 reduced high-risk spending by 25% (Gambling Commission, 2021).

Advertising regulations also play a role. Norway restricts gambling ads to late-night hours, while Spain mandates warnings akin to tobacco products (Planzer et al., 2014). However, enforcement remains challenging due to the global nature of online platforms. A 2022 study by Kim et al. highlighted the need for international cooperation to regulate cross-border gambling sites, which often circumvent national laws.

Ethical concerns arise regarding industry self-regulation. While gaming companies like Epic Games have introduced "spending limits" for in-game purchases, critics argue these measures are insufficient without governmental oversight (Clark et al.,

2022). Policymakers must balance innovation with consumer protection, particularly for emerging technologies like virtual reality casinos.

8. ADVANCING PERSONALIZED MEDICINE FOR ADDICTION TREATMENT

Genetic and epigenetic treatments for addiction are innovative approaches aimed at understanding and intervening in the biological mechanisms behind addictive behaviors (Hiroi & Agatsuma, 2005). Genetic treatment involves modifying genes that regulate the brain's response to addictive substances, such as DA receptors or proteins related to synaptic plasticity, in order to reduce dependence (Nestler et al. 2019). Drug use causes epigenetic modifications, and similarly, environmental changes can promote addiction through epigenetic alterations. Epigenetic mechanisms include DNA methylation and post-translational modifications such as methylation, acetylation, phosphorylation, ubiquitylation, sumoylation, dopaminylation, crotonylation of histones, and ADP-ribosylation (Koijam et al., 2024). Non-coding RNAs also play a role in inducing epigenetic changes. This review explores these mechanisms and emphasizes the need to investigate epidrugs as an alternative and adjunctive treatment, considering the limited success of current addiction therapies (Koijam et al., 2024). Epigenome editing complexes have recently proven effective in eukaryotic systems. Targeted DNA cleavage technologies like the CRISPR-Cas9 system, CRISPR-dCas9 complexes, transcription activator-like effector nucleases (TALENs), and zinc-finger nucleases (ZFNs) have been used as platforms for DNA recognition or anchoring, combined with epigenetic writer or eraser proteins and delivered through transfection or transduction methods (Wang et al., 2016). The efficacy of epidrugs has been observed in various neuropsychiatric conditions, with remarkable initial results in addiction treatment using model organisms. Epidrugs present a promising alternative treatment for addiction.

However, third-wave therapies such as Mindfulness-Based Relapse Prevention (MBRP), Mindfulness-Oriented Recovery Enhancement (MORE), and Acceptance and Commitment Therapy (ACT) have been developed to improve addiction treatment (Rosenthal et al., 2021). Mindfulness is a practice of present-moment awareness without judgment. Initially used for chronic pain, it has been integrated into medical and psychiatric therapies, including addiction treatment. MBIs have shown positive effects and are used in therapeutic approaches such as Dialectical Behavior Therapy (DBT) and ACT. Several studies and meta-analyses evaluate their effectiveness in treating addictions (Rosenthal et al., 2021).

Studies show that mindfulness and MBIs reduce brain responses to addiction-related cues (e.g., in the ventral striatum and medial PFC and increase responses to healthy natural rewards, indicating a restructuring of brain reward processes. Furthermore, research on opioid users has shown that the more program reduces opioid consumption, cue reactivity to drugs, and improves responses to natural rewards. This supports the idea that these approaches shift the valuation of substances toward healthier rewards, thus reducing addictive behavior (Rosenthal et al., 2021). MBIs (MBIs) help reduce negative affect and stress reactivity, key factors in addictive disorders. They improve positive affect, increase self-control, and reduce cravings for substances. MBIs also decrease the avoidance of negative emotions, a behavior often linked to addiction. By changing how individuals react to addiction cues, these interventions promote abstinence and emotional regulation, thereby reducing the risk of relapse (Rosenthal et al., 2021).

Large-scale, robust, and controlled clinical trials are needed to draw conclusions on the effectiveness as well as the cognitive and neurobiological mechanisms underlying mindfulness as an interventional approach in addictive disorders. Research in the field of behavioral addictions is still limited. However, in light of this study, we believe the future of MBIs in addiction treatment looks promising. With their ability to intervene in brain circuits related to reward and emotional regulation, these approaches could offer more sustainable and tailored solutions to treat addiction and reduce long-term relapse risks.

CONCLUSION

Behavioral addictions represent a significant challenge, with profound neurobiological, psychological, and societal implications. Understanding the neural mechanisms, including neurotransmitter imbalances and reward system dysfunctions, is crucial for effective intervention. Various forms of behavioral addictions, such as gambling, gaming, and food addiction, require precise diagnostic tools, including clinical criteria, psychometric assessments, and neuroimaging techniques. Treatment approaches range from psychotherapeutic methods, like CBT and mindfulness, to pharmacological interventions targeting neurotransmitter systems. However, challenges such as stigma, underdiagnosis, and co-occurring mental health conditions complicate treatment. Prevention and public health strategies, including awareness campaigns and industry regulations, are essential to reducing addiction risks. Future research should focus on personalized medicine and innovative diagnostic tools to enhance treatment efficacy. Addressing behavioral addictions requires a multidisciplinary and evidence-based approach to mitigate their growing impact on individuals and society.

REFERENCES

Adu-Akoh, P. J. (2022). Problem Gambling Correlates and Their Effects on Study Habits of Students" Sport Bettors in the University of Cape Coast (Doctoral dissertation, University of Cape Coast).

Albrecht, U., Kirschner, N. E., & Grüsser, S. M. (2007). Diagnostic instruments for behavioural addiction: an overview. GMS Psycho-Social Medicine, 4.

Amemiya, S., Takao, H., & Abe, O. (2024). Resting-State fMRI: Emerging Concepts for Future Clinical Application. *Journal of Magnetic Resonance Imaging*, *59*(4), 1135–1148. DOI: 10.1002/jmri.28894 PMID: 37424140

American Psychiatric Association (APA). (2013). *Diagnostic and Statistical Manual of Mental Disorders* (5th ed.). American Psychiatric Publishing.

Arrigoni, C. L. E. (2019). Are loot boxes gambling? A crate start for a new gambling framework.

Baer, R. A., & Huss, D. B. (2008). Mindfulness-and acceptance-based therapy. Twenty-first century psychotherapies: Contemporary approaches to theory and practice, 123-166.

Baik, J. H. (2020). Stress and the dopaminergic reward system. *Experimental & Molecular Medicine*, *52*(12), 1879–1890. DOI: 10.1038/s12276-020-00532-4 PMID: 33257725

Bautovich, A. (2017). Pharmacological Management of Problem Gambling. In C. McIntosh & K. O'Neill, Evidence-Based Treatments for Problem Gambling (p. 85-93). Springer International Publishing. DOI: 10.1007/978-3-319-62485-3_9

Belujon, P., & Grace, A. A. (2017). Dopamine system dysregulation in major depressive disorders. *The International Journal of Neuropsychopharmacology*, *20*(12), 1036–1046. DOI: 10.1093/ijnp/pyx056 PMID: 29106542

Bickel, W. K., Mellis, A. M., Snider, S. E., Athamneh, L. N., Stein, J. S., & Pope, D. A. (2018). 21st century neurobehavioral theories of decision making in addiction: Review and evaluation. *Pharmacology, Biochemistry, and Behavior*, *164*, 4–21. DOI: 10.1016/j.pbb.2017.09.009 PMID: 28942119

Billieux, J., Schimmenti, A., Khazaal, Y., Maurage, P., & Heeren, A. (2015). Are we overpathologizing everyday life? A tenable blueprint for behavioral addiction research. *Journal of Behavioral Addictions*, *4*(3), 119–123. DOI: 10.1556/2006.4.2015.009 PMID: 26014667

Bowen, S., Chawla, N., Grow, J., & Marlatt, G. A. (2021). Mindfulness-based relapse prevention for addictive behaviors. Guilford Publications. https://books.google.com/books?hl=fr&lr=&id=nOj3DwAAQBAJ&oi=fnd&pg=PP1

Brand, M., Antons, S., Bőthe, B., Demetrovics, Z., Fineberg, N. A., Jimenez-Murcia, S., King, D. L., Mestre-Bach, G., Moretta, T., Müller, A., Wegmann, E., & Potenza, M. N. (2025). Current Advances in Behavioral Addictions : From Fundamental Research to Clinical Practice. *The American Journal of Psychiatry*, *182*(2), 155–163. DOI: 10.1176/appi.ajp.20240092 PMID: 39659159

Breault, A. A. (2020). *L'hyperphagie boulimique et la dépendance alimentaire: comparaison des profils* (Doctoral dissertation, Université Laval).

Brewer, J. A., & Potenza, M. N. (2008). The neurobiology and genetics of impulse control disorders : Relationships to drug addictions. *Biochemical Pharmacology*, *75*(1), 63–75. DOI: 10.1016/j.bcp.2007.06.043 PMID: 17719013

Camardese, G., Leone, B., Walstra, C., Janiri, L., & Guglielmo, R. (2015). Pharmacological Treatment of Internet Addiction. In Montag, C., & Reuter, M. (Eds.), *Internet Addiction* (pp. 151–165). Springer International Publishing., DOI: 10.1007/978-3-319-07242-5_10

Campana, B., Brasiel, P. G., de Aguiar, A. S., & Dutra, S. C. P. L. (2019). Obesity and food addiction: Similarities to drug addiction. *Obesity Medicine*, *16*, 100136. DOI: 10.1016/j.obmed.2019.100136

Ceceli, A. O., King, S. G., McClain, N., Alia-Klein, N., & Goldstein, R. Z. (2023). The neural signature of impaired inhibitory control in individuals with heroin use disorder. *The Journal of Neuroscience : The Official Journal of the Society for Neuroscience*, *43*(1), 173–182. DOI: 10.1523/JNEUROSCI.1237-22.2022 PMID: 36396402

Chakravarthy, S., Balasubramani, P. P., Mandali, A., Jahanshahi, M., & Moustafa, A. A. (2018). The many facets of dopamine: Toward an integrative theory of the role of dopamine in managing the body's energy resources. *Physiology & Behavior*, *195*, 128–141. DOI: 10.1016/j.physbeh.2018.06.032 PMID: 30031088

Chanda, C., & Surepalli, S. (2019). Dopaminergic dysfunction in neuropsychiatric disorders. Pathophysiology, current therapeutics, and future perspectives. *Neuropsychiatria i Neuropsychologia/Neuropsychiatry and Neuropsychology, 14*(1), 39-47.

Chen, J., Li, X., Zhang, Q., Zhou, Y., Wang, R., Tian, C., & Xiang, H. (2021). Impulsivity and response inhibition related brain networks in adolescents with internet gaming disorder: A preliminary study utilizing resting-state fMRI. *Frontiers in Psychiatry, 11*, 618319. DOI: 10.3389/fpsyt.2020.618319 PMID: 33519558

Chen, M., Sun, Y., Lu, L., & Shi, J. (2017). Similarities and differences in neurobiology. Substance and Non-substance Addiction, 45-58.

Clark, L., Smith, T., & Johnson, R. (2022). Ethical game design: Industry promises and consumer realities. *Journal of Behavioral Addictions, 11*(3), 456467.

Colledge, F., Sattler, I., Schilling, H., Gerber, M., Pühse, U., & Walter, M. (2020). Mental disorders in individuals at risk for exercise addiction–A systematic review. *Addictive Behaviors Reports, 12*, 100314. DOI: 10.1016/j.abrep.2020.100314 PMID: 33364322

Collins, A. L., & Saunders, B. T. (2020). Heterogeneity in striatal dopamine circuits: Form and function in dynamic reward seeking. *Journal of Neuroscience Research, 98*(6), 1046–1069. DOI: 10.1002/jnr.24587 PMID: 32056298

Da Silva, F. L. (2023). EEG: origin and measurement. In *EEG-fMRI: physiological basis, technique, and applications* (pp. 23–48). Springer International Publishing.

Dalley, J. W., & Ersche, K. D. (2019). Neural circuitry and mechanisms of waiting impulsivity: relevance to addiction. *Philosophical Transactions of the Royal Society B, 374*(1766), 20180145.

Dingemans, A., Danner, U., & Parks, M. (2017, November 22). Emotion Regulation in Binge Eating Disorder: A Review. *Nutrients, 9*(11), 1274. DOI: 10.3390/nu9111274 PMID: 29165348

Dom, G., & Moggi, F. (Eds.). (2015). *Co-occurring Addictive and Psychiatric Disorders : A Practice-Based Handbook from a European Perspective*. Springer Berlin Heidelberg., DOI: 10.1007/978-3-642-45375-5

Domoff, S. E., Harrison, K., Gearhardt, A. N., Gentile, D. A., Lumeng, J. C., & Miller, A. L. (2019). Development and validation of the Problematic Media Use Measure: A parent report measure of screen media "addiction" in children. *Psychology of Popular Media Culture, 8*(1), 2–11. DOI: 10.1037/ppm0000163 PMID: 30873299

Dowling, N. A., Cowlishaw, S., Jackson, A. C., Merkouris, S. S., Francis, K. L., & Christensen, D. R. (2015). Prevalence of psychiatric co-morbidity in treatment-seeking problem gamblers : A systematic review and meta-analysis. *The Australian and New Zealand Journal of Psychiatry, 49*(6), 519–539. DOI: 10.1177/0004867415575774 PMID: 25735959

Dunlop, S., Freeman, B., & Perez, D. (2016). Exposure to internet-based tobacco advertising and branding: Results from population surveys of Australian youth 2010-2013. *Journal of Medical Internet Research, 18*(6), e104. DOI: 10.2196/jmir.5595 PMID: 27338761

Ekhtiari, H., Sangchooli, A., Carmichael, O., Moeller, F. G., O'Donnell, P., Oquendo, M. A., & Brady, K. (2024). Neuroimaging biomarkers of addiction. *Nature Mental Health*, •••, 1–20. PMID: 39281741

Esparza-Reig, J., Guillén-Riquelme, A., Martí-Vilar, M., & González-Sala, F. (2021). A reliability generalization meta-analysis of the south oaks gambling screen (SOGS). *Psicothema, 33*(3), 490–499. DOI: 10.7334/psicothema2020.449 PMID: 34297680

Feleke, N., Mihretu, A., Habtamu, K., Amare, B., & Teferra, S. (2024). Validation of the Amharic version of Internet Addiction Test-20: A cross-sectional study. *Frontiers in Psychiatry, 14*, 1243035. DOI: 10.3389/fpsyt.2023.1243035 PMID: 38264639

Ferracci, S., Manippa, V., D'Anselmo, A., Bovolon, L., Guagnano, M. T., Brancucci, A., Porcelli, P., & Conti, C. (2024). The role of impulsivity and binge eating in out-patients with overweight or obesity: An EEG temporal discounting study. *Journal of Eating Disorders, 12*(1), 130. DOI: 10.1186/s40337-024-01080-2 PMID: 39227881

Ferrer-Pérez, C., Montagud-Romero, S., & Blanco-Gandía, M. C. (2024). Neurobiological Theories of Addiction: A Comprehensive Review. *Psychoactives, 3*(1), 35–47. DOI: 10.3390/psychoactives3010003

Ferris, J., & Wynne, H. (2001). L'indice canadien du jeu excessif. Ottawa, Canada: Centre canadien de lutte contre l'alcoolisme et les toxicomanies.

Fineberg, N. A., Menchón, J. M., Hall, N., Dell'Osso, B., Brand, M., Potenza, M. N., Chamberlain, S. R., Cirnigliaro, G., Lochner, C., Billieux, J., Demetrovics, Z., Rumpf, H. J., Müller, A., Castro-Calvo, J., Hollander, E., Burkauskas, J., Grünblatt, E., Walitza, S., Corazza, O., & Zohar, J. (2022). Advances in problematic usage of the internet research–A narrative review by experts from the European network for problematic usage of the internet. *Comprehensive Psychiatry, 118*, 152346. DOI: 10.1016/j.comppsych.2022.152346 PMID: 36029549

Firat, R. B. (2019). Opening the "Black Box": Functions of the frontal lobes and their implications for sociology. *Frontiers in Sociology, 4*, 3. DOI: 10.3389/fsoc.2019.00003 PMID: 33869331

First, M. B., Gaebel, W., Maj, M., Stein, D. J., Kogan, C. S., Saunders, J. B., Poznyak, V. B., Gureje, O., Lewis-Fernández, R., Maercker, A., Brewin, C. R., Cloitre, M., Claudino, A., Pike, K. M., Baird, G., Skuse, D., Krueger, R. B., Briken, P., Burke, J. D., & Reed, G. M. (2021). An organization-and category-level comparison of diagnostic requirements for mental disorders in ICD-11 and DSM-5. *World Psychiatry; Official Journal of the World Psychiatric Association (WPA)*, *20*(1), 34–51. DOI: 10.1002/wps.20825 PMID: 33432742

First, M. B., Reed, G. M., Hyman, S. E., & Saxena, S. (2015). The development of the ICD-11 clinical descriptions and diagnostic guidelines for mental and behavioural disorders. *World Psychiatry; Official Journal of the World Psychiatric Association (WPA)*, *14*(1), 82–90. DOI: 10.1002/wps.20189 PMID: 25655162

Galea, S., Nandi, A., & Vlahov, D. (2004). The social epidemiology of substance use. *Epidemiologic Reviews*, *26*(1), 36–52. DOI: 10.1093/epirev/mxh007 PMID: 15234946

Gambling Commission. (2020). *Evaluating the impact of the Bet Regret campaign*. UK Gambling Commission.

Gambling Commission. (2021). *Credit card ban evaluation report*. UK Gambling Commission.

García-Castro, J., Cancela, A., & Cárdaba, M. A. (2023). Neural cue-reactivity in pathological gambling as evidence for behavioral addiction: A systematic review. *Current Psychology (New Brunswick, N.J.)*, *42*(32), 28026–28037. DOI: 10.1007/s12144-022-03915-0 PMID: 36373116

Gearhardt, A. N., White, M. A., & Potenza, M. N. (2011, September). Binge eating disorder and food addiction. *Current Drug Abuse Reviews*, *4*(3), 201–207. DOI: 10.2174/1874473711104030201 PMID: 21999695

German, D. C., & Manaye, K. F. (1993, May 15). Midbrain dopaminergic neurons (nuclei A8, A9, and A10): Three-dimensional reconstruction in the rat. *The Journal of Comparative Neurology*, *331*(3), 297–309. DOI: 10.1002/cne.903310302 PMID: 8514911

Ghallab, Y. K., & Elassal, O. S. (2024). Biochemical and Neuropharmacology of Psychiatric Disorders. In *Nutrition and Psychiatric Disorders: An Evidence-Based Approach to Understanding the Diet-Brain Connection* (pp. 25–47). Springer Nature Singapore. DOI: 10.1007/978-981-97-2681-3_2

Giel, K. E., Bulik, C. M., Fernandez-Aranda, F., Hay, P., Keski-Rahkonen, A., Schag, K., Schmidt, U., & Zipfel, S. (2022). Binge eating disorder. *Nature Reviews. Disease Primers*, *8*(1), 16. DOI: 10.1038/s41572-022-00344-y PMID: 35301358

Ginley, M. K., Zajac, K., Rash, C. J., & Petry, N. M. (2019). Pharmacological treatment of behavioral addictions. https://psycnet.apa.org/record/2019-20159-028

Gjoneska, B. B\Hothe, B., Potenza, M. N., Szabo, A., & Demetrovics, Z. (2024). Epidemiology of Behavioral Addictions. The Sage Handbook of Addiction Psychology, 47.

Gongora, M., Teixeira, S., Martins, L., Marinho, V., Velasques, B., Moraes, L., & Ribeiro, P. (2019). Neurobiological evidences, functional and emotional aspects associated with the amygdala: From "What is it?" to "What's to be done?". *Neuropsychiatry*, *9*(3), 749–751.

Goulet-Kennedy, J., Labbe, S., & Fecteau, S. (2016). The involvement of the striatum in decision making. *Dialogues in Clinical Neuroscience*, *18*(1), 55–63. DOI: 10.31887/DCNS.2016.18.1/sfecteau PMID: 27069380

Gouveia, A. (2024). On the concept, taxonomy, and transculturality of disordered grief. *Frontiers in Psychology*, *14*, 1165421. DOI: 10.3389/fpsyg.2023.1165421 PMID: 38374931

Grant, J. E., & Chamberlain, S. R. (2016). Expanding the definition of addiction: DSM-5 vs. ICD-11. *CNS Spectrums*, *21*(4), 300–303. DOI: 10.1017/S1092852916000183 PMID: 27151528

Grant, J. E., & Chamberlain, S. R. (2020). Gambling and substance use: Comorbidity and treatment implications. *Progress in Neuro-Psychopharmacology & Biological Psychiatry*, *99*, 109852. DOI: 10.1016/j.pnpbp.2019.109852 PMID: 31881248

Grant, J. E., Ioannidis, K., & Chamberlain, S. R. (2024). Defining treatment response in gambling disorder. *Journal of Psychiatric Research*, *180*, 382–386. DOI: 10.1016/j.jpsychires.2024.11.006 PMID: 39522449

Grant, J. E., Odlaug, B. L., Chamberlain, S. R., Potenza, M. N., Schreiber, L. R., Donahue, C. B., & Kim, S. W. (2013). A randomized, placebo-controlled trial of N-acetylcysteine plus imaginal desensitization for nicotine-dependent pathological gamblers. *The Journal of Clinical Psychiatry*, *74*(1), 16833. PMID: 24345329

Grant, J. E., Potenza, M. N., Weinstein, A., & Gorelick, D. A. (2010). Introduction to behavioral addictions. *The American Journal of Drug and Alcohol Abuse*, *36*(5), 233–241. DOI: 10.3109/00952990.2010.491884 PMID: 20560821

Greenwood, B. N. (2019). The role of dopamine in overcoming aversion with exercise. *Brain Research*, *1713*, 102–108. DOI: 10.1016/j.brainres.2018.08.030 PMID: 30171838

Hausenblas, H. A., & Giacobbi, P. R.Jr. (2004). Relationship between exercise dependence symptoms and personality. *Personality and Individual Differences*, *36*(6), 1265–1273. DOI: 10.1016/S0191-8869(03)00214-9

He, X., Chen, S., Yu, Q., Yang, P., & Yang, B. (2024). Correlations between problematic internet use and suicidal behavior among Chinese adolescents: A systematic review and meta-analysis. *Frontiers in Psychiatry*, *15*, 1484809. DOI: 10.3389/fpsyt.2024.1484809 PMID: 39588549

Hiroi, N., & Agatsuma, S. (2005). Genetic susceptibility to substance dependence. *Molecular Psychiatry*, *10*(4), 336–344. DOI: 10.1038/sj.mp.4001622 PMID: 15583701

Hultman, R., Mague, S. D., Li, Q., Katz, B. M., Michel, N., Lin, L., Wang, J., David, L. K., Blount, C., Chandy, R., Carlson, D., Ulrich, K., Carin, L., Dunson, D., Kumar, S., Deisseroth, K., Moore, S. D., & Dzirasa, K. (2016). Dysregulation of prefrontal cortex-mediated slow-evolving limbic dynamics drives stress-induced emotional pathology. *Neuron*, *91*(2), 439–452. DOI: 10.1016/j.neuron.2016.05.038 PMID: 27346529

Ioannidis, K., Huneke, N. T., Solly, J. E., Veronesi, G. F., Tzagarakis, C., Parlatini, V., Westwood, S. J., Del Giovane, C., Baldwin, D. S., & Grant, J. E. (2024). Placebo and nocebo effects in gambling disorder pharmacological trials : A meta-analysis. *Acta Neuropsychiatrica*, •••, 1–11. PMID: 39563187

İzci, F., Sağlam, N. G. U., & Ergelen, M. (2022). Neurobiology and Genetics of Behavioral Addictions: A Brief Review. *Bağimlik Dergisi*, *23*(2), 233–241. DOI: 10.51982/bagimli.991533

Jawad, L., Aboufatima, R., Aicha, O., Bezza, K., El Gabbas, Z., Mehdi, A. L., Fatimazahra, M., Aaziz, K., & Chait, A. (2019). Behavioral and histological characterization of the effects of cigarette smoke inhalation and withdrawal in rats. *Toxicological and Environmental Chemistry*, *101*(1-2), 129–147. DOI: 10.1080/02772248.2019.1628236

Johnson, M. E., Salvatore, M. F., Maiolo, S. A., & Bobrovskaya, L. (2018). Tyrosine hydroxylase as a sentinel for central and peripheral tissue responses in Parkinson's progression: Evidence from clinical studies and neurotoxin models. *Progress in Neurobiology*, *165*, 1–25. DOI: 10.1016/j.pneurobio.2018.01.002 PMID: 29331395

Kalon, E., Hong, J. Y., Tobin, C., & Schulte, T. (2016). Psychological and neurobiological correlates of food addiction. *International Review of Neurobiology*, *129*, 85–110. DOI: 10.1016/bs.irn.2016.06.003 PMID: 27503449

Kbah, S. N. S., Tan, T. S., Sheikh, J., Al-Qazzaz, N. K., Salim, M. I. M., Hum, Y. C., & Qiu, F. (2025). Review on Fundamental of Electroencephalography and Detection Techniques in Substance and Behavioral Addiction. *Journal of Human Centered Technology*, *4*(1), 78–85. DOI: 10.11113/humentech.v4n1.98

King, D., & Delfabbro, P. (2019). Video game monetization: Psychological impacts. *Current Addiction Reports*, *6*(3), 323–330.

Koijam, A. S., Singh, K. D., Nameirakpam, B. S., Haobam, R., & Rajashekar, Y. (2024). Drug addiction and treatment: An epigenetic perspective. *Biomedicine and Pharmacotherapy*, *170*, 115951. DOI: 10.1016/j.biopha.2023.115951 PMID: 38043446

Koo, C., Wati, Y., Lee, C. C., & Oh, H. Y. (2011). Internet-addicted kids and South Korean government efforts: Boot-camp case. *Cyberpsychology, Behavior, and Social Networking*, *14*(6), 391–394. DOI: 10.1089/cyber.2009.0331 PMID: 21204693

Koob, G. F., & Volkow, N. D. (2016). Neurobiology of addiction: A neurocircuitry analysis. *The Lancet. Psychiatry*, *3*(8), 760–773. DOI: 10.1016/S2215-0366(16)00104-8 PMID: 27475769

Kroemer, N. B., Lee, Y., Pooseh, S., Eppinger, B., Goschke, T., & Smolka, M. N. (2019). L-DOPA reduces model-free control of behavior by attenuating the transfer of value to action. *NeuroImage*, *186*, 113–125. DOI: 10.1016/j.neuroimage.2018.10.075 PMID: 30381245

Kumar, M., & Jha, A. K. (2024). Adolescent Brain Development: Limbic System and Emotions. In *Encyclopedia of Religious Psychology and Behavior* (pp. 1–10). Springer Nature Switzerland. DOI: 10.1007/978-3-031-38971-9_10-1

Kuss, D. J., & Griffiths, M. D. (2017). Internet and gaming addiction: A systematic literature review of neuroimaging studies. *Brain Sciences*, *7*(5), 46. PMID: 28441336

Kuss, D. J., & Lopez-Fernandez, O. (2016). Internet addiction and problematic Internet use: A systematic review of clinical research. *World Journal of Psychiatry*, *6*(1), 143. DOI: 10.5498/wjp.v6.i1.143 PMID: 27014605

Laskowski, C. (2022). *Impacts of reward schedules and a dopamine agonist on dopamine receptor expression in an animal model of gambling addiction* (Doctoral dissertation, University of Lethbridge (Canada)).

Lechan, R. M., & Toni, R. (2016). *Functional anatomy of the hypothalamus and pituitary*. Endotext. [Internet]

Lee, J. H. (2023). Understanding Parkinson's Disorders: Classification and Evaluation Methods, Movement Disorders, and Treatment Methods. *International Journal of Advanced Culture Technology*, *11*(3), 9–17.

Lee, J. H.. (2014). Neurobiological mechanisms of compulsive buying: A review of the literature. *Journal of Psychiatric Research*, *57*, 79–86.

Lemmens, J. S., Valkenburg, P. M., & Peter, J. (2023). Psychosocial causes and consequences of pathological gaming. *Computers in Human Behavior*, *103*, 118–124.

Lerner, T. N., Holloway, A. L., & Seiler, J. L. (2021). Dopamine, updated: Reward prediction error and beyond. *Current Opinion in Neurobiology*, *67*, 123–130. DOI: 10.1016/j.conb.2020.10.012 PMID: 33197709

Lezhari, E. (2020). Addictions and tensions: the Psychomotor rehabilitation regarding the regulation of stress and anxiety among people suffering from addiction.

Li, B., Nguyen, T. P., Ma, C., & Dan, Y. (2020). Inhibition of impulsive action by projection-defined prefrontal pyramidal neurons. *Proceedings of the National Academy of Sciences of the United States of America*, *117*(29), 17278–17287. DOI: 10.1073/pnas.2000523117 PMID: 32631999

Lichtenstein, M. B., Hinze, C. J., Emborg, B., Thomsen, F., & Hemmingsen, S. D. (2017). Compulsive exercise: Links, risks and challenges faced. *Psychology Research and Behavior Management*, *10*, 85–95. DOI: 10.2147/PRBM.S113093 PMID: 28435339

Lind, K., Marionneau, V., Järvinen-Tassopoulos, J., & Salonen, A. H. (2021). Sociodemographics, gambling participation, gambling settings, and addictive behaviors associated with gambling modes: A population-based study. *Journal of Gambling Studies*, *38*(4), 1–16. DOI: 10.1007/s10899-021-10074-7 PMID: 34623554

Liu, X., Zheng, Y., Niculescu, M., Liang, Q., Yang, A., Dong, G., Gao, Z., Lin, P., Liu, Y., Chen, L., & Xu, D. (2023). The involvement of spontaneous brain activity in natural recovery from internet gaming disorder: A resting-state fMRI study. *Frontiers in Psychiatry*, *14*, 1093784. DOI: 10.3389/fpsyt.2023.1093784 PMID: 36896348

Martini, F., Fregna, L., Bosia, M., Perrozzi, G., & Cavallaro, R. (2022). Substance-related disorders. In *Fundamentals of Psychiatry for Health Care Professionals* (pp. 263–295). Springer International Publishing. DOI: 10.1007/978-3-031-07715-9_9

Matar, R., & Abdelfattah, N. (2023). Neurobiological underpinnings of compulsive buying disorder: A multimodal imaging study. *Archives of Clinical Psychiatry, 50*(5).

Matheson, F. I., Hamilton-Wright, S., Hahmann, T., McLuhan, A., Tacchini, G., Wendaferew, A., & Dastoori, P. (2022). Filling the GAP: Integrating a gambling addiction program into a shelter setting for people experiencing poverty and homelessness. *PLoS One, 17*(3), e0264922. DOI: 10.1371/journal.pone.0264922 PMID: 35290379

Minarini, A., Ferrari, S., Galletti, M., Giambalvo, N., Perrone, D., Rioli, G., & Galeazzi, G. M. (2017). N -acetylcysteine in the treatment of psychiatric disorders: Current status and future prospects. *Expert Opinion on Drug Metabolism & Toxicology, 13*(3), 279–292. DOI: 10.1080/17425255.2017.1251580 PMID: 27766914

Monaghan, S., & Blaszczynski, A. (2009). *Internet-based interventions for the treatment of problem gambling*. Centre for Addiction and Mental Health., https://www.academia.edu/download/30708795/InternetTreatmentforProblemGambli ngCAMH2009_Final.pdf

Müller, A., & Mitchell, J. E. (2011). Overview of Treatment for Compulsive Buying. In *Compulsive Buying* (pp. 145–164). Routledge., https://www.taylorfrancis.com/chapters/edit/10.4324/9780203840962-18/overview-treatment-compulsive-buying DOI: 10.4324/9780203840962

Naassila, M. (2014). Chapitre 3. Neurobiologie de l'addiction. Dans Benyamina, A. (dir.), Addictions et comorbidités. (p. 25 -54). Dunod.

Napier, T. C., Kirby, A., & Persons, A. L. (2020). The role of dopamine pharmacotherapy and addiction-like behaviors in Parkinson's disease. *Progress in Neuro-Psychopharmacology & Biological Psychiatry, 102*, 109942. DOI: 10.1016/j.pnpbp.2020.109942 PMID: 32272129

National Eating Disorders Association. (2022). *National Eating Disorders Awareness Week: Expanding the scope*. https://www.nationaleatingdisorders.org

Nestler, E. J., & Lüscher, C. (2019). The molecular basis of drug addiction: Linking epigenetic to synaptic and circuit mechanisms. *Neuron, 102*(1), 48–59. DOI: 10.1016/j.neuron.2019.01.016 PMID: 30946825

Oberoi, T. (2024). *Common Mechanisms of Change in Mindfulness-Based Cognitive Therapy (MBCT) and Traditional Cognitive Behavioral Therapy (CBT)*. Implications for Therapeutic Effectiveness.

Pallanti, S., Marras, A., & Makris, N. (2021). A research domain criteria approach to gambling disorder and behavioral addictions: Decision-making, response inhibition, and the role of cannabidiol. *Frontiers in Psychiatry*, *12*, 634418. DOI: 10.3389/fpsyt.2021.634418 PMID: 34603091

Panksepp, J., & Wilson, C. G. (2016). Brain SEEKING circuitry in neuroeconomics: a unifying hypothesis for the role of dopamine-energized arousal of the medial forebrain bundle in enthusiasm-guiding decision-making. *Neuroeconomics*, 231-252.

Pascoli, V., Terrier, J., & Lüscher, C. (2016). Addiction par stimulation des neurones dopaminergiques mésolimbiques. *médecine/sciences, 32*(8-9), 692-696.

Peng, Z., Jia, Q., Mao, J., Luo, X., Huang, A., Zheng, H., Jiang, S., Ma, Q., Ma, C., & Yi, Q. (2025). Neurotransmitters crosstalk and regulation in the reward circuit of subjects with behavioral addiction. *Frontiers in Psychiatry*, *15*, 1439727. DOI: 10.3389/fpsyt.2024.1439727 PMID: 39876994

Pessoa, L. (2017). A network model of the emotional brain. *Trends in Cognitive Sciences*, *21*(5), 357–371. DOI: 10.1016/j.tics.2017.03.002 PMID: 28363681

Petry, N. M., Ginley, M. K., & Rash, C. J. (2017). A systematic review of treatments for problem gambling. *Psychology of Addictive Behaviors*, *31*(8), 951–961. DOI: 10.1037/adb0000290 PMID: 28639817

Pinna, F. E. D. E. R. I. C. A., Dell'Osso, B., Di Nicola, M., Janiri, L., Altamura, A. C., Carpiniello, B. E. R. N. A. R. D. O., & Hollander, E. (2015). Behavioural addictions and the transition from DSM-IV-TR to DSM-5. *Journal of Psychopathology*, *21*(4), 380–389.

Planzer, S., Gray, H. M., & Shaffer, H. J. (2014). Associations between national gambling policies and disordered gambling prevalence rates within Europe. *International Journal of Law and Psychiatry*, *37*(2), 217–229. DOI: 10.1016/j.ijlp.2013.11.002 PMID: 24370209

Potenza, M. N. (2014). Non-substance addictive behaviors in the context of DSM-5. *Addictive Behaviors*, *39*(1), 1–2. DOI: 10.1016/j.addbeh.2013.09.004 PMID: 24119712

Potenza, M. N. (2017). Clinical neuropsychiatric considerations regarding nonsubstance or behavioral addictions. *Dialogues in Clinical Neuroscience*, *19*(3), 281–291. DOI: 10.31887/DCNS.2017.19.3/mpotenza PMID: 29302225

Qi-Lytle, X., Sayers, S., & Wagner, E. J. (2023). Current Review of the Function and Regulation of Tuberoinfundibular Dopamine Neurons. *International Journal of Molecular Sciences*, *25*(1), 110. DOI: 10.3390/ijms25010110 PMID: 38203281

Quinones, M. P., & Kaddurah-Daouk, R. (2009). Metabolomics tools for identifying biomarkers for neuropsychiatric diseases. *Neurobiology of Disease*, *35*(2), 165–176. DOI: 10.1016/j.nbd.2009.02.019 PMID: 19303440

Raimo, S., Cropano, M., Trojano, L., & Santangelo, G. (2021). The neural basis of gambling disorder: An activation likelihood estimation meta-analysis. *Neuroscience and Biobehavioral Reviews*, *120*, 279–302. DOI: 10.1016/j.neubiorev.2020.11.027 PMID: 33275954

Ratković, D., Knežević, V., Dickov, A., Fedrigolli, E., & Čomić, M. (2023, April). Comparison of binge-eating disorder and food addiction. *The Journal of International Medical Research*, *51*(4), 3000605231171016. DOI: 10.1177/03000605231171016 PMID: 37115520

Remon, H. (2024). Online Addiction: A New Form of Mental Health Issue. *Science Insights*, *44*(3), 1291–1300. DOI: 10.15354/si.24.re938

Renard, J., Rushlow, W. J., & Laviolette, S. R. (2018). Effects of adolescent THC exposure on the prefrontal GABAergic system: Implications for schizophrenia-related psychopathology. *Frontiers in Psychiatry*, *9*, 281. DOI: 10.3389/fpsyt.2018.00281 PMID: 30013490

Ricciutti, N. M., & Zhang, S. (2024). A pilot study of the behavioral addictions knowledge survey: Ensuring students' knowledge about process/behavioral addictions. *Journal of Addictions & Offender Counseling*, *45*(2), 205–220. DOI: 10.1002/jaoc.12132

Rolls, E. T. (2019). The cingulate cortex and limbic systems for emotion, action, and memory. *Brain Structure & Function*, *224*(9), 3001–3018. DOI: 10.1007/s00429-019-01945-2 PMID: 31451898

Rosenberg, K. P. (2014). *Behavioral addictions : Criteria, evidence, and treatment*. Academic Press.

Rosenthal, A., Levin, M. E., Garland, E. L., & Romanczuk-Seiferth, N. (2021). Mindfulness in treatment approaches for addiction—Underlying mechanisms and future directions. *Current Addiction Reports*, *8*(2), 282–297. DOI: 10.1007/s40429-021-00372-w

Royse, S. K., Lopresti, B. J., Mathis, C. A., Tollefson, S., & Narendran, R. (2023). Beyond monoamines: II. Novel applications for PET imaging in psychiatric disorders. *Journal of Neurochemistry*, *164*(3), 401–443. DOI: 10.1111/jnc.15657 PMID: 35716057

Rueda, C. (2020). Neuroeducation: Teaching with the brain. *Journal of Neuroeducation*, *1*(1), 108–113. DOI: 10.1344/joned.v1i1.31657

Sancho, M., De Gracia, M., Rodriguez, R. C., Mallorquí-Bagué, N., Sánchez-González, J., Trujols, J., Sánchez, I., Jiménez-Murcia, S., & Menchón, J. M. (2018). Mindfulness-based interventions for the treatment of substance and behavioral addictions: A systematic review. *Frontiers in Psychiatry*, *9*, 95. DOI: 10.3389/fpsyt.2018.00095 PMID: 29651257

Sandua, d. (2024). Overcoming addictions: strategies for breaking free from compulsive patterns.

Sayin, H. U. (2019). Getting high on dopamine: Neuro scientific aspects of pleasure. *SexuS J*, *4*, 883–906.

Schultz, W. (2015, July). Neuronal Reward and Decision Signals: From Theories to Data. *Physiological Reviews*, *95*(3), 853–951. DOI: 10.1152/physrev.00023.2014 PMID: 26109341

Schwebel, F. J., Korecki, J. R., & Witkiewitz, K. (2020). Addictive Behavior Change and Mindfulness-Based Interventions: Current Research and Future Directions. *Current Addiction Reports*, *7*(2), 117–124. DOI: 10.1007/s40429-020-00302-2 PMID: 33585158

Sears, S. M., & Hewett, S. J. (2021). Influence of glutamate and GABA transport on brain excitatory/inhibitory balance. *Experimental Biology and Medicine*, *246*(9), 1069–1083. DOI: 10.1177/1535370221989263 PMID: 33554649

Šimić, G., Tkalčić, M., Vukić, V., Mulc, D., Španić, E., & Šagud, M. & R. Hof, P. (. (2021). Understanding emotions: Origins and roles of the amygdala. *Biomolecules*, *11*(6), 823. DOI: 10.3390/biom11060823 PMID: 34072960

Singh, S., Khanna, D., & Kalra, S. (2020). Role of neurochemicals in schizophrenia. *Current Psychopharmacology*, *9*(2), 144–161. DOI: 10.2174/2211556009666200401150756

Singha, R. (2025). Neuroeconomic Insights on Addiction: Integrating the Multidimensional Addiction Behaviour Scale for Treatment, Prevention, and Holistic Well-Being. In Behavioral Economics and Neuroeconomics of Health and Healthcare (p. 181-212). IGI Global. https://www.igi-global.com/chapter/neuroeconomic-insights-on-addiction/356626

Sinha, R. (2024). Stress and substance use disorders: Risk, relapse, and treatment outcomes. *The Journal of Clinical Investigation*, *134*(16), e172883. DOI: 10.1172/JCI172883 PMID: 39145454

Soriano-Molina, E., Limiñana-Gras, R. M., Patró-Hernández, R. M., & Rubio-Aparicio, M. (2024). The Impact of Internet Addiction on Adolescents Mental Health: A Meta-analytic Review.

Spicer, S. G., Nicklin, L. L., Uther, M., Lloyd, J., Lloyd, H., & Close, J. (2022). Loot boxes, problem gambling and problem video gaming: A systematic review and meta-synthesis. *New Media & Society*, *24*(4), 1001–1022. DOI: 10.1177/14614448211027175

Stein, D. J., Szatmari, P., Gaebel, W., Berk, M., Vieta, E., Maj, M., de Vries, Y. A., Roest, A. M., de Jonge, P., Maercker, A., Brewin, C. R., Pike, K. M., Grilo, C. M., Fineberg, N. A., Briken, P., Cohen-Kettenis, P. T., & Reed, G. M. (2020). Mental, behavioral and neurodevelopmental disorders in the ICD-11: An international perspective on key changes and controversies. *BMC Medicine*, *18*(1), 1–24. DOI: 10.1186/s12916-020-1495-2 PMID: 31983345

Stevens, M. W., Dorstyn, D., Delfabbro, P. H., & King, D. L. (2021). Global prevalence of gaming disorder: A systematic review and meta-analysis. *The Australian and New Zealand Journal of Psychiatry*, *55*(6), 553–568. DOI: 10.1177/0004867420962851 PMID: 33028074

Stevens, M. W. R., King, D. L., Dorstyn, D., & Delfabbro, P. H. (2019). Cognitive–behavioral therapy for Internet gaming disorder: A systematic review and meta-analysis. *Clinical Psychology & Psychotherapy*, *26*(2), 191–203. DOI: 10.1002/cpp.2341 PMID: 30341981

Su, H., Ye, T., Cao, S., & Hu, C. (2024). Understanding the shift to compulsion in addiction: Insights from personality traits, social factors, and neurobiology. *Frontiers in Psychology*, *15*, 1416222. DOI: 10.3389/fpsyg.2024.1416222 PMID: 39315036

Subramanian, A., Chitlangia, S., & Baths, V. (2022). Reinforcement learning and its connections with neuroscience and psychology. *Neural Networks*, *145*, 271–287. DOI: 10.1016/j.neunet.2021.10.003 PMID: 34781215

Teicher, M. H., Samson, J. A., Anderson, C. M., & Ohashi, K. (2016). The effects of childhood maltreatment on brain structure, function and connectivity. *Nature Reviews. Neuroscience*, *17*(10), 652–666. DOI: 10.1038/nrn.2016.111 PMID: 27640984

Throuvala, M. A., Griffiths, M. D., Rennoldson, M., & Kuss, D. J. (2019). School-based prevention for adolescent internet addiction: Prevention is the key. A systematic literature review. *Current Neuropharmacology*, *17*(6), 507–525. DOI: 10.2174/1570159X16666180813153806 PMID: 30101714

Tracy, K., & Wallace, S. P. (2016). Benefits of peer support groups in the treatment of addiction. *Substance Abuse and Rehabilitation*, *7*, 143–154. DOI: 10.2147/SAR.S81535 PMID: 27729825

Tran, L. T., Wardle, H., Colledge-Frisby, S., Taylor, S., Lynch, M., Rehm, J., Volberg, R., Marionneau, V., Saxena, S., Bunn, C., Farrell, M., & Degenhardt, L. (2024). The prevalence of gambling and problematic gambling: A systematic review and meta-analysis. *The Lancet. Public Health*, *9*(8), e594–e613. DOI: 10.1016/S2468-2667(24)00126-9 PMID: 39025095

Trivedi, R. H., & Teichert, T. (2018). Attitudes, beliefs and impulsivity in online gambling addiction. *International Gambling Studies*, *18*(2), 327–342. DOI: 10.1080/14459795.2018.1466188

Uhl, G. R., Koob, G. F., & Cable, J. (2019). The neurobiology of addiction. *Annals of the New York Academy of Sciences*, *1451*(1), 5–28. DOI: 10.1111/nyas.13989 PMID: 30644552

Ünübol, B., Ünsalver, B. Ö., Ünübol, H., & Sayar, G. H. (2022, January 3). The prevalence and psychological relation of problem shopping: Data from a large-scale sample from Turkey. *BMC Psychology*, *10*(1), 1. DOI: 10.1186/s40359-021-00711-6 PMID: 34980253

van Timmeren, T., Jansen, J. M., Caan, M. W., Goudriaan, A. E., & van Holst, R. J. (2017). White matter integrity between left basal ganglia and left prefrontal cortex is compromised in gambling disorder. *Addiction Biology*, *22*(6), 1590–1600. DOI: 10.1111/adb.12447 PMID: 27612435

Vasile, D., & Vasiliu, O. (2021). Evidence-based pharmacological strategies for gambling disorder. Psihiatru. ro, 66(3).

Vecchio, L. M. (2016). *Investigating Monoamine Regulation: The Transport Of The Dopamine Transporter To Striatal Terminals And The Effects Of Tyrosine Hydroxylase Overexpression On Dopaminergic and Noradrenergic-Related Phenotypes*. University of Toronto.

Veit, R., Schag, K., Schopf, E., Borutta, M., Kreutzer, J., Ehlis, A. C., Zipfel, S., Giel, K. E., Preissl, H., & Kullmann, S. (2021). Diminished prefrontal cortex activation in patients with binge eating disorder associates with trait impulsivity and improves after impulsivity-focused treatment based on a randomized controlled IMPULS trial. *NeuroImage. Clinical*, *30*, 102679. DOI: 10.1016/j.nicl.2021.102679 PMID: 34215149

Vinberg, M., Wetterborg, D., & Enebrink, P. (2021). Gambling at work: A qualitative study of Swedish elite athletes, coaches, and managers. *Journal of Gambling Studies*, *37*(4), 1197–1217. DOI: 10.1007/s10899-021-10007-4 PMID: 33527302

Volkow, N. D., Michaelides, M., & Baler, R. (2019). The neuroscience of drug reward and addiction. *Physiological Reviews*, *99*(4), 2115–2140. DOI: 10.1152/physrev.00014.2018 PMID: 31507244

Volkow, N. D., Wang, G. J., Fowler, J. S., Tomasi, D., Telang, F., & Baler, R. (2010, September). Addiction: Decreased reward sensitivity and increased expectation sensitivity conspire to overwhelm the brain's control circuit. *BioEssays*, *32*(9), 748–755. DOI: 10.1002/bies.201000042 PMID: 20730946

Volkow, N. D., Wise, R. A., & Baler, R. (2017). The dopamine motive system: Implications for drug and food addiction. *Nature Reviews. Neuroscience*, *18*(12), 741–752. DOI: 10.1038/nrn.2017.130 PMID: 29142296

Von Deneen, K. M., Hussain, H., Waheed, J., Xinwen, W., Yu, D., & Yuan, K. (2022). Comparison of frontostriatal circuits in adolescent nicotine addiction and internet gaming disorder. *Journal of Behavioral Addictions*, *11*(1), 26–39. DOI: 10.1556/2006.2021.00086 PMID: 35049521

Wakefield, J. C. (2013). DSM-5: An overview of changes and controversies. *Clinical Social Work Journal*, *41*(2), 139–154. DOI: 10.1007/s10615-013-0445-2

Wang, H., La Russa, M., & Qi, L. S. (2016). CRISPR/Cas9 in genome editing and beyond. *Annual Review of Biochemistry*, *85*(1), 227–264. DOI: 10.1146/annurev-biochem-060815-014607 PMID: 27145843

Weinstein, A., & Lejoyeux, M. (2020). Neurobiological mechanisms underlying internet gaming disorder. *Dialogues in Clinical Neuroscience*, *22*(2), 113–126. DOI: 10.31887/DCNS.2020.22.2/aweinstein PMID: 32699511

Williams, W. A., Grant, J. E., Winstanley, C. A., & Potenza, M. N. (2008). Current concepts in the classification, treatment, and modeling of pathological gambling and other impulse control disorders. Animal and translational models for CNS drug discovery, 317-357.

World Health Organization. (2024). *Clinical descriptions and diagnostic requirements for ICD-11 mental, behavioural and neurodevelopmental disorders*. World Health Organization.

Xie, L., Zhao, J., Li, Y., & Bai, J. (2024). PET brain imaging in neurological disorders. *Physics of Life Reviews*. PMID: 38574584

Yılmazer, E. (2024). Hormonal Underpinnings of Emotional Regulation: Bridging Endocrinology and Psychology. *The Journal of Neurobehavioral Sciences, 11*(2), 60–75.

Young, K. S. (2009). Internet addiction test. Center for on-line addictions.

Young, P. A. (2023). *Investigating the Role of the Lateral Nigrostriatal Pathway in Modulating Voluntary Movement* (Doctoral dissertation).

Zack, M., George, R. S., & Clark, L. (2020). Dopaminergic signaling of uncertainty and the aetiology of gambling addiction. *Progress in Neuro-Psychopharmacology & Biological Psychiatry, 99*, 109853. DOI: 10.1016/j.pnpbp.2019.109853 PMID: 31870708

Zeng, X., Sun, Y. H., Gao, F., Hua, L., Xu, S., & Yuan, Z. (2024). Concurrent behavioral modeling and multimodal neuroimaging reveals how feedback affects the performance of decision making in internet gaming disorder. *NeuroImage, 297*, 120726. DOI: 10.1016/j.neuroimage.2024.120726 PMID: 38986794

Zhang, J., Wang, E., Zhang, L., & Chi, X. (2024). Internet addiction and depressive symptoms in adolescents: Joint trajectories and predictors. *Frontiers in Public Health, 12*, 1374762. DOI: 10.3389/fpubh.2024.1374762 PMID: 38894983

Chapter 2
Unraveling Internet Addiction:
Clinical Perspectives, Implications, and Interventions

Joselyn Barnhart
https://orcid.org/0009-0006-2517-7509
University of Texas Rio Grande Valley, USA

Leslie Reyes
https://orcid.org/0009-0002-4095-1639
University of Texas Rio Grande Valley, USA

Cameron Lacy Ortega
https://orcid.org/0000-0003-0827-2070
University of Texas Rio Grande Valley, USA

ABSTRACT

Internet addiction (IA) is a growing public health concern, particularly among adolescents and those with psychological vulnerabilities. As digital connectivity expands, excessive internet use is linked to social isolation, mental health issues, and cognitive impairment. This chapter explores the demographic, psychological, and environmental factors contributing to IA, emphasizing impulsivity, emotional distress, and social influences. It examines IA's neurobiological basis, drawing parallels with substance use disorders, focusing on dopamine dysregulation and reward processing. Cultural perspectives show how societal norms and technology access shape IA prevalence. Peer pressure, family dynamics, and socioeconomic disparities are analyzed as risk factors. Effective treatments are reviewed, including cognitive-behavioral therapy (CBT), motivational interviewing (MI), family ther-

DOI: 10.4018/979-8-3373-0518-9.ch002

apy, and exercise-based interventions. The chapter highlights relapse prevention, advocacy, and policy recommendations to promote responsible technology use and support affected individuals.

CHAPTER OVERVIEW

Internet addiction (IA) has emerged as a significant public health concern, particularly among vulnerable populations such as adolescents and individuals with pre-existing psychological conditions. As digital connectivity continues to expand, excessive internet use has been linked to negative consequences, including social isolation, mental health disorders, and impaired cognitive and emotional functioning. This chapter explores the demographic, psychological, and environmental factors contributing to IA, highlighting the role of impulsivity, emotional distress, and social influences in the development of compulsive internet use.

The chapter also examines the neurobiological underpinnings of IA, drawing parallels between internet addiction and substance use disorders, with a focus on dopamine dysregulation and altered reward processing. Additionally, it explores cultural perspectives on IA, illustrating how societal norms, values, and access to technology influence attitudes and prevalence rates across various populations. The impact of peer pressure, family dynamics, and socioeconomic disparities on the risk of IA is analyzed, emphasizing the need for tailored interventions.

Treatment approaches, including cognitive-behavioral therapy (CBT), motivational interviewing (MI), family-centered therapy, and exercise-based interventions, are explored as effective strategies for mitigating symptoms of IA. The chapter further underscores the importance of relapse prevention, community outreach, and advocacy in addressing the broader implications of IA. By fostering awareness and promoting evidence-based interventions, this research aims to inform policies and therapeutic strategies that support individuals struggling with internet addiction while encouraging responsible technology use in an increasingly digital world.

UNRAVELING INTERNET ADDICTION: CLINICAL PERSPECTIVES, IMPLICATIONS, AND INTERVENTIONS

In recent years, internet addiction (IA) has become an increasingly significant issue, reflecting the rapid advancement of technology and the deep integration of the internet into our daily lives. The exponential growth of digital connectivity and online platforms has transformed social interactions, educational practices, and work environments. However, this widespread presence also has a darker side: an addiction that can significantly impact individual well-being and societal dynamics.

Internet addiction can be defined as a compulsive behavior characterized by an excessive preoccupation with internet use, which negatively impacts personal, social, educational, or occupational functioning (American Psychological Association [APA], 2015). This issue goes beyond merely excessive usage; it encompasses a range of behaviors and experiences that can lead to significant impairment in various aspects of life (APA, 2015). As internet use continues to expand, it is essential to understand the nuances of internet addiction.

The signs and symptoms of internet addiction can vary from one individual to another, but they often include withdrawal symptoms, increased tolerance, and continued use despite facing negative consequences. Those affected may struggle to reduce their internet usage, which can lead to neglecting important relationships or responsibilities. Recognizing these signs is crucial for those directly affected, as well as for the communities and systems that often deal with the repercussions of this challenge.

For nearly two decades, researchers have been investigating internet addiction and its various aspects. This complex topic has undergone significant evolution over time (Pan et al., 2020). The concept of internet addiction disorder was first introduced by Kimberly Young in a landmark paper published in 1996 (Reuter et al., 2017). She argued that internet addiction (IA) should be considered for inclusion in the Diagnostic and Statistical Manual of Mental Disorders (DSM), Fourth Edition (Zhu et al., 2023). Research on internet addiction has not been fully incorporated into the DSM-5 due to inconsistent diagnostic criteria, leading to varied reports on frequency, progression, and treatment (Andic & Durak Batigun, 2019). Although internet addiction is not currently recognized in the DSM-5, a related condition called internet gaming disorder (IGD) has been acknowledged as a disorder that requires further analysis and research (APA, 2015). Young's recommendations opened up new avenues for inquiry into internet addiction, prompting additional investigations.

IA is recognized as a public health concern in countries like China and South Korea, where there is advocacy for more research as well as improved education and treatment for internet addiction (Reuter et al., 2017). In the United States, however, there is a lack of governmental recognition or response to internet addiction disorder (IAD) (Reuter et al., 2017). Despite this, numerous studies are being conducted to understand the various elements of internet addiction and their impact on individuals' mental and physical health.

The accessibility of the internet has increased significantly in recent decades, with daily usage rising rapidly. For instance, a 2015 study in Germany reported that 44.5 million people accessed the internet daily, which represented a 3.5 million increase from the previous year (Leménager et al., 2018). The COVID-19 pandemic likely further amplified global internet usage. During the pandemic, lockdowns and quarantines led to increased reliance on the internet for education, work, social interaction, and entertainment (Onukwuli et al., 2023). Social distancing measures and stay-at-home regulations contributed to the prolonged time individuals spent online (Onukwuli et al., 2023). The pandemic also caused financial stress and social isolation for many, leading individuals to turn to the internet for coping, which likely resulted in increased usage (Masaeli & Farhadi, 2021). As face-to-face interactions were replaced by virtual ones, online time continued to rise. The combination of increased internet usage and the uncertainty surrounding the pandemic created an environment conducive to the development of internet addiction (Onukwuli et al., 2023).

Understanding internet addiction is crucial due to its prevalence and potential long-term impact on society. As technology evolves, it fosters new forms of interaction that can lead to addictive behaviors. A comprehensive exploration of this addiction can help inform interventions, policy-making, and public health strategies aimed at mitigating its effects. Recognizing internet addiction as a significant mental health concern enables stakeholders to address the issue holistically, promoting healthier habits and lifestyles.

COGNITIVE AND BEHAVIORAL INDICATORS

Problematic internet use is often characterized by compulsive behavior, withdrawal symptoms, and tolerance, all of which stem from an individual's inability to control their internet usage. This can lead to emotional distress and functional difficulties, resulting in various social and health-related challenges (Liu et al., 2022). Key indicators of problematic internet use include an excessive preoccupation with the internet, prolonged online time, increased tolerance for internet activities, and unsuccessful attempts to reduce or limit internet usage.

Excessive internet use impairs individuals by interfering with their daily activities, relationships, and responsibilities (Zhu et al., 2023). Individuals who develop internet dependencies may use online engagement to avoid personal issues or alleviate negative moods (Tang et al., 2024). This behavior can jeopardize personal relationships, hinder job performance, and interfere with educational goals, making it difficult for individuals to reduce their internet time (Zeidi et al., 2020). Additionally, individuals exhibiting Internet Addiction (IA) may engage in behaviors that threaten their relationships, including deceit. In adolescents, excessive internet use not only affects their behavior but can also impede the formation of a personal identity, which is vital during this developmental stage (Leménager et al., 2018). When offline, they may experience withdrawal symptoms, emotional distress, and cognitive issues (Leménager et al., 2018). Common signs of IA include tension, mood swings, sleep disruptions, irritability, agitation, and fluctuations in weight (either gain or loss) (Chang & Lee, 2024; Wang et al., 2022). Other consequences may include social isolation and even substance abuse. IA affects various aspects of an individual's life and has a significant impact on their overall mental and physical health. Recognizing the effects of internet addiction can help determine the best approaches for providing adequate care and treatment for those affected.

An example of compulsive internet use is when a person eagerly awaits their next opportunity to access the internet. They may constantly reminisce about past moments of online engagement, even when offline (Chadha et al., 2024). The level of attention and focus devoted to internet usage can influence an individual's tolerance for online activities (Reuter et al., 2017). This could lead to an increase in the frequency of online interactions and more intensive internet use to achieve the same satisfaction they previously experienced. Many individuals might use the internet as a way to escape from personal issues or to cope with negative emotions such as feelings of powerlessness, shame, stress, or depression (Baloğlu et al., 2020).

People with problematic internet usage often spend excessive amounts of time online (Baloğlu et al., 2020). They can lose track of time and stay online longer than intended. This excessive use may lead to neglecting responsibilities, such as work or school (Baloğlu et al., 2020). Chronic internet usage can strain interpersonal relationships, potentially causing conflicts with family, friends, and romantic partners. Individuals might even resort to deceptive tactics to conceal the extent of their online activity (Reuter et al., 2017). Despite the negative consequences, these individuals may continue to engage in excessive internet use, which can lead to further issues in their relationships, as well as in their academic or career pursuits, and health concerns (Baloğlu et al., 2020).

The inability to regulate internet usage can manifest in various behaviors and experiences, often signaling compulsive conduct associated with problematic internet use. Such behaviors may cause significant distress and functional impairment, driven by an overwhelming urge to remain online at all times (Liu et al., 2022).

Several key aspects of compulsive behaviors related to problematic internet use are worth noting. A primary compulsive behavior among those affected is the uncontrollable urge to use the internet. This intense compulsion can make it extremely difficult for individuals to resist the desire to be online (Ge et al., 2023). This uncontrollable craving might manifest as a constant checking of online activities, such as frequently refreshing social media accounts or emails in search of new information (Pettorruso et al., 2020). Individuals with problematic internet use often struggle to end their online sessions once they have logged in. They may even be hesitant to disconnect from the internet, fearing the need to return to their online engagements.

CULTURAL AND SOCIETAL INFLUENCE

The differences in cultures among individuals significantly impact views on internet addiction. Cultural values, social norms, and access to technology all influence the perception and acceptability of internet addiction. Some cultures consider internet addiction a serious problem, while others do not (Reuter et al., 2017). By analyzing various cultural factors, including the prevalence of internet addiction, cultural attitudes, and cultural adaptation, we can gain valuable insights into this phenomenon.

The prevalence of internet addiction varies widely across different cultures. Research indicates that Eastern populations often report higher rates of internet addiction compared to Western populations (Baloğlu et al., 2020). A study conducted across eleven European countries found that the overall prevalence of problematic internet use among adolescents was 4.4% (Lopez-Fernandez, 2015). Globally, the prevalence rate for Internet addiction (IA) is 3.05%, with European countries reporting a lower prevalence rate at 2.7% compared to Asian countries at 5.1% (Chang & Lee, 2024). Internet usage in the United States has surged over the past twenty years. By 2015, 95% of youth and 84% of adults were online (Rosenthal et al., 2018). As of March 2021, approximately three in ten American adults reported using the internet “almost constantly.” Additionally, over 53% of American adults increased their screen time during the COVID-19 pandemic (Khubchandani et al., 2021). Research has shown that male adolescents are more likely to experience internet addiction than female adolescents, attributed to higher engagement in activities such as gaming and cybersex (Zhou et al., 2018). In China, 14% of students were identified as heavy internet users, while only 4% of students in the United States fell into this category (Błachnio et al., 2019). The Philippines reported a problematic internet use rate of 51%, Japan 48%, and China 17% (Błachnio et al., 2019). These studies highlight that internet addiction is a global issue, with cultural differences significantly influencing internet usage rates.

Cultural attitudes and norms play a critical role in how internet addiction is perceived and whether it is recognized as a problem within specific cultures (WANG et al., 2024). In some cultures, internet addiction may be viewed as shameful due to prevailing cultural standards, leading individuals to hide or downplay their internet usage (Błachnio et al., 2019). This stigma can complicate efforts to assess the extent of internet addiction (Błachnio et al., 2019). For instance, in regions like China, internet addiction is now recognized as a disorder and regarded as a serious concern (Reuter et al., 2017). Parents' perspectives on internet usage can also influence their children's attitudes; if a parent views the internet positively, a child is more likely to adopt that same view. As a result, if this child later develops internet addiction, it may go unrecognized as a problem due to these shared attitudes. This underscores how cultural values and attitudes strongly influence internet usage, technology adoption, and related outcomes (Baloğlu et al., 2020; Lukavská et al., 2022). A study comparing internet use in the United States, Africa, and China found that internet addiction may develop in stages, with variations depending on cultural access to and familiarity with technology (Chen & Nath, 2016). Other research has shown that individuals lacking emotional support or those dissatisfied with their lives are more vulnerable to developing problematic internet use or internet addiction (Błachnio et al., 2019). Cultural attitudes and norms significantly shape the perception and acceptability of internet addiction, impacting how it manifests across the globe.

When evaluating perceptions of internet addiction, cultural adaptation is also an important factor. Cultural adaptation refers to an individual's ability to adjust to an online culture (Yue et al., 2024). According to the theory of cross-cultural adaptation, individuals who encounter a cultural environment different from their own may go through psychological adjustments (Yue et al., 2024). Adolescents, for instance, face a variety of online cultures, and if they lack effective adaptation strategies, they may experience cultural shock. This shock can lead to unconscious bias, negative emotions, and illogical online behaviors (Yue et al., 2024). This theory is relevant in the context of internet use, and adaptation has been shown to have a substantial impact on internet addiction (Yue et al., 2024).

Understanding how cultural differences impact internet addiction is crucial for developing culturally sensitive prevention and intervention measures. Ignoring these cultural factors can result in ineffective treatment for individuals with internet addiction and hinder efforts to address the social and cultural underpinnings of this issue.

INTERNET ADDICTION AMONG VULNERABLE POPULATIONS

In the digital era, internet addiction (IA) has become a significant public health concern, particularly impacting vulnerable populations such as adolescents and individuals with pre-existing psychological conditions. As technology becomes increasingly integrated into everyday life, excessive internet use continues to rise, worsening mental health issues, social isolation, and developmental challenges. Understanding the demographic, psychological, and environmental factors contributing to IA is essential for developing effective prevention and intervention strategies.

Demographic variables, including age, gender, race/ethnicity, and socioeconomic status, play a crucial role in shaping the prevalence of internet addiction. Adolescents are particularly vulnerable due to their developmental stage, which involves identity exploration and increased exposure to digital platforms. Research indicates that older adolescents exhibit higher rates of IA, likely due to greater access to technology and an intensified need for social interaction (Malak, 2018; Chang &

Lee, 2024). Variations in internet accessibility have a significant impact on internet addiction rates (Khubchandani et al., 2021). During the pandemic, severe internet addiction was higher in urban areas (16%) than in rural (13%) and suburban areas (8%) (Khubchandani et al., 2021). Studies also indicate gender differences, with boys more prone to general internet addiction and girls to excessive social media use (Harsej et al., 2021; Kolaib et al., 2020). A cross-national study involving college students from the United States, China, and Singapore revealed that male students exhibited a higher rate of internet addiction at 6.0% compared to 5.0% for female students (Tang et al., 2017). This finding highlights significant gender differences in the types of internet-related addiction (Tang et al., 2017). Race and ethnicity are also demographic variables that may influence the development of internet addiction. A study conducted on U.S. adults during the COVID-19 pandemic found notable variations in the prevalence of definite or severe internet addiction by race and ethnicity (Khubchandani et al., 2021). Specifically, Asians displayed a prevalence rate of 23%, Hispanics at 19%, Whites at 13%, and African Americans at 11% (Khubchandani et al., 2021). Furthermore, socioeconomic factors play a role in influencing internet addiction patterns, as individuals from lower-income backgrounds may resort to the internet as a coping mechanism for social and economic stressors.

Beyond demographics, psychological factors play a significant role in the development of IA. Impulsivity—defined as acting without forethought—has been consistently linked to excessive internet use, as individuals with high impulsivity often use online activities to escape underlying psychological distress, including anxiety and depression (Ge et al., 2023; Chung et al., 2019; Arzani-Birgani et al., 2021). This issue is particularly concerning for adolescents with Attention-Deficit/Hyperactivity Disorder (ADHD), as they may struggle with self-regulation and exhibit compulsive digital media use. Karen et al. (2018) found that prolonged digital exposure can exacerbate ADHD symptoms, impairing attention and behavioral control, which in turn creates a cycle of dependency on online interactions.

The relationship between IA and mental health is well-documented, with studies indicating that individuals with psychiatric disorders are more likely to develop internet addiction (Yar et al., 2019). Social isolation further heightens the risk of IA, as lonely adolescents often turn to the internet for companionship, unintentionally reinforcing their sense of detachment from real-world interactions (Ge et al., 2023). This paradox highlights the internet's dual role: it provides a connection, yet it also contributes to worsening social well-being.

Environmental influences, including family dynamics and peer pressure, also shape internet usage behaviors. Adolescents from dysfunctional family backgrounds face a higher risk of IA, while positive family interactions serve as a protective factor (Harsej et al., 2021; Nwufo et al., 2022; Xin et al., 2018). Parental attitudes toward digital media play a crucial role in determining children's internet habits;

discrepancies between parents' perceptions and adolescents' actual social media use can lead to ineffective interventions (Patra et al., 2021). Open parent-child communication about online engagement has been shown to mitigate feelings of loneliness and anxiety among adolescents (Chen et al., 2025).

Peer influence is another significant factor, as adolescents often conform to social norms surrounding digital consumption. Studies indicate that peer pressure can lead to excessive internet use, making IA more socially acceptable and increasing its prevalence (Reuter et al., 2017; Chung et al., 2019). Furthermore, the widespread availability of smartphones and digital devices has facilitated constant connectivity, fostering compulsive usage patterns that disrupt academic, social, and emotional well-being (Colder Carras et al., 2024; Reuter et al., 2017; Wei et al., 2025; Kamate et al., 2019). The nature of online content, such as social media and gaming, further contributes to these compulsive behaviors.

Cultural perspectives also shape attitudes toward IA, influencing how societies recognize and address this issue. Research suggests that cultural norms regarding social interactions and digital engagement lead to varying IA prevalence rates across different ethnic groups (Błachnio et al., 2019). Ethnic minorities often face socioeconomic challenges that heighten IA risks, including limited access to mental health resources and cultural stigmas surrounding psychological treatment. These factors can lead individuals to engage in excessive internet use as a means of coping with social isolation and discrimination (Sharma & Palanichamy, 2018; Tang et al., 2024). While the internet can offer a sense of belonging, it can also reinforce isolation from real-world social interactions, creating a paradoxical dependence on digital connections (Yar et al., 2019). The prevalence of internet addiction demonstrates the need for comprehensive strategies to address this issue across various demographic, psychological, and environmental contexts.

THE NEUROBIOLOGY OF INTERNET ADDICTION

The reward pathways in the brain, particularly those associated with the mesolimbic dopamine system, play a vital role in the development of addictive behaviors, including Internet addiction (IA). Research has shown that individuals with IA exhibit altered activation patterns in brain regions associated with reward processing, including the striatum and the prefrontal cortex. For instance, Li et al. (2020) demonstrated decreased functional connectivity in the brains of adolescents with IA, indicating that the neural circuits involved in reward processing are compromised. This finding supports the notion that IA may share similar neurobiological characteristics with substance use disorders, where the dysregulation of the dopamine system is a common feature (Brahma & Brahma, 2023).

Dopamine is a crucial neurotransmitter in the brain's reward system, playing a significant role in the context of IA. Findings suggest that individuals with IA had notably lower levels of dopamine D2 receptors in the striatum (Lu, 2023; Wang et al., 2023). This reduction inversely correlated with the severity of their addiction. A decrease in receptor availability indicates that the dopaminergic system may respond less effectively to rewarding stimuli, which could drive individuals to seek more intense or frequent internet use to achieve the same level of satisfaction (Chang & Lee, 2024; Wang et al., 2023). Dopamine dysregulation is a key feature of IA, characterized by reduced receptor availability and altered levels of the dopamine transporter. Yaunin et al. (2019) reported that individuals with IA also experience dysfunction in the serotonin system, highlighting the complex interactions between multiple neurotransmitter systems in the context of addiction. This dysregulation can lead to compulsive internet use, as individuals seek to compensate for the decreased reward response by engaging in behaviors that provide immediate gratification.

EFFECTS OF DIFFERENT ONLINE ACTIVITIES

Gaming is one of the most studied behaviors associated with IA. Research indicates that excessive gaming activates the brain's reward pathways, similar to substance addiction. Lu (2023) reported a finding that individuals with IA exhibited reduced levels of dopamine D2 receptors in the striatum, which is crucial for reward processing. This reduction suggests that people with IA may have a diminished capacity for experiencing pleasure, leading them to seek more intense gaming experiences to achieve the same level of satisfaction (Chang & Lee, 2024; Wang et al., 2022). Moreover, Chang and Lee (2024) reported microstructural changes in neuronal pathways among individuals with intracranial aneurysms (IA). This finding indicates that prolonged gaming can lead to alterations in brain structure, potentially affecting cognitive functions and emotional regulation. These results highlight the potential for gaming not only to activate reward pathways but also to induce structural changes in the brain that could exacerbate addictive behaviors.

Social media use also significantly impacts neurobiological responses. Studies have shown that social media can trigger dopamine release, reinforcing compulsive behaviors similar to those observed in substance use disorders (Andreassen et al., 2017). For example, Andreassen et al. noted that excessive social media use is characterized by an uncontrollable urge to log on, which can impair other important areas of life (Andreassen et al., 2017). This compulsive behavior is often driven by the immediate rewards associated with social media interactions, such as likes and comments, leading to heightened dopamine activity in the brain's reward circuitry (Wang et al., 2022; Wang et al., 2023).

Understanding the neurobiological responses associated with specific internet behaviors has significant implications for treatment, particularly for individuals with IA, especially those engaged in excessive gaming or social media use. Treatment strategies may need to be tailored to address the underlying neurobiological mechanisms. Cognitive-behavioral therapy (CBT) has shown promise in treating IA by helping individuals develop healthier coping strategies and improve emotional regulation (Alavi et al., 2021).

INTERVENTION AND TREATMENT APPROACHES

Internet addiction remains a significant issue across various age groups, prompting numerous studies to examine its adverse effects and symptoms on individuals and their daily lives. Given that internet use has become essential for everyday activities, including work, the ideal treatment outcome for this disorder is for clients to achieve a controlled use of the Internet while avoiding applications that hinder full recovery (Sharma & Palanichamy, 2018).

Currently, no single intervention or treatment approach is considered the most effective. However, several strategies have been researched and shown promise in treating internet addiction. Notable among these are cognitive behavioral therapy (CBT) and motivational enhancement therapy (MET) (Sharma & Palanichamy, 2018). Additionally, family-based therapy has been incorporated into treatment interventions. This approach helps foster a supportive family environment, which can be crucial for individuals struggling with internet addiction (WANG et al., 2024).

Once clients learn to identify the problems and consequences associated with internet addiction, they can set treatment goals. This enables the introduction of recovery and relapse prevention strategies, such as harm reduction techniques, which are typically part of the third phase in CBT for internet addiction (Xu et al., 2021).

Cognitive Behavioral Therapy (CBT)

Cognitive Behavioral Therapy (CBT) is designed to educate clients and help them challenge their thoughts, which ultimately aids in regulating their behavior (Zeidi et al., 2020). This therapeutic approach has been studied and implemented as a treatment for internet addiction (IA) across various age groups, as it focuses on assisting individuals in understanding the feelings associated with addiction and the behaviors that stem from it (Antoniac et al., 2024). A key component of CBT is teaching clients to identify and control unproductive thinking patterns, which can lead to recovery and equip them with skills to manage cravings and prevent relapse (Zeidi et al., 2020).

Unlike substance use addiction, where the primary goal is complete abstinence, treating internet addiction requires a different perspective. Given that technology and media are integral parts of our daily lives, a complete disconnection from the Internet is impractical. Instead, the intended outcome of treatment for IA is to achieve "moderate and controlled use" of the Internet while aiming to eliminate harmful behaviors associated with excessive use of specific applications (Antoniac et al., 2024; Sharma & Palanichamy, 2018). To achieve this, a specific form of CBT known as CBT-IA has been developed.

Dr. Kimberly Young introduced CBT for internet addiction (CBT-IA), which encompasses a three-phase process designed to help clients minimize and regulate their daily Internet usage, transform cognitive patterns that contribute to harmful use, and address any underlying issues through harm reduction (Pluhar et al., 2019; Antoniac et al., 2024; Reuter et al., 2017).

The first phase involves behavior modification, where clients work with therapists to establish strategies and set goals for limiting their online time (Pluhar et al., 2019; WANG et al., 2024). The second phase is cognitive restructuring, which helps clients challenge negative thought processes or emotions contributing to their internet-related problems (Pluhar et al., 2019). The final phase focuses on harm reduction, highlighting any underlying issues that may contribute to problematic Internet use, thereby reducing the potential for misuse and relapse (Pluhar et al., 2019).

While further research is necessary to determine the most effective intervention, CBT-IA has shown significant efficacy in reducing internet usage among clients, especially in group settings for students (Zeidi et al., 2020). However, a limitation of CBT-IA and group CBT is the lack of comprehensive research on the long-term effects of these interventions for IA (Reuter et al., 2017).

In addition to CBT-IA, different forms or techniques of motivational interventions may also be utilized alongside other therapies. These motivational interventions expand the therapeutic process to accommodate a broader range of age groups and address the motivations and issues underlying problematic internet usage (Ong et al., 2024). By employing one or more of these techniques, clients can develop healthier internet usage habits and address the core issues that have contributed to their internet addiction (Colder Carras et al., 2024).

Motivational Interventions

An intervention that falls within the category of motivational approaches and is used for Internet Addiction (IA) is Motivational Interviewing (MI). Motivational Interviewing is a client-centered therapeutic approach that emphasizes collaboration between the therapist and the client (Dieris-Hirche et al., 2021). During sessions, the therapist strives to be empathetic and affirming, employs reflective listening, asks open-ended questions, and remains receptive to the client's input. This creates a safe environment for clients to explore their internal motivations and consider changing their behaviors (Dieris-Hirche et al., 2021; Sharma & Palanichamy, 2018; Zeidi et al., 2020). Additionally, MI helps clients identify the effects of their Internet use and examines their ambivalence toward it, assisting them in overcoming this ambivalence (Sharma & Palanichamy, 2018). For IA, MI can be applied in-person or through an online-based motivational program (OMPRIS), which combines MI techniques with elements of Cognitive Behavioral Therapy (CBT) (Dieris-Hirche et al., 2021).

OMPRIS has shown efficacy in improving behaviors associated with various addictive disorders. Given its incorporation of CBT elements, which has been effectively studied and utilized in treating IA, this therapeutic approach offers educational therapy and social counseling. Thus, it is considered a promising intervention for IA (Dieris-Hirche et al., 2021). Essentially, OMPRIS operates through a browser-based platform that enables clients to become aware of their problematic media use. Through the therapeutic process, they develop achievable goals by emphasizing their strengths and adopting new behaviors using MI techniques (Dieris-Hirche et al., 2021; Niemann et al., 2023). While further studies are needed to explore the effectiveness and long-term outcomes of MI in treating IA, it is likely to succeed in future treatments when combined with additional therapeutic approaches (Dieris-Hirche et al., 2021).

A similar approach to MI is Motivational Enhancement Therapy (MET), which also involves a collaborative, non-confrontational dynamic between the therapist and the client (Sharma & Palanichamy, 2018). In this approach, the client and therapist collaborate to create a personalized plan for addressing IA and setting achievable goals (Sharma & Palanichamy, 2018). MET helps clients understand their emotions and how these feelings contribute to excessive Internet use, as well as how they use these emotions to justify their problematic behaviors (Sharma & Palanichamy, 2018).

As with MI, MET can be combined with other interventions such as CBT. While CBT focuses on educating the client and examining their thoughts and behaviors, MET and motivational interventions concentrate on exploring the client's motivations and identifying positive factors to encourage commitment to change (Sharma & Palanichamy, 2018; Zeidi et al., 2020).

Family-Centered Therapeutic Approaches

Although internet addiction (IA) may arise from a client's personal issues, thoughts, and behaviors, it can also develop due to family-related factors. These factors include, but are not limited to, a lack of support or attention from family members or parents, poor relationships between parents and children or among siblings, and childhood trauma (Hua et al., 2022; Tang et al., 2024). Because IA can either be a consequence of or a contributing factor to family dysfunction and childhood trauma, studies suggest that incorporating family-based therapy as an intervention may lead to improvements in various areas, rather than solely focusing on changing the client's behavior (Hua et al., 2022).

Family-based therapy views every family member as part of a system, each playing a role in the family's dynamics. When these dynamics are not functioning correctly, therapy can help bring about positive change and create a supportive environment, provided all family members are willing to participate (Tang et al., 2024). Ultimately, family-based therapy aims to help families develop and maintain effective communication skills that benefit everyone involved. Good communication enables family members to express and explore their challenges, which can boost children's self-esteem (Zeidi et al., 2020).

Exercised-Based Interventions

Interventions to enhance dopamine function, such as exercise-based therapies, may offer significant benefits. Research indicates that physical activity has a positive influence on neurobiology and can alleviate some symptoms of Internet Addiction (IA) by enhancing dopamine receptor sensitivity (Li et al., 2020). Moreover, engaging in daily physical activity can have psychological benefits for clients. Exercise may also address other diagnoses that contribute to the development of IA, such as anxiety or depression (Koçak, 2018). It can be a rewarding intervention on its own or with other tailored treatment approaches (Li et al., 2020).

Exercise acts as a natural reward, facilitating neurobiological regulation by influencing the dopamine system related to the nigrostriatal pathway. Stimulating this pathway can increase dopamine release (Li et al., 2020). Higher dopamine levels enhance various aspects of an individual's life, including motivation and habit formation, creating a positive reward cycle (Li et al., 2020). Ultimately, exercise impacts reward stimulation and helps reduce impulsive behaviors by affecting the prefrontal cortex, which plays a role in dysregulated factors observed in individuals with IA (Liu et al., 2019).

In addition to improving physical health, physical activity boosts self-esteem and overall well-being, thereby lowering the likelihood of developing depression or other mental health issues (Li et al., 2020). Increased self-esteem may reduce the need for online acceptance or self-satisfaction through internet use, leading to lower rates of IA or problematic internet behavior (Li et al., 2023). Regular exercise can help individuals with IA reduce their internet usage over time (Koçak, 2018). Establishing a routine through regular exercise enables individuals to manage their social lives, physical health, and emotions, which may be impacted by internet use (Koçak, 2018).

Different exercise-based interventions can address IA and effectively combine with other therapeutic techniques or theories to enhance treatment success. For instance, cognitive behavioral therapy (CBT) is often paired with movement-based interventions, such as yoga, which can benefit young adults and adolescents by reducing stress and fostering mindfulness regarding their behaviors while promoting relaxation (Tadpatrikar et al., 2023). Other therapies incorporating exercise include mixed or motor skill activities. Open-skill exercises, such as basketball, require quick responses to external stimuli, providing a platform for individuals to express negative emotions through movement, which can help alleviate the discomfort of remaining passive on social media (Li et al., 2023). In contrast, closed-skill exercises, such as swimming, require continuous practice, allowing individuals to focus on the activity rather than turning to social media as an escape (Li et al., 2023). Although both open and closed-skill exercises are practical when practiced separately, their combined use has shown the most tremendous success in preventing or minimizing the impacts of IA (Li et al., 2023).

Relapse Prevention and Harm Reduction

Using various interventions or therapeutic approaches can significantly aid clients in preparing for relapse prevention. Typically, relapse prevention is integrated within the interventions utilized during therapy sessions, especially in the termination phase of OMPRIS, which incorporates CBT techniques (Dieris-Hirche et al., 2021). One effective technique is self-monitoring, where clients track and recognize triggers that may lead them to engage in problematic internet behaviors (Dieris-Hirche et al., 2021). Clients must learn to regulate the emotions that drive excessive internet use. Once they develop the ability to manage their emotions, they can acquire skills to navigate situations that might tempt them to relapse (Dieris-Hirche et al., 2021).

In addition to working on relapse prevention strategies, it is essential to address the underlying issues that contribute to internet addiction, such as a client's loneliness, to avoid potential relapse triggers in the future (Chen et al., 2025). Research suggests that expecting complete abstinence from the internet may not be the most favorable outcome for therapy, as moderate use could be beneficial for some clients. If abstinence is viewed as the sole solution, the risk of relapse may increase (Colder Carras et al., 2024). Several factors must be considered for effective relapse prevention, with one of the most crucial being the therapist's role in referring clients to additional treatment options. This helps ensure clients maintain progress and minimize the chance of reverting to problematic behaviors (Dieris-Hirche et al., 2021).

IMPLICATIONS FOR PRACTICE AND COMMUNITY OUTREACH

For treatment of internet addiction (IA) to be effective, practitioners must have a thorough understanding of the addiction, the technology associated with it, and the root causes for each client. Additionally, they should possess the knowledge and skills to employ various interventions that can aid in treatment. Neglecting these considerations may lead to ineffective therapy and could potentially harm clients rather than help them overcome their addiction. Practitioners must be culturally competent and take into account the diverse backgrounds and values of their clients, as internet addiction can affect individuals across all demographics (Reuter et al., 2017). By becoming culturally competent, practitioners can consider the unique cultural norms, beliefs, and needs of each client, enabling them to provide tailored and effective therapy.

Beyond individual therapy, outreach programs are vital for helping individuals understand internet addiction and learn how to prevent problematic behaviors (Reuter et al., 2017). Providing resources and support to underserved communities is crucial, as these populations may lack access to necessary help or cannot afford treatment. Outreach initiatives can target youth, families, or groups that are at a higher risk of developing IA, taking into account various factors in their lives. Practitioners can advocate for their clients or marginalized populations by promoting treatment policies that include outreach programs, such as digital literacy initiatives or expanding insurance coverage (Lo et al., 2020).

Professional Competencies

There may be many challenges that therapists face when helping clients manage excessive internet usage or addiction, as internet addiction (IA) can arise from various factors in a client's life rather than a single cause. Factors that may contribute to IA and can influence one another include social influences, family dynamics, socio-economic status, and other psychological aspects (Chen et al., 2025). Practitioners must understand these factors in their clients' lives to provide effective treatment and reduce the risk of relapse (Chen et al., 2025).

In addition to identifying the root causes of IA for each client, practitioners need to be skilled in therapeutic techniques to address any psychological issues and effectively treat internet addiction. Important clinical competencies include assessing and diagnosing clients (Reuter et al., 2017). During the assessment phase, practitioners should utilize tools such as the Internet Addiction Test (IAT) or Young's Internet Addiction Scale (YIAS), which help identify symptoms aligned with IA (Antoniac et al., 2024; Reuter et al., 2017). Through thorough assessment, practitioners can also identify other psychological issues that the client may be facing alongside IA, enabling the development of a more effective treatment plan (Reuter et al., 2017).

Considering culturally diverse clients is essential as practitioners gain skills and knowledge over time. Clients from different backgrounds may experience internet addiction differently and may require therapy that reflects the unique values of their cultures (Liu et al., 2024). For example, a study highlights differences between Asian and European countries in terms of excessive internet use, which may stem from varying social norms and environmental influences (Reuter et al., 2017). Therefore, it is crucial for practitioners to understand how IA is perceived in different cultures and to assess clients based on their cultural beliefs.

Cultural perspectives on addiction can significantly affect how clients receive therapy or diagnoses. Practitioners need to apply various therapeutic interventions that take into account the client's cultural background. For instance, some cultures prioritize family unity in addressing issues, while others may emphasize individual independence (Lo et al., 2020). Flexibility in treatment approaches that consider the client's beliefs, needs, values, and culture is vital for successful therapy (Lo et al., 2020).

To continuously improve as professionals, therapists should stay informed about new research and developments in interventions. This ongoing learning enhances their skills and addresses the needs of culturally diverse clients effectively (Reuter et al., 2017). Being knowledgeable and adaptable contributes to a more ethical and effective therapeutic process for all clients, especially those from diverse backgrounds.

Community Outreach and Prevention Initiatives

Accessing help and affording support is a privilege that many in lower socioeconomic populations do not have. Therefore, it is essential to incorporate community outreach into mental health services and preventive initiatives for those who are unable to seek help due to economic disadvantages. Promoting awareness and providing support for young children, families, and other at-risk groups is crucial for both treating and preventing IA. Community outreach facilitates education, awareness, and the provision of strategies and support for individuals affected by IA (Reuter et al., 2017). Additionally, it empowers communities with resources to assist vulnerable populations in preventing IA (Jain et al., 2024).

Engaging with communities, particularly those with limited access to education compared to higher socioeconomic groups, is crucial in preventing IA and providing support to those who are less fortunate. Community outreach programs for IA can encompass campaigns, community-based services, mental health programs, and other strategies designed to foster resilience and awareness (Jain et al., 2024; Reuter et al., 2017). For example, campaigns such as "Smart Off" can make a significant impact.

Advocacy and Policy Support

Professionals in the behavioral health field play a vital role in advocating for their clients, particularly those affected by Internet Addiction (IA). It is crucial to support policies that enhance treatment for IA, especially for clients who may struggle to afford therapy. By promoting wellness, recovery, and prevention efforts, practitioners help create a less stigmatizing environment and foster more comprehensive support across various healthcare services (van Namen et al., 2024).

Community outreach programs are essential for raising awareness and offering support to diverse populations. Behavioral health professionals should advocate for these programs, as they play a significant role in educating young people and families (Colder Carras et al., 2024). Initiatives that promote digital literacy and workshops led by professionals are effective ways to support different communities (Chadha et al., 2024; Colder Carras et al., 2024). Teaching digital literacy helps inform individuals about healthy internet usage and recognize signs of excessive use that could lead to IA, effectively raising awareness in various populations (Colder Carras et al., 2024).

Additionally, professionals need to consider that many individuals may not have the financial means to access therapy or treatment for IA. An example of successful advocacy is the Massachusetts Child Psychiatry Access Program for Moms (MCPAP), where professionals worked to secure funding due to its high cost and its importance in treating untreated cases, particularly in light of concerning mortality rates (King et al., 2025). If professionals can effectively advocate for insurance coverage, it could significantly improve access to treatment for numerous communities.

Furthermore, investing in the ongoing training of behavioral health professionals in the area of IA is essential for delivering effective treatment. This training not only helps professionals understand their clients better but also fosters empathy (Jain et al., 2024; van Namen et al., 2024). While training for behavioral health professionals is vital, it is equally important to educate other professionals, such as physicians and social workers, to ensure comprehensive and inclusive treatment that supports IA recovery (van Namen et al., 2024). Overall, practitioners should prioritize advocacy and inclusion for communities and individuals from various backgrounds and cultures.

REFERENCES

Alavi, S. S., Ghanizadeh, M., Mohammadi, M. R., Jannatifard, F., Esmaeeli Alamooti, S., & Farahani, M. (2021). The effects of cognitive-behavioral group therapy on reducing the symptoms of internet addiction disorder and promoting the quality of life and mental health. *Trends in Psychiatry and Psychotherapy*, *43*(1). Advance online publication. DOI: 10.47626/2237-6089-2020-0010 PMID: 33681908

American Psychological Association. (2015). *APA Dictionary of Psychology* (2nd ed.). American Psychological Association.

Andic, S., & Durak Batigun, A. (2019). *Development of Internet Addiction Scale Based on DSM-5 Diagnostic Criteria: An Evaluation in Terms of Internet Gaming Disorder*. Turkish Journal of Psychiatry., DOI: 10.5080/u23194

Antoniac, L.-D., Hu ul, T.-D., Karner-Hu uleac, A., & Hu ul, A. (2024). Addressing Internet Addiction Among Adolescents: A Literature Review and a Proposal of Guidelines for Psychotherapists and Mental Health Workers. *The American Journal of Family Therapy*, *1*(16). Advance online publication. DOI: 10.1080/01926187.2024.2434850

Arzani-Birgani, A., Zarei, J., Favaregh, L., & Ghanaatiyan, E. (2021). Internet addiction, mental health, and sleep quality in students of medical sciences, Iran: A cross-sectional study. *Journal of Education and Health Promotion*, *10*(1), 409. DOI: 10.4103/jehp.jehp_1506_20 PMID: 35071615

Baloğlu, M., Şahin, R., & Arpaci, I. (2020). A review of recent research in problematic internet use: Gender and cultural differences. *Current Opinion in Psychology*, *36*, 124–129. DOI: 10.1016/j.copsyc.2020.05.008 PMID: 32629412

Błachnio, A., Przepiórka, A., Gorbaniuk, O., Benvenuti, M., Ciobanu, A. M., Senol-Durak, E., Durak, M., Giannakos, M. N., Mazzoni, E., Pappas, I. O., Popa, C., Seidman, G., Wu, A. M. S., Yu, S., & Ben-Ezra, M. (2019). Cultural Correlates of Internet Addiction. *Cyberpsychology, Behavior, and Social Networking*, *22*(4), 258–263. DOI: 10.1089/cyber.2018.0667 PMID: 30958038

Brahma, A., & Brahma, M. C. (2023). An overview of internet pornography addiction. *Eastern Journal of Psychiatry*, *20*(1), 3–6. DOI: 10.5005/EJP-20-1-3

Chadha, Y., Patil, R., Toshniwal, S., & Sinha, N. (2024). Internet Addiction Management: A Comprehensive Review of Clinical Interventions and Modalities. *Cureus*, *16*(3). Advance online publication. DOI: 10.7759/cureus.55466 PMID: 38571828

Chang, M. L., & Lee, I. O. (2024). Functional connectivity changes in the brain of adolescents with internet addiction: A systematic literature review of imaging studies. *PLOS Mental Health*, *1*(1), e0000022. Advance online publication. DOI: 10.1371/journal.pmen.0000022

Chen, L., & Nath, R. (2016). Understanding the underlying factors of Internet addiction across cultures: A comparison study. *Electronic Commerce Research and Applications*, *17*, 38–48. DOI: 10.1016/j.elerap.2016.02.003

Chen, W., Gao, Y., Ren, R., Bi, Y., & Liao, Y. (2025). Socioeconomic status and internet addiction: Double-mediated moderation. *BMC Public Health*, *25*(1), 48. Advance online publication. DOI: 10.1186/s12889-024-21153-w PMID: 39762803

Chung, S., Lee, J., & Lee, H. K. (2019). Personal Factors, Internet Characteristics, and Environmental Factors Contributing to Adolescent Internet Addiction: A Public Health Perspective. *International Journal of Environmental Research and Public Health*, *16*(23), 4635. DOI: 10.3390/ijerph16234635 PMID: 31766527

Colder Carras, M., Aljuboori, D., Shi, J., Date, M., Karkoub, F., Ortiz, K. G., Abreha, F. M., & Thrul, J. (2024). Prevention and Health Promotion Interventions for Young People in the Context of Digital Well-Being: Rapid Systematic Review. *Journal of Medical Internet Research*, *26*, e59968. Advance online publication. DOI: 10.2196/59968 PMID: 39693138

Dieris-Hirche, J., Bottel, L., Pape, M., te Wildt, B. T., Wölfling, K., Henningsen, P., Timmesfeld, N., Neumann, A., Neusser, S., Beckers, R., & Herpertz, S. (2021). Effects of an online-based motivational intervention to reduce problematic internet use and promote treatment motivation in internet gaming disorder and internet use disorder (OMPRIS): Study protocol for a randomised controlled trial. *BMJ Open*, *11*(8), e045840. DOI: 10.1136/bmjopen-2020-045840 PMID: 34344675

Ge, M.-W., Hu, F.-H., Jia, Y.-J., Tang, W., Zhang, W.-Q., Zhao, D.-Y., Shen, W.-Q., & Chen, H.-L. (2023). The relationship between loneliness and internet or smartphone addiction among adolescents: A systematic review and meta-analysis. *Psychological Reports*, *128*(3), 1429–1451. DOI: 10.1177/00332941231180119 PMID: 37261719

Harsej, Z., Mokhtari Lakeh, N., Sheikholeslami, F., & KazemnezhadLeili, E. (2021). Internet addiction and its relationship with family functioning in high school students. *Journal of Holistic Nursing and Midwifery*, *31*(1), 44–52. DOI: 10.32598/jhnm.31.1.2025

Hua, Y., Wang, W., Shi, J., Wang, H., Xu, K., Shi, G., Guo, L., & Lu, C. (2022). Childhood trauma and internet addiction among Chinese adolescents: The mediating role of coping styles. *Current Psychology (New Brunswick, N.J.)*, *42*(19), 16507–16517. DOI: 10.1007/s12144-022-02862-0

Jain, N., Adams, E. A., Joyes, E. C., McLellan, G., Burrows, M., Paisi, M., McGowan, L. J., Iafrate, L., Landes, D., Watt, R., Sniehotta, F. F., Kaner, E., & Ramsay, S. E. (2024). Engagement and access to support for oral health, substance use, smoking and diet by people with severe and multiple disadvantage: A qualitative study. *PLoS One*, *19*(12), e0315254. Advance online publication. DOI: 10.1371/journal.pone.0315254 PMID: 39693306

Kamate, R., Baliga, S., & Mallapur, M. D. (2019). Internet addiction among engineering students in Belagavi city: Cross sectional study. *International Journal of Community Medicine and Public Health*, *6*(4), 1488. DOI: 10.18203/2394-6040.ijcmph20191372

Khubchandani, J., Sharma, S., & Price, J. H. (2021). COVID-19 Pandemic and the Burden of Internet Addiction in the United States. *Psychiatry International*, *2*(4), 402–409. DOI: 10.3390/psychiatryint2040031

King, C., Hayes, M., Maldonado, L., Monter, E., Aujla, R., Phlegar, E., Smith, C., Parker, L., Blome, K., Sandford, A., Douglas, E., & Guille, C. (2025). A perinatal psychiatry access program to address rural and medically underserved populations using telemedicine. *BMC Women's Health*, *25*(1), 30. Advance online publication. DOI: 10.1186/s12905-025-03561-1 PMID: 39838366

Koçak, Ç. V. (2018). How does regular exercise affect internet addiction level in university students? *Physical Education of Students*, *23*(4), 186–190. DOI: 10.15561/20755279.2019.0404

Kolaib, A. M. A., Al-Hazmi, A. H., & Kulaib, M. M. A. (2020). Prevalence of internet addiction and its associated factors among medical students at Taiba University, Saudi Arabia. *Journal of Family Medicine and Primary Care*, *9*(9), 4797. DOI: 10.4103/jfmpc.jfmpc_655_20 PMID: 33209802

Leménager, T., Hoffmann, S., Dieter, J., Reinhard, I., Mann, K., & Kiefer, F. (2018). The links between healthy, problematic, and addicted internet use regarding comorbidities and self-concept-related characteristics. *Journal of Behavioral Addictions*, *7*(1), 31–43. DOI: 10.1556/2006.7.2018.13 PMID: 29444606

Li, S., Wu, Q., Tang, C., Chen, Z., & Liu, L. (2020). Exercise-Based Interventions for Internet Addiction: Neurobiological and Neuropsychological Evidence. *Frontiers in Psychology, 11*, 1296. Advance online publication. DOI: 10.3389/fpsyg.2020.01296 PMID: 32670157

Li, Z., Xia, X., Sun, Q., & Li, Y. (2023). Exercise intervention to reduce mobile phone addiction in adolescents: A systematic review and meta-analysis of randomized controlled trials. *Frontiers in Psychology, 14*, 1294116. Advance online publication. DOI: 10.3389/fpsyg.2023.1294116 PMID: 38192396

Liu, S., Xiao, T., Yang, L., & Loprinzi, P. D. (2019). Exercise as an alternative approach for treating smartphone addiction: A systematic review and meta-analysis of random controlled trials. *International Journal of Environmental Research and Public Health, 16*(20), 3912. DOI: 10.3390/ijerph16203912 PMID: 31618879

Liu, S., Xu, B., Zhang, D., Tian, Y., & Wu, X. (2022). Core symptoms and symptom relationships of problematic internet use across early, middle, and late adolescence: A network analysis. *Computers in Human Behavior, 128*, 107090. DOI: 10.1016/j.chb.2021.107090

Liu, Y., Duan, L., Shen, Q., Xu, L., & Zhang, T. (2024). The relationship between childhood psychological abuse and depression in college students: Internet addiction as mediator, different dimensions of alexithymia as moderator. *BMC Public Health, 24*(1), 2744. Advance online publication. DOI: 10.1186/s12889-024-20232-2 PMID: 39379902

Lo, C. K. M., Yu, L., Cho, Y. W., & Chan, K. L. (2020). A qualitative study of practitioners' views on family involvement in treatment process of adolescent internet addiction. *International Journal of Environmental Research and Public Health, 18*(1), 86. DOI: 10.3390/ijerph18010086 PMID: 33374348

Lu, R. (2023). Adolescents' internet addiction: Influence factors, risks, and neuroscience connectivity. *Journal of Education. Humanities and Social Sciences, 8*, 483–490. DOI: 10.54097/ehss.v8i.4293

Lukavská, K., Hrabec, O., Lukavský, J., Demetrovics, Z., & Király, O. (2022). The associations of adolescent problematic internet use with parenting: A meta-analysis. *Addictive Behaviors, 135*, 107423. DOI: 10.1016/j.addbeh.2022.107423 PMID: 35933287

Malak, M. Z. (2018). *Internet addiction and cognitive behavioral therapy*. Cognitive Behavioral Therapy and Clinical Applications., DOI: 10.5772/intechopen.71277

Masaeli, N., & Farhadi, H. (2021). Prevalence of internet-based addictive behaviors during COVID-19 pandemic: A systematic review. *Journal of Addictive Diseases*, *39*(4), 1–27. DOI: 10.1080/10550887.2021.1895962 PMID: 33749537

Niemann, A., Hillerich, V., Wasem, J., Dieris-Hirche, J., Bottel, L., Pape, M., Herpertz, S., Timmesfeld, N., Basten, J., Theodor, B., Wölfling, K., Beckers, R., Henningsen, P., Neusser, S., & Neumann, A. (2023). Health Economic Evaluation of an online-based motivational program to reduce problematic media use and promote treatment motivation for internet use disorder—Results of the OMPRIS study. *International Journal of Environmental Research and Public Health*, *20*(24), 7144. DOI: 10.3390/ijerph20247144 PMID: 38131696

Nwufo, J. I., Ike, O. O., Nwoke, M. B., Eze, J., Chukwuorji, J. C., & Kanu, G. C. (2022). Social anxiety and internet addiction among adolescent students in a sub-Saharan African country: Does family functioning make a difference? *South African Journal of Psychology. Suid-Afrikaanse Tydskrif vir Sielkunde*, *53*(2), 275–285. DOI: 10.1177/00812463221140224

Ong, R. H. S., Sim, H. S., Bergman, M. M., How, C. H., Png, C. A. L., Lim, C. S., Peh, L. H., & Oh, H. C. (2024). Prevalence and associations of problematic smartphone use with smartphone activities, psychological well-being, and sleep quality in a household survey of Singapore adults. *PLoS One*, *19*(12), e0315364. Advance online publication. DOI: 10.1371/journal.pone.0315364 PMID: 39693321

Onukwuli, V. O., Onyinye, E. N., Udigwe, I. B., Umeh, U. M., Enebe, J. T., & Umerah, A. T. (2023). Internet addiction during the COVID-19 pandemic among adolescents in southeast Nigeria and implications for adolescent care in the post-pandemic era: A cross-sectional study. *SAGE Open Medicine*, *11*, 205031212311527–20503121 2311527. DOI: 10.1177/20503121231152763 PMID: 36860685

Pan, Y.-C., Chiu, Y.-C., & Lin, Y.-H. (2020). Systematic Review and Meta-Analysis of Epidemiology of Internet Addiction. *Neuroscience and Biobehavioral Reviews*, *118*(1), 612–622. Advance online publication. DOI: 10.1016/j.neubiorev.2020.08.013 PMID: 32853626

Pettorruso, M., Valle, S., Cavic, E., Martinotti, G., & Grant, J. E. (2020). Problematic Internet use (PIU), personality profiles and emotion dysregulation in a cohort of young adults: Trajectories from risky behaviors to addiction. *Psychiatry Research*, *289*, 113036. DOI: 10.1016/j.psychres.2020.113036 PMID: 32450451

Pluhar, E., Kavanaugh, J. R., Levinson, J. A., & Rich, M. (2019). Problematic interactive media use in teens: Comorbidities, assessment, and treatment. *Psychology Research and Behavior Management*, *12*, 447–455. DOI: 10.2147/PRBM.S208968 PMID: 31308769

Reuter, M., & Montag, C. (2017). *Internet addiction neuroscientific approaches and therapeutical implications including smartphone addiction*. Springer International Publishing.

Rosenthal, S. R., Cha, Y., & Clark, M. A. (2018). The Internet Addiction Test in a Young Adult U.S. Population. *Cyberpsychology, Behavior, and Social Networking*, *21*(10), 661–666. DOI: 10.1089/cyber.2018.0143 PMID: 30334654

Sharma, M. K., & Palanichamy, T. S. (2018). Psychosocial interventions for technological addictions. *Indian Journal of Psychiatry*, *60*(8), 541. DOI: 10.4103/psychiatry.IndianJPsychiatry_40_18 PMID: 29540928

Tadpatrikar, A., Sharma, S., Sharma, M. K., Bhargav, H., Anand, N., & Mishra, P. (2023). An integrated yoga and cognitive behavioral therapy intervention for managing excessive use of internet among the youth: A case series. *International Journal of Yoga*, *16*(1), 56–60. DOI: 10.4103/ijoy.ijoy_47_23 PMID: 37583538

Tang, C. S.-K., Koh, Y. W., & Gan, Y. (2017). Addiction to Internet Use, Online Gaming, and Online Social Networking Among Young Adults in China, Singapore, and the United States. *Asia-Pacific Journal of Public Health*, *29*(8), 673–682. DOI: 10.1177/1010539517739558 PMID: 29191049

Tang, H., Li, Y., Dong, W., Guo, X., Wu, S., Chen, C., & Lu, G. (2024). The relationship between childhood trauma and internet addiction in adolescents: A meta-analysis. *Journal of Behavioral Addictions*, *13*(1), 36–50. DOI: 10.1556/2006.2024.00001 PMID: 38340148

van Namen, D. M., Hilberink, S. R., de Vries, H., Nagelhout, G. E., & van Staa, A. (2024). “Please, see me”; Informal and professional support of students with relatives with addiction problems: A three-year longitudinal qualitative study. *BMC Public Health*, *24*(1), 3092. Advance online publication. DOI: 10.1186/s12889-024-20531-8 PMID: 39516781

Wang, H., Li, X., Lok, G. K. I., Meng, C., Tan, Y., Lee, U. M., & Chan, N. (2024). Family-based therapy for internet addiction among adolescents and young adults: A meta-analysis. *Journal of Behavioral Addictions*, *13*(2), 295–312.

Wang, Y., Qin, Y., Li, H., Yao, D., Sun, B., Gong, J., Dai, Y., Wen, C., Zhang, L., Zhang, C., Luo, C., & Zhu, T. (2023). Acupuncture modulates the functional connectivity among the subcortical nucleus and fronto-parietal network in adolescents with internet addiction. *Brain and Behavior*, *13*(11), e3241. Advance online publication. DOI: 10.1002/brb3.3241 PMID: 37721727

Wang, Z., Potenza, M. N., Song, K., Dong, G., Fang, X., & Zhang, J. (2022). Subgroups of internet gaming disorder based on addiction-related resting-state functional connectivity. *Addiction (Abingdon, England)*, *118*(2), 327–339. DOI: 10.1111/add.16047 PMID: 36089824

Wei, Z., Hassan, N. C., Hassan, S. A., Ismail, N., Gu, X., & Dong, J. (2025). Psychometric validation of Young's Internet Addiction Test among Chinese undergraduate students. *PLoS One*, *20*(4), e0320641. Advance online publication. DOI: 10.1371/journal.pone.0320641 PMID: 40273278

Xin, M., Xing, J., Pengfei, W., Houru, L., Mengcheng, W., & Hong, Z. (2018). Online activities, prevalence of internet addiction and risk factors related to family and school among adolescents in China. *Addictive Behaviors Reports*, *7*, 14–18. DOI: 10.1016/j.abrep.2017.10.003 PMID: 29450251

Xu, L., Wu, L., Geng, X., Wang, Z., Guo, X., Song, K., Liu, G., Deng, L., Zhang, J., & Potenza, M. N. (2021). A review of psychological interventions for internet addiction. *Psychiatry Research*, *302*, 114016. DOI: 10.1016/j.psychres.2021.114016 PMID: 34087672

Yar, A., Gündoğdu, Ö. Y., Tural, Ü., & Memik, N. Ç. (2019). Prevalance of internet addiction among adolescents with psychiatric disorders. *Archives of Neuropsychiatry*. DOI: 10.29399/npa.23045

Yaunin, Y., Darwin, E., Yanwirasti, Y., Nurdin, A., Yetti, H., & Liza, R. (2019). The difference of dopamine transporter and serotonin transporter level between addicted and non-addicted internet user experiencing stress in senior high school students in Padang, Indonesia. *Proceedings of the Proceedings of the 1st EAI International Conference on Medical and Health Research, ICoMHER November 13-14th*. DOI: 10.4108/eai.13-11-2018.2283690

Yue, Y., Jun, Z., Yao, N., Yanwen, F., Yiting, Z., & Yiting, F. (2024). The influence of adolescents' internet adaptation on internet addiction: The mediating role of internet cultural adaptation. *Frontiers in Psychiatry*, *14*, 1338343. Advance online publication. DOI: 10.3389/fpsyt.2023.1338343 PMID: 38260791

Zeidi, I. M., Divsalar, S., Morshedi, H., & Alizadeh, H. (2020). The effectiveness of group cognitive-behavioral therapy on general self-efficacy, self-control, and internet addiction prevalence among medical university students. *Social Health and Behavior, 3*(3), 93–102. DOI: 10.4103/SHB.SHB_20_20

Zhou, N., Cao, H., Li, X., Zhang, J., Yao, Y., Geng, X., Lin, X., Hou, S., Liu, F., Chen, X., & Fang, X. (2018). Internet addiction, problematic internet use, nonproblematic internet use among Chinese adolescents: Individual, parental, peer, and sociodemographic correlates. *Psychology of Addictive Behaviors, 32*(3), 365–372. DOI: 10.1037/adb0000358 PMID: 29771562

Zhu, Y., Chen, H., Li, J., Mei, X., & Wang, W. (2023). Effects of different interventions on internet addiction: A systematic review and network meta-analysis. *BMC Psychiatry, 23*(1), 921. Advance online publication. DOI: 10.1186/s12888-023-05400-9 PMID: 38066462

KEY TERMS AND DEFINITIONS

Closed-Skill Exercises: Repetitive activities performed in a controlled environment (e.g.,swimming).

Cognitive Behavioral Therapy (CBT): A structured psychotherapy that helps individuals identify and modify maladaptive thoughts and behaviors.

Cognitive Behavioral Therapy for Internet Addiction (CBT-IA): A phased treatment approach focused on reducing excessive internet use and promoting balanced digital habits.

Culturally Competent: An approach that acknowledges and integrates clients' diverse values, beliefs, and backgrounds into treatment.

Dopamine Dysregulation: An imbalance in dopamine activity, often linked to addiction and impaired reward processing.

Dopamine: A neurotransmitter essential for motivation, pleasure, and reinforcement learning.

Family-Based Therapy: A therapeutic approach that enhances communication and problem solving within families to support mental health.

Internet Addiction (IA): A compulsive reliance on internet use, leading to significant impairment in daily life.

Motivational Enhancement Therapy (MET): A structured, client-driven approach that strengthens motivation for change through goal-setting and self-reflection.

Motivational Interviewing (MI): A client-centered therapy that fosters behavioral change through collaborative and goal-oriented conversations.

Movement-Based Intervention: A therapy using physical activities, such as yoga, to reduce stress and improve emotional well-being.

Online-Based Motivational Program (OMPRIS): A digital intervention combining motivational interviewing (MI) and cognitive behavioral therapy (CBT) techniques.

Open-Skill Exercises: Dynamic activities requiring adaptation to unpredictable external stimuli (e.g., basketball).

Prefrontal Cortex: A brain region involved in decision-making, impulse control, and emotional regulation, often implicated in behavioral dysregulation.

Problematic Internet Use: Difficulty in regulating internet use, resulting in negative personal, social, or occupational consequences.

Reward Pathways: Neural circuits, primarily involving the mesolimbic dopamine system, that reinforce behaviors and contribute to addiction.

Self-Monitoring: A strategy where individuals track behaviors and triggers to increase self awareness and regulate problematic habits.

Striatum: A brain region central to reward processing and habit formation.

Chapter 3
Exploring the Digital Abyss:
The Consequences of Problematic Social Media Use on Mental Wellbeing

Elaine Mora
https://orcid.org/0009-0002-1355-5091
University of Texas Rio Grande Valley, USA

ABSTRACT

This chapter explores the impact of problematic social media use on mental well-being, examining its diverse effects across various age groups and demographics, including individuals with disabilities. It synthesizes empirical research and practical insights and intends to create awareness regarding the detriments of excessive social media engagement, while also offering effective strategies for treatment and intervention. The chapter delves into the symptoms of social media addiction, like excessive use and withdrawal, and outlines treatment options, including Cognitive Behavioral Therapy (CBT), group therapy, and the promotion of digital literacy. By integrating robust case studies, empirical research, and relevant statistical analyses, this chapter aims to clarify the underlying issues surrounding problematic social media use, highlight its varied implications, and propose effective strategies for treatment and intervention.

DOI: 10.4018/979-8-3373-0518-9.ch003

INTRODUCTION

Over the last two decades, social media has profoundly reshaped how individuals connect, communicate, and perceive the world around them. Platforms like Facebook, Myspace, Instagram, LinkedIn, X (formerly Twitter), Pinterest, Snapchat, YouTube, WhatsApp, Reddit, and TikTok have become ubiquitous, prompting widespread conversations concerning their influence on mental health. The chapter provides a comprehensive overview of social media and its effects on individuals, highlighting its potential for both positive and negative outcomes. Although these digital spaces offer unprecedented opportunities for connection and information sharing, they have also contributed to the emergence of behavioral addictions, often characterized by compulsive platform use, which can have detrimental consequences for personal, social, and professional spheres (Tang et al., 2017). This chapter examines the complex phenomenon of social media addiction, investigating its manifestations across diverse populations, encompassing adolescents, adults, older adults, and individuals with disabilities. The increasing integration of social media into everyday life has fueled significant debate regarding its effects on mental well-being. While providing tools for instantaneous connection and global communication, social media environments can also inadvertently encourage excessive engagement, leading to potentially harmful behaviors and outcomes (Blackwell et al., 2017).

According to the Pew Research Center (2021), approximately 69% of U.S. adults and an overwhelming 84% of adolescents report using social media regularly, raising significant concerns about mental health and addiction-related behaviors. The Pew Research Center's survey also revealed significant differences across age groups, gender, and ethnicity in social media platform usage. For example, they found that age significantly correlated with platform preference and engagement, with YouTube usage high across all age groups (93% of 18–29-year-olds). Similarly, Facebook usage was prevalent among this group (68%). Instagram and Snapchat, according to the Pew Research Center (2024), were more popular among younger adults, decreasing with age, with only 19% of those 65+ using Instagram and 4% using Snapchat. The Pew Research Center (2024) also found that gender influenced social media habits, with women reporting higher use of Facebook (78%) than men (61%). Women also tended to use Instagram, Pinterest, and TikTok more than men. Men, however, used Reddit and X (formerly Twitter) more than women (Pew Research Center, 2024).

Therefore, it is essential to consider these findings in the context of developing effective strategies to promote digital literacy and responsible social media use among diverse user groups. By integrating robust case studies, empirical research, and relevant statistical analyses, this chapter aims to clarify the underlying issues surrounding problematic social media use, highlight its varied implications, and propose effective strategies for treatment and intervention.

IMPORTANCE OF UNDERSTANDING SOCIAL MEDIA ADDICTION

Social media addiction has emerged as a significant form of online addiction, impacting individuals globally due to the increasing integration of digital technologies into daily life and the widespread use of smartphones and internet access (Guedes et al., 2016). According to Kuss & Griffiths (2011), online addiction, alternatively labeled as internet addiction, embodies the compulsive behavior of devoting excessive amounts of time to online activities, detrimentally impacting various facets of life including social interactions, personal pursuits, and professional responsibilities. They further explain how this condition mirrors other addictive patterns, as individuals may encounter withdrawal symptoms, a loss of interest in alternative activities, and difficulty managing their internet usage. This demonstrates that internet addiction has been a recognized concern for well over a decade, particularly as problematic social media use has emerged as a significant factor contributing to this ongoing issue.

Social media platforms like Facebook, Instagram, and TikTok, with their billions of active users worldwide, are designed to stimulate reward mechanisms within the brain, making them inherently addictive (Guedes et al., 2016; Tamir & Mitchel, 2012). The continuous stream of updates, likes, and comments can lead to a compulsive need to check these platforms, often at the expense of real-life commitments and relationships. Overuse of the internet, often facilitated by social media, can have serious negative consequences on an individual's mental health, relationships, and overall wellbeing (Alavi et al., 2011; Lebni et al., 2020), including feelings of isolation (Beyari, 2023; Cash et al., 2012; Tateno et al., 2019), depression (Ye et al., 2023), anxiety (Abu Khait et al., 2022), and even physical health problems like eye strain and fatigue due to extended periods of sedentary behavior (Aziz et al., 2024; Chu et al., 2023; Daniyal et al., 2022; Wacks & Weinstein, 2021).

The design of social media, characterized by instant communication, rapid information dissemination, and the potential for social validation, creates a powerful draw (Guedes et al., 2016). Sharing information about oneself on these platforms activates the brain's reward system, producing a pleasurable experience akin to natural rewards like food or sex (Tamir & Mitchel, 2012). The ability to curate and present an idealized self-further intensifies this effect, creating a cycle of seeking validation and approval that can contribute to addictive behavior (Amichai-Hamburger & Vinitzky, 2010). Individuals may turn to social media to escape negative emotions like loneliness or anxiety, and experience withdrawal symptoms when unable to access these platforms (Tang et al., 2017). Consequently, dependence on social media can manifest as mood swings, obsessive preoccupation, tolerance (requiring increased use to achieve the same satisfaction), and significant conflicts in real-life relationships (Andreassen et al., 2012). As research continues to evolve, social media addiction is increasingly recognized as a serious concern with substantial implications for mental health and overall well-being (Guedes et al., 2016).

Understanding the psychological underpinnings of problematic social media use is paramount. This knowledge is crucial for equipping mental health professionals and educators with the tools to effectively address the symptoms, risks, and potential solutions associated with this behavior. This approach acknowledges the addictive nature of problematic social media use, drawing parallels to both substance-related addictions (e.g., drug dependence) and behavioral addictions (e.g., pathological gambling) by highlighting common indicators (Andreassen & Pallesen, 2015). Emerging research increasingly demonstrates a link between addictive social media use and heightened levels of anxiety, depression, and loneliness (Zhou et al., 2021). These findings underscore the need for further investigation into the intricacies of this addiction, exploring its underlying causes, diverse manifestations, and broader impacts. This overview aims to clarify and synthesize the complex relationships between social media usage patterns and mental health outcomes, thus laying the groundwork for the development of robust prevention and intervention strategies.

SCOPE OF THE PROBLEM

Defining Social Media Addiction

Social media addiction, often used interchangeably with terms like Social Networking Site (SNS) addiction or problematic social media use, is a complex phenomenon that has gained increasing attention due to the pervasive integration of social media into daily life (Andreassen & Pallesen, 2015). The core of this addiction lies in an individual's excessive preoccupation and compulsive engagement with online social platforms, leading to negative repercussions across personal, social, and emotional domains. Studies indicate that excessive social media use correlates with heightened risks of social isolation (McHugh et al., 2018), depression (Sujarwoto & Yumarni, 2023), and body image disturbances (Roberts et al., 2022). Such findings highlight the need for a comprehensive examination of how social media addiction manifests differently across age groups and among individuals with disabilities. The consequence is a detrimental impact on various facets of life, including social activities, academic or professional performance, relationships, and overall psychological health and well-being (Andreassen & Pallesen, 2015).

Building upon the consequences of social media use and its multifaceted impacts on people's lives, it becomes evident that reliance on these platforms can lead to significant psychological challenges. Research indicates that heightened social media engagement is closely associated with various mental health issues, including anxiety, depression, and low self-esteem (Twenge et al., 2018). Additionally, social media's role in promoting externalizing behaviors cannot be overlooked. The constant exposure to negative interactions, cyberbullying, or harmful content can provoke aggressive behaviors as a means of self-defense or expression of frustration (Machado et al., 2024). This outcome underscores the importance of understanding social media not merely as a benign space for interaction, but as a complex environment that can shape and influence behaviors in both positive and negative ways.

RISKS ASSOCIATED WITH PROBLEMATIC USAGE

The effects of excessive social media use are significant and complex, impacting emotional well-being, social connections, and self-image. These risks encompass heightened social isolation, distorted body image, sleep disturbances, and the detrimental impact of cyberbullying and negative online interactions (Ajewumi et al., 2024).

Social Isolation

Despite social media's intent to foster connections, excessive use can lead to increased feelings of isolation. This paradox occurs when individuals become more engaged with virtual conversations rather than face-to-face interactions (Primack et al., 2017). For instance, a teenager might spend hours scrolling through Instagram feeds, participating in "likes" and comments, but they may neglect to meet friends in person or join group activities. This behavior can intensify feelings of loneliness and anxiety, contributing to depressive symptoms. In a world where social validation is often dependent on likes or comments, those who primarily rely on social media for social interactions can find themselves feeling more disconnected than ever, particularly during times of significant life transitions, such as starting college or entering the workforce (Ajewumi et al., 2024).

Body Image and Self Esteem Disturbances

Social media often showcases idealized images of beauty, success, and lifestyle, which can adversely affect self-esteem. For example, a young woman may frequently encounter photos of influencers flaunting "perfect" bodies and lifestyles, leading her to compare herself unfavorably. This constant comparison may result in body dissatisfaction and a skewed self-image (Roberts et al., 2022). Such perceptions can trigger harmful behaviors, such as excessive dieting or even eating disorders, as she strives to mirror the unattainable ideals seen online. Research indicates that individuals who develop a habit of engaging with such content are more likely to report feelings of inadequacy and decrease self-worth due to these unrealistic benchmarks (Sadagheyani & Tatari, 2021).

However, the connection between social media and body image remains a contentious issue, particularly as it pertains to young women. With that said, Roberts et al. (2022) conducted a study revealing that adolescents dedicating excessive time to social media exhibits concerning body image disturbances, leading to self-esteem issues. This study demonstrated how 60% of the teenage girls surveyed admitted that they often feel self-conscious about their appearances due to comparing themselves to influencers and peers. The implications of this are vast, leading to physical manifestations such as eating disorders and psychological distress (Roberts et al., 2022).

Interestingly, while much focus is placed on young women's experiences, it is crucial to note that social media also impacts young men. A significant finding reveals that approximately 20% of young men report feelings of inadequacy and pressure related to their body image due to social media influence, highlighting that the struggle with body image is not limited to one gender (Choudhury & Ali, 2020). This indicates a broader societal concern about how social media cultivates unattainable standards of beauty and success, affecting individuals across the gender spectrum. As discussions around body image evolve, it is essential to recognize the diverse experiences and challenges young people face in relation to social media, encouraging healthier conversations and practices to empower all users.

Sleep Disturbances

The engagement with social media doesn't just disrupt day-to-day activities; it significantly impacts sleep quality. The urge to check notifications or scroll through feeds right before bed often leads to late-night usage, resulting in insufficient sleep. For instance, a high school student may stay up late interacting with friends online, thinking it enhances their social life, but this behavior undermines their sleep schedule. Lack of proper rest can lead to impaired cognitive functions, increased irritability, and lower emotional resilience (Twenge et al., 2018). Over time, these disturbances contribute not only to physical health issues but also to the exacerbation of anxiety and mood disorders, creating a detrimental feedback loop where poor sleep negatively impacts mental well-being (Twenge et al., 2018).

Cyberbullying and Negative Online Interactions

The anonymity and reach of social media also create an environment where cyberbullying can thrive (McHugh et al., 2018). For instance, a young user might share a personal story online, only to be met with negative comments or harassment from peers. This experience can lead to significant emotional distress, including heightened anxiety, depression, and an amplified sense of isolation. The consequences of cyberbullying are profound and can result in lasting psychological effects, leaving victims feeling powerless and deeply affected by their online experiences. Such long-term impacts underline the importance of fostering a safe digital environment and educating users about the repercussions of their online behaviors (Machado et al., 2024).

Overall, the link between problematic social media use and adverse mental health outcomes is becoming increasingly evident (Ajewumi et al., 2024). Continuous exposure to distressing or negative content can perpetuate a cycle of low self-esteem and heightened anxiety. Understanding these dynamics is crucial for creating effective mental health interventions and promoting healthier online practices among users.

IMPLICATIONS FOR VARIOUS AGE GROUPS

Adolescents

The vulnerability of problematic social media use can be particularly pronounced during adolescence, a developmental period marked by significant emotional and social changes (Heller & Casey, 2016; Roberts et al., 2019). Adolescents are navigating identity formation and peer relationships and, as such, may turn to social media for validation and connection. However, this reliance can spiral into compulsive behaviors, where they may feel compelled to check notifications incessantly or spend excessive time curating their online personas. Adolescents may resort to online platforms as a coping mechanism for the stressors they face, such as academic pressures, social conflicts, and familial issues (Frison & Eggermont, 2015).

While social media can provide a sense of belonging and offer an outlet for expression, it often does so in a maladaptive manner. For instance, the propensity to seek reassurance through likes or comments can momentarily alleviate feelings of distress but may lead to increased reliance on external validation rather than fostering internal coping strategies (Nesi & Prinstein, 2015). As a result, adolescents may find themselves caught in a cycle where they neglect essential responsibilities and face escalating emotional challenges, creating a detrimental feedback loop that adversely affects their overall well-being (Twenge et al., 2019). The following example will provide a nuanced exploration of the challenges faced by adolescents as they navigate the complexities of social media, offering a detailed examination of the ways in which problematic social media use can have a profound impact on their mental and emotional well-being.

Case Example: Mary Ann's Struggle for Identity

Mary Ann, a 16-year-old high school student, grew up in a low-income household with a single mother working multiple jobs to make ends meet. After experiencing bullying and social exclusion in middle school, Mary Ann found solace in social media, where she could curate a perfect online persona and connect with others who shared similar interests. However, her online engagement soon became an all-consuming force in her life. Mary Ann's social media usage statistics reveal a troubling trend:

- **Impact on Self-Esteem:** Mary Ann spends an average of 4 hours daily on social media, often comparing her life to the highlight reels of her peers, leading to feelings of inadequacy and low self-esteem.
- **Online Relationships:** Mary Ann has over 8,000 followers, but only 5 close friends in real life, highlighting the disconnect between her online and offline relationships.
- **Social Media Habits:** Mary Ann posts at least 3 times a day, often sharing provocative content to garner likes and attention, which has led to online harassment and cyberbullying.

Research from Berryman et al. (2018) suggests that adolescents like Mary Ann, who experience social isolation and trauma, are more vulnerable to the negative effects of social media, including decreased self-esteem, increased anxiety, and depression. In addition, Mary Ann's experiences highlight the particularly strong emotional impact of social media on young people. For Mary Ann, seeking validation through likes and comments has unfortunately fueled her social anxiety, making it harder for her to connect with people in real life. To mitigate the detrimental effects of social media on her well-being and that of her peers, a multifaceted strategy should prioritize empathy-driven education, nuanced social media literacy, accessible mental health resources, and mindful online practices that encourage a balanced and authentic online experience. By doing so, we can empower individuals like Mary Ann to cultivate a more positive self-image and develop healthier relationships with technology.

Adults

Adults often engage with social media in diverse ways, but the potential negative impacts remain a shared concern. Many individuals turn to these platforms for escapism (Coyne et al., 2020), stress reduction, and social connection (Bae, 2023). Prolonged use, however, can lead to a disconnect from real-life relationships and diminished well-being. The following example will delve deeper into the phenomenon, illustrating how adults may engage in problematic social media use characterized by escapism, self-validation, and self-comparison, highlighting the often-overlooked ways in which these behaviors can negatively impact mental health and real-life relationships.

Case Example: Javid's Digital Sanctuary

Javid, a 28-year-old artist, grew up in a household with traditional values, where his identity as a gay man was not openly embraced. This created feelings of isolation and self-doubt for him. Upon discovering social media, he found a sense of belonging and the ability to freely express himself within online LGBTQ+ communities. However, his reliance on social media evolved, presenting both benefits and challenges:

- **Escapism**: Javid spent hours scrolling through Instagram and X (formerly known as Twitter), using social media as an escape from the trauma of his past and the stress of living in a society that often marginalized him. This excessive use of social media became a coping mechanism, diverting his attention away from the negative emotions that arose from his experiences.
- **Self-Validation**: Javid found himself constantly seeking validation through likes, comments, and followers, which further eroded his self-esteem and made him feel like he was living vicariously through his online persona. The more he craved validation online, the more disconnected he became from genuine, face-to-face interactions and meaningful connections in his life.
- **Social Comparison**: Javid compared his life to the curated highlight reels of his online friends, feeling like he fell short and was inadequate. As a result, he began to experience anxiety, depression, and a sense of discontent in his own life, perpetuating a cycle of self-doubt and dissatisfaction.

According to Abreu and Kenny (2018), LGBTQ+ youth are more likely to experience cyberbullying and online harassment, which can exacerbate feelings of isolation, lower self-esteem, depression, and even suicidal ideation. By examining Javid's experiences and behaviors, this case example aims to shed light on how problematic social media use can affect mental health, relationships, and overall well-being, and to provide a deeper understanding of the need for responsible social media use and the cultivation of healthy online habits.

Older Adults

As older adults increasingly join the digital world, they face unique challenges in navigating social media platforms. While some may experience feelings of FoMo (fear of missing out) due to the constant stream of information, many struggle to connect with others online (Pontes et al., 2018; Zainab et al., 2022). Limited media literacy skills and digital competencies hinder their ability to fully engage with mediated spaces, leading to feelings of isolation and exclusion.

Moreover, the lack of formal adult media literacy programs exacerbates these issues, leaving many seniors to rely on self-taught learning or informal assistance (Zainab et al., 2022). The following will illustrate the impact of these challenges on a specific individual, highlighting the practical consequences of limited media literacy in the context of modern social participation.

Case Example: Estella's Digital Connection

Estella, a 72-year-old widow of Bolivian heritage, lives alone in the United States. With her children and grandchildren residing in Bolivia, maintaining close relationships has always been a priority. Initially hesitant about technology, Estella gradually embraced video calling and Facebook to stay connected. While these platforms brought immense joy, they also presented unexpected challenges:

- **The Weight of Constant Connection**: Estella valued the ability to see her grandchildren's faces and share stories in real-time. However, the constant stream of updates and the perceived need to respond immediately led to feelings of pressure and exhaustion. The digital world, while connecting her, also seemed to demand a constant presence that sometimes overshadowed her need for quiet time.
- **The Language Barrier and Cultural Nuances**: Though fluent in both Spanish and English, Estella sometimes found it difficult to fully convey her thoughts and feelings through written messages or translate complex cultural jokes made by her younger family. The lack of nonverbal cues in online interactions also led to misunderstandings.
- **The Fear of Missing Out (FoMo)**: While Estella cherished the glimpses into her family's daily lives shared through posts and photos, she also found herself experiencing a sense of FoMo (Blackwell et al., 2017; Oberst et al., 2017). The constant exposure to social events and activities in which she could not participate in Bolivia occasionally intensified her feelings of loneliness.

This case example underscores the complex relationship older adults have with digital platforms. Understanding these challenges is critical to ensuring technology serves as a bridge, rather than a barrier, for older adults like Estella. Furthermore, it highlights the essential need for inclusive media literacy programs designed specifically for older adults. Such programs would empower them to develop the necessary skills to effectively participate in digital spaces, overcome the barriers to online connection, and navigate the complexities of social media with confidence and ease.

Individuals with Disabilities

Social media presents a complex and often contradictory space for individuals with disabilities. While offering unprecedented opportunities for connection, community building, and information access (Sweet et al., 2019), these platforms can also exacerbate existing vulnerabilities, leading to feelings of isolation, inadequacy, and, in some cases, problematic usage patterns. In addition, studies show that individuals with learning disabilities are at greater risks of cyberbullying, financial and sexual exploitation, and grooming (Bannon et al., 2015; Buijs et al., 2017; Lough & Fisher, 2016). The following case studies explores the nuanced experiences of two individuals – one with a visible disability and one with an invisible disability – within a framework that considers the interplay of disability, cultural context, and the potential for both positive and negative social media impacts.

Case Example: Aisha's Experience

Aisha is a 25-year-old woman with cerebral palsy, living in a diverse urban community. Her family is originally from Pakistan, and her cultural values emphasize family, community, and respect. Aisha has always navigated societal challenges, including ableism, with grace. She utilizes a wheelchair for mobility. Aisha primarily uses Instagram and TikTok. Initially, she found immense value in connecting with other disabled individuals, particularly within the South Asian diaspora. These platforms have enabled her to connect with others and engage in meaningful discussions about culture and disability.

- **Positive Aspects**: Aisha uses Instagram to showcase her art, which is inspired by Pakistani and South Asian culture. She promotes body positivity and inclusion of all races. Her Instagram account has become a space to combat negative stereotypes and to share her life experiences and advocate for disability rights within her community.
- **Problematic Use**: Over time, Aisha found herself spending excessive amounts of time on her accounts. She constantly compared her body and physical ap-

pearance to those she followed. She was also experiencing "doom-scrolling" due to the large amount of hate comments and threats she received from people online (Satici et al., 2023).

- **Cultural Competency**: Aisha's experience highlights the intersection of disability, cultural identity, and social media. Her use of the platforms has created a space for her cultural experience, and her ability to reach other South Asian women with disabilities and create a community.

Case Example: Kristopher's Experience

Kristopher is a 30-year-old man with bipolar disorder. He grew up in a low-income Hispanic neighborhood where mental health issues were stigmatized, and resources were limited. He works a desk job and often feels misunderstood. His diagnosis is often a struggle, and the symptoms can be challenging to manage. Kristopher primarily uses X (formally twitter) and Facebook. He initially found these platforms useful to keep in touch with friends and family. He has found support communities for mental illness, with others that experience the same struggles as him.

- **Positive Aspects**: X (formally twitter) offers a sense of community, particularly around mental health. Kristopher follows mental health professionals and support groups on social media. He finds these platforms a place to share his experiences with others, and he feels that others relate to him.
- **Problematic Use**: Social media exacerbated his depression and contributed to manic episodes (Pontes et al., 2018). He was feeling the need to constantly be present and post, which he found hard to do. He isolated himself from his friends and family. His social media interactions led him to feel inadequate. The constant comparisons to others' "perfect" lives contributed to feelings of isolation. Kristopher also experiences the pressure of "performing" happiness online, which is not genuine.
- **Cultural Competency**: Kristopher's case illuminates the unique challenges faced by individuals with invisible disabilities, especially in communities where mental health stigma is prevalent. He can now advocate for himself and use this platform to encourage others to reach out for mental health support.

Thus, as social media continues to evolve, its impact on individuals with disabilities becomes increasingly complex, necessitating a deeper understanding of both its benefits and potential harms. By learning about the experiences of people with both visible and invisible disabilities, using a framework that is sensitive to cultural differences, we can get a complete view of the difficulties and benefits linked with social media

SYMPTOMS OF PROBLEMATIC SOCIAL MEDIA USE

Engagement with social networking sites (SNS) can become excessive, leading to a range of adverse outcomes that mirror the hallmarks of established addiction models (Andreassen & Pallesen, 2015; Pontes et al., 2018). This section will delve into the key characteristics of problematic social media use, providing a comprehensive understanding of its complexities.

Excessive Engagement

Excessive engagement is a clear indicator of problematic social media use, characterized by the disproportionate amount of time dedicated to SNSs at the expense of other essential aspects of life. The process often begins with "salience," where an individual's thoughts become dominated by social networking and the desire to increase their online activity (Andreassen & Pallesen, 2015). This can manifest in a compulsion to constantly check social media, a form of salience where thoughts and behaviors are dominated by the online world (Pontes et al., 2018). Individuals may sacrifice sleep, neglect work or studies, and damage interpersonal relationships. A simple yet effective strategy to mitigate this issue is to establish phone-free periods, allowing users to disconnect and engage in other activities.

Withdrawal Symptoms

Individuals struggling with problematic social media use often experience withdrawal symptoms when access to SNSs is limited or denied (Pontes et al., 2018). These symptoms can manifest as feelings of stress, restlessness, irritability, anxiety, or even physical symptoms like headaches (Andreassen & Pallesen, 2015). These aversive experiences drive the individual to seek out social media, thus reinforcing the cycle of problematic use.

Cravings for Online Engagement

Cravings for online engagement are a critical component of problematic social media use. These cravings are not simply a desire to check one's accounts, but rather an intense and often uncontrollable urge to engage with SNSs. The power of these cravings can be so strong that users may continue using social media even when they are aware of the negative consequences, highlighting the addictive nature of the behavior (Andreassen & Pallesen, 2015).

Emotional Sensitivity

Problematic social media use is often linked to emotional sensitivity, with individuals using SNSs for mood modification and to regulate their emotions (Andreassen & Pallesen, 2015). They may turn to social media to alleviate feelings of anxiety, depression, boredom, or loneliness. Social media can become a primary coping mechanism, creating a cycle of dependence. Recognizing and addressing underlying emotional needs is crucial in breaking this cycle.

Conflict and Tolerance

"Conflict" is a defining feature of problematic social media use, with SNSs often taking precedence over essential activities. This can manifest in neglecting hobbies, academic pursuits, or work responsibilities, and damaging relationships with family and friends (Andreassen & Pallesen, 2015). Prioritizing online interactions over face-to-face communication can lead to feelings of isolation and loneliness, despite being constantly connected. Problematic social media users may also develop "tolerance," needing to spend increasing amounts of time online to achieve the same level of satisfaction or emotional response (Andreassen & Pallesen, 2015). This escalating pattern further reinforces the cycle of problematic use, as the individual becomes trapped in a constant pursuit of online engagement.

Beyond the core features of addiction, other contributing factors play a crucial role in the development of problematic social media use. Fear of missing out (FoMo) (Blackwell et al., 2017; Oberst et al., 2017) is a significant driver, reflecting a persistent apprehension that others are having rewarding experiences from which one is absent. Maladaptive cognitions, or distorted and unhelpful thoughts and beliefs about social media, are also critical. Furthermore, the impact on psychiatric distress should not be overlooked, with problematic social media use often exacerbating existing mental health issues, such as depression, anxiety, and poor psychological functioning (Pontes et al., 2018; Tang & Koh, 2017).

TREATMENT OPTIONS

While there is a growing body of research addressing treatment options for teens, young adults, and individuals with disabilities regarding social media addiction, older adults remain an underrepresented demographic in this discourse. However, the therapeutic interventions developed for younger populations can often be adapted to suit older adults, acknowledging the unique challenges they face with problematic social media use (Chen et al., 2022). As the prevalence of social media addiction continues to rise, it is increasingly important to investigate effective treatment strategies that are tailored to different age groups.

In this discussion, we will explore a range of treatment options, from self-help strategies to community-based interventions, and highlight how these approaches can be modified to meet the needs of older adults. By understanding that the same foundational principles of intervention can apply across age demographics, we can develop comprehensive solutions that not only address social media addiction but also enhance the overall well-being of older adults. The following sections will outline these treatments, paving the way for a broader understanding of how to support individuals struggling with social media usage, regardless of their age or life circumstances.

Self-Help Strategies

Self-help strategies, such as the use of apps to limit social media use, setting time limits, and modifying thought patterns, may prove useful (Andreassen & Pallesen, 2015). Furthermore, a holistic approach that integrates technological training with psychological support, fostering both digital competence and emotional well-being, is key. This strategy empowers individuals to navigate the digital landscape with greater confidence and resilience. This approach is exemplified by the case of Sonia, whose journey demonstrates a positive transformation:

Case Example: Sonia's Digital Detox

Sonia, a 26-year-old college senior, was feeling overwhelmed by the constant stream of notifications and updates on social media. As a psychology major and an avid user of social media platforms like Instagram and TikTok, she often found herself comparing her life to the curated online profiles of her peers. Born and raised in a close-knit Indian community in Oregon, Sonia valued her cultural heritage and the importance of family and social connections. However, she realized that her excessive social media use was affecting her relationships with her family and friends, as well as her academic performance.

- **App-Based Time Limits**: Sonia downloaded an app that allowed her to set daily limits for each social media platform. She started with one hour per day and gradually reduced it to 30 minutes, allocating the time saved to her studies and hobbies.
- **Digital "No-Go" Zones**: She established "no-phone zones" in her life, such as during family dinners and when practicing yoga, to promote mindful presence and improve her overall well-being.

- **Mindfulness Practices**: Sonia began incorporating mindfulness techniques like deep breathing and short meditation sessions, inspired by her grandmother's teachings on traditional Indian meditation practices. She used these techniques to manage the urge to check her phone and to become more aware of her emotional responses to social media content.
- **Offline Activities**: She increased her involvement in cultural events and community activities, such as volunteering at a local Indian cultural center and participating in traditional dance classes. By replacing time spent online with meaningful offline activities, Sonia was able to reconnect with her cultural roots and build stronger relationships with her family and friends.

Employing these tactics can empower individuals to regain control over their social media consumption, allowing them to cultivate healthier online habits and allocate more time to offline activities that foster meaningful connections and personal growth. By harnessing the potential of these self-help tools, individuals can develop a more balanced and intentional approach to social media use, ultimately leading to improved mental wellbeing and a reduced risk of addiction (Mousa, 2023). Furthermore, the adoption of these strategies offers a proactive means of addressing the early stages of problematic social media use before it escalates into a more severe and debilitating addiction, highlighting the importance of early intervention and self-awareness.

Cognitive Behavioral Therapy (CBT)

Cognitive Behavioral Therapy (CBT) serves as a highly effective therapeutic intervention for those struggling with problematic social media use. Rooted in the understanding of how thoughts, feelings, and actions are interconnected, CBT aims to help people cultivate healthier behavioral patterns and enhance overall well-being (Zhou et al., 2021). For those experiencing social media addiction, CBT provides a framework to identify and modify the cognitive distortions, or biased thought patterns, that often drive compulsive online behavior (Mousa, 2023). This approach is particularly beneficial for youth, who are often the most vulnerable demographic to the negative effects of social media addiction.

A key element of CBT is cognitive restructuring, which challenges the distorted thinking patterns that often contribute to problematic social media use. Individuals may, for instance, overestimate the importance of being constantly connected or have an intense fear of missing out (FoMO), which can lead to relentless checking of their feeds (Pontes et al., 2018). CBT empowers individuals to critically assess these thoughts and substitute them with more rational perspectives (Mousa, 2023).

This includes developing the skill to recognize and differentiate between social media addiction and healthy SNS usage patterns (Zhou et al., 2021).

CBT also emphasizes the importance of emotional regulation, assisting individuals in managing the emotions that often fuel their addiction (Pontes et al., 2018). By enhancing emotional control, individuals can adopt behaviors and thought patterns that aid in their recovery from social media addiction. Furthermore, CBT recognizes and addresses the social and familial influences that can contribute to the development and maintenance of addiction (Mousa, 2023). These are all vital components of CBT, leading to a comprehensive approach.

Case Example: Joey's Journey to Balanced Social Media Use

These CBT principles can be seen in practice through real-world examples. Consider the case of Joey, a 17-year-old high school student, who exemplifies the application of CBT. Joey, an otherwise active and outgoing individual, discovered that he was spending an excessive amount of time on social media, which was negatively impacting his academic performance and social life. His parents, who placed a high value on education, held expectations that added further pressure. Joey also felt significant pressure to maintain a perfect online persona, experiencing anxiety related to comparison and the desire for validation.

- **Cognitive Restructuring and Behavior Modification:** To manage his issues, Joey underwent CBT, including cognitive restructuring, and behavioral strategies (Corey, 2017). During his therapy sessions, Joey worked with a therapist to identify and challenge the cognitive distortions underlying his problematic social media use. Specifically, he learned to challenge the idea that his self-worth was directly tied to the number of "likes" and comments he received. By questioning the validity of this thought pattern, he began to focus on his intrinsic value and personal accomplishments, fostering a healthier self-image independent of online validation.
- **Behavioral Strategies and Coping Mechanisms:** Furthermore, Joey implemented structured plans to limit his social media consumption. He utilized applications to track his time on social media, set daily time limits, and developed specific schedules for engagement. He also explored alternative behaviors and coping strategies to manage the anxiety and stress that prompted his social media use, including deep breathing exercises, mindfulness practices, and increased engagement in his extracurricular activities.

After undergoing CBT, Joey developed a greater understanding of his social media use and the triggers that prompted him to spend excessive time online. He was able to manage his anxiety and stress in healthier ways. Through CBT, he regained control over his social media use, ultimately improving his academic performance and enhancing his overall well-being. This case underscores how the multifaceted approach of CBT, involving cognitive restructuring, behavioral strategies, and emotional regulation, can be a powerful tool in addressing problematic social media use.

Group Therapy

Group counseling provides a structured setting where individuals facing similar challenges can come together, share experiences, and learn from one another. This therapeutic modality, often facilitated by a trained counselor, offers a unique blend of support, insight, and accountability (Corey, 2017). Within the group environment, participants feel less isolated, realizing they are not alone in their struggles. They can observe how others cope with social media use, learn new strategies, and gain a fresh perspective on their own behavior (Mooy et al., 2024). The following case will demonstrate how group counseling provides support to individuals with disabilities struggling with social media addiction.

Case Example: Analee Navigating Social Media and Disability

Analee, a 35-year-old software engineer, was diagnosed with multiple sclerosis (MS) over 9 years ago. While she had adapted to life with the disability, she recently began to use social media as a coping mechanism for increased MS symptoms and emotional distress. She joined a group therapy program designed to support individuals adjusting to acquired disabilities. This group was led by a therapist experienced in working with individuals with MS and the unique challenges they face. As a culturally sensitive approach, the therapist ensured that the group's discussions and activities addressed the specific needs and concerns of individuals with MS, such as navigating ableism and language barriers.

- **Fostering Community and Addressing Emotional Needs:** The group sessions provided Analee with a safe and supportive environment to share her experiences and connect with others facing similar challenges (Corey, 2023). This shared experience reduced feelings of isolation and provided validation for her struggles. The group focused on developing healthy coping mechanisms to manage MS symptoms and emotional challenges.
- **Collaborative Problem-Solving and Peer Support:** Together, the group members developed strategies to promote healthier online behaviors. They

shared tips for setting boundaries, managing notifications, and practicing mindful social media use. They also discussed ways to resist the urge to compare themselves to others and to focus on their individual strengths and accomplishments. Group members provided emotional support and held each other accountable for their goals. This mutual support was crucial in maintaining motivation and progress (Corey, 2023).

- **Group Dynamics and Skill-Building:** Through group therapy, Analee and the other members learned a range of skills, including cognitive restructuring, behavioral techniques, mindfulness, and assertive communication (Corey, 2023). The group setting encouraged skill practice and provided valuable feedback, fostering a sense of empowerment and control. The group experience helped Analee, and others, develop healthier boundaries with technology, fostering a more balanced and fulfilling life.

The benefits of group counseling in addressing social media addiction are multifaceted. It combats feelings of isolation, which are often associated with addiction, by connecting individuals with others who understand their struggles (Menon et al., 2023). The group environment facilitates deeper self-reflection, allowing participants to identify triggers and patterns of behavior (Mooy et al., 2024). Participants learn and practice practical coping strategies for managing cravings, setting healthy boundaries, and engaging in fulfilling activities (Ulfatari et al., 2022). The group encourages commitment to goals and mutual support (Mooy et al., 2024). Moreover, group counseling is often a more affordable and accessible treatment option than individual therapy (Corey, 2023), expanding its reach and impact.

DIGITAL LITERACY AND SELF-REGULATION STRATEGIES

To effectively address problematic social media use, particularly for individuals with disabilities, treatment strategies must prioritize digital literacy. This crucial skill, encompassing the ability to critically evaluate and navigate the digital world, is no longer optional but rather a cornerstone of responsible social media use. As highlighted by Pradana et al. (2024), digital literacy forms the bedrock of successful interventions in today's rapidly evolving digital landscape. The constant flow of information demands these skills to empower individuals and mitigate the potential harms of excessive social media engagement.

1. **Combatting the Viral Nature of Misinformation**: One significant challenge is the accelerated spread of false or misleading information, with hoaxes often outpacing the dissemination of truth (Vosoughi et al., 2018). Digital literacy

interventions should equip individuals to identify and combat misinformation. When people can discern truthful news, they can reduce the time they spend online. This becomes a crucial skill in battling addiction. Digital literacy empowers users to be more discerning about content that supports their emotional well-being.

2. **Strengthening Critical Analysis**: Essential to digital literacy is the development of critical thinking skills. By analyzing information, we can evaluate the reliability of sources, identify biases, and separate fact from opinion (Tandoc, 2020). When we can better see the value in what we consume, we will find it easier to engage less in addiction. By incorporating critical thinking exercises into social media addiction interventions, the user can improve those skills.
3. **Breaking Free from "Echo Chambers"**: Social media algorithms often create "echo chambers," where users are primarily exposed to information confirming their existing beliefs (Cinelli & Morales, 2021). This can exacerbate harmful content, including misinformation. Through media literacy, we can find ways to broaden our scope of knowledge. Intervention approaches can also help social media users increase their willingness to engage with different perspectives. This is an effective method for those dealing with addiction, helping users reduce their need to have a constant stream of information.
4. **Demonstrating the Effectiveness of Targeted Training**: Several studies have found that the structured nature of digital literacy training can reduce the belief in misinformation (Guess & Munger, 2023; Orosz et al., 2024). This makes them ideal for social media addiction. Interventions can address this issue by providing individuals with the skills and knowledge to identify unreliable sources, assess information critically, and make informed decisions about their online engagement.
5. **Enhancing Self-Control through Digital Literacy**: Digital literacy provides a more critical framework for evaluating information. It can help individuals develop self-control. When confronted with information, individuals can think about how to use it. This is particularly critical for diminishing the damaging effects of false content in a social media context (Mahendra et al., 2024).

DISCUSSION AND FUTURE DIRECTIONS

The exploration of problematic social media use reveals significant risks impacting diverse populations. By examining the nuanced dynamics of social media use across various demographics, we can better understand the urgent need for targeted interventions and preventative measures.

Preventative Measures

Preventative measures are crucial in mitigating the negative effects of excessive social media use, as highlighted in the observations outlined in this chapter. Implementing preventative strategies is key, such as educational initiatives in schools that encourage open discussions about mental health and promote self-regulation and responsible social media use among younger demographics. Similarly, workplaces can play a role by establishing formal guidelines for technological use during work hours, which can help employees strike a balance between their responsibilities and provide opportunities for real-time connection and enrichment without the constant distraction of social media. By taking such measures, a balanced culture surrounding social media can be created, enabling individuals to cultivate healthier relationships with technology.

Promoting Healthy Digital Experiences

Cultivating balanced online environments is crucial for enhancing mental well-being, and it is only by initiating this conversation that we can begin to address the growing concerns surrounding problematic social media use. Through a more informed understanding of the nuanced impact of social media, educators, mental health professionals, and researchers can develop proactive strategies to mitigate its negative effects. By engaging with communities and fostering digital environments that prioritize respect, connection, and emotional intelligence, we can lay the groundwork for a society that promotes healthier digital interactions. This proactive approach is essential, given the significant and far-reaching consequences of problematic social media use.

Continued Research

The persistent challenge of problematic social media use necessitates a commitment to understanding its long-term effects, particularly within a context of rapidly changing technologies. Future research should focus on longitudinal studies that examine mental health outcomes in relation to both evolving platform designs and algorithms. Importantly, investigations into the experiences of marginalized communities will be pivotal to developing targeted, effective interventions. This ongoing adaptation will be critical; and it will drive advances in education, therapy, and advocacy, ensuring that these efforts remain relevant and beneficial as the digital world continues to transform.

CONCLUSION

The exploration within this chapter has illuminated the wide-ranging effects of excessive social media consumption, demonstrating its multifaceted impact on various groups and highlighting the pressing need for strategies to combat its negative consequences. Given the rapid evolution of digital technology, adopting a balanced approach to online engagement, one that places mental well-being at the forefront, is paramount. Ultimately, by confronting the intricate challenges of problematic social media use head-on, we can cultivate a future where online spaces nurture mental well-being and empower positive human connection.

REFERENCES

Abreu, R. L., & Kenny, M. C. (2018). Cyberbullying and LGBTQ youth: A systematic literature review and recommendations for prevention and intervention. *Journal of Child & Adolescent Trauma, 11*(1), 81–97. DOI: 10.1007/s40653-017-0175-7 PMID: 32318140

Abu Khait, A., Mrayyan, M. T., Al-Rjoub, S., Rababa, M., & Al-Rawashdeh, S. (2023). Cyberchondria, anxiety sensitivity, hypochondria, and internet addiction: Implications for mental health professionals. *Current Psychology (New Brunswick, N.J.), 42*(31), 27141–27152. DOI: 10.1007/s12144-022-03815-3 PMID: 36254213

Ajewumi, O. E., Magbagbeola, V., Kalu, O. C., Ike, R. A., Folajimi, O., & Diyaolu, C. O. (2024). The impact of social media on mental health and well-being. *World Journal of Advanced Research and Reviews, 24*(1), 107–121. DOI: 10.30574/wjarr.2024.24.1.3027

Alavi, S. S., Maracy, M. R., Jannatifard, F., & Eslami, M. (2011). The effect of psychiatric symptoms on the internet addiction disorder in Isfahan's University students. *Journal of Research in Medical Sciences : the Official Journal of Isfahan University of Medical Sciences, 16*(6), 793. PMID: 22091309

Amichai-Hamburger, Y., & Vinitzky, G. (2010). Social network use and personality. *Computers in Human Behavior, 26*(6), 1289–1295. DOI: 10.1016/j.chb.2010.03.018

Andreassen, C. S. (2015). Online social network site addiction: A comprehensive review. *Current Addiction Reports, 2*(2), 175–184. DOI: 10.1007/s40429-015-0056-9

Andreassen, C. S., Torsheim, T., Brunborg, G. S., & Pallesen, S. (2012). Development of a Facebook Addiction Scale. *Psychological Reports, 110*(2), 501–517. DOI: 10.2466/02.09.18.PR0.110.2.501-517 PMID: 22662404

Aziz, M., Chemnad, K., Al-Harahsheh, S., Abdelmoneium, A. O., Bagdady, A., Hassan, D. A., & Ali, R. (2024). The influence of adolescents essential and non-essential use of technology and Internet addiction on their physical and mental fatigues. *Scientific Reports, 14*(1), 1745. DOI: 10.1038/s41598-024-51655-x PMID: 38242916

Bae, M. (2023). Coping strategies initiated by COVID-19-related stress, individuals' motives for social media use, and perceived stress reduction. *Internet Research, 33*(1), 124–151. DOI: 10.1108/INTR-05-2021-0269

Bannon, S., McGlynn, T., McKenzie, K., & Quayle, E. (2015). The Internet and young people with Additional Support Needs (ASN): Risk and safety. *Computers in Human Behavior*, *53*, 495–503. DOI: 10.1016/j.chb.2014.12.057

Berryman, C., Ferguson, C. J., & Negy, C. (2018). Social media use and mental health among young adults. *The Psychiatric Quarterly*, *89*(2), 307–314. DOI: 10.1007/s11126-017-9535-6 PMID: 29090428

Beyari, H. (2023). The relationship between social media and the increase in mental health problems. *International Journal of Environmental Research and Public Health*, *20*(3), 2383. DOI: 10.3390/ijerph20032383 PMID: 36767749

Blackwell, D., Leaman, C., Tramposch, R., Osborne, C., & Liss, M. (2017). Extraversion, neuroticism, attachment style and fear of missing out as predictors of social media use and addiction. *Personality and Individual Differences*, *116*, 69–72. DOI: 10.1016/j.paid.2017.04.039

Buijs, P., Boot, E., Shugar, A., Fung, W. L. A., & Bassett, A. S. (2017). Internet safety issues for adolescents and adults with intellectual disabilities. *Journal of Applied Research in Intellectual Disabilities*, *30*(2), 416–418. DOI: 10.1111/jar.12250 PMID: 26914835

Caplan, S. E. (2006). Relations among loneliness, social anxiety, and problematic Internet use. *Cyberpsychology & Behavior*, *10*(2), 234–242. DOI: 10.1089/cpb.2006.9963 PMID: 17474841

Cash, H. D., Rae, C. H., Steel, A., & Winkler, A. (2012). Internet addiction: A brief summary of research and practice. *Current Psychiatry Reviews*, *8*(4), 292–298. DOI: 10.2174/157340012803520513 PMID: 23125561

Chen, E., Wood, D., & Ysseldyk, R. (2022). Online social networking and mental health among older adults: A scoping review. *Canadian Journal on Aging*, *41*(1), 26–39. DOI: 10.1017/S0714980821000040 PMID: 33736725

Choudhury, M., & Ali, A. (2020). Social media addiction among youth: A gender comparison. *International Journal of Indian Psychology*, *8*(3), 740–748.

Chu, G. C., Chan, L. Y., Do, C. W., Tse, A. C., Cheung, T., Szeto, G. P., So, B. C. L., Lee, R. L. T., & Lee, P. H. (2023). Association between time spent on smartphones and digital eye strain: A 1-year prospective observational study among Hong Kong children and adolescents. *Environmental Science and Pollution Research International*, *30*(20), 58428–58435. DOI: 10.1007/s11356-023-26258-0 PMID: 36991204

Cinelli, M., De Francisci Morales, G., Galeazzi, A., Quattrociocchi, W., & Starnini, M. (2021). The echo chamber effect on social media. *Proceedings of the National Academy of Sciences of the United States of America, 118*(9), e2023301118. DOI: 10.1073/pnas.2023301118 PMID: 33622786

Corey, G. (2017). *Theory and practice of counselling and psychotherapy*. Cengage Learning.

Corey, G. (2023). *Theory & practice of group counseling*. Cengage.

Coyne, S. M., Rogers, A. A., Zurcher, J. D., Stockdale, L., & Booth, M. (2020). Does time spent using social media impact mental health?: An eight year longitudinal study. *Computers in Human Behavior, 104*, 106160. DOI: 10.1016/j.chb.2019.106160

Daniyal, M., Javaid, S. F., Hassan, A., & Khan, M. A. (2022). The relationship between cellphone usage on the physical and mental wellbeing of university students: A cross-sectional study. *International Journal of Environmental Research and Public Health, 19*(15), 9352. DOI: 10.3390/ijerph19159352 PMID: 35954709

Frison, E., & Eggermont, S. (2016). Exploring the relationships between different types of Facebook use, perceived online social support, and adolescents' depressed mood. *Social Science Computer Review, 34*(2), 153–171. DOI: 10.1177/0894439314567449

Guedes, E., Nardi, A. E., Guimarães, F. M. C. L., Machado, S., & King, A. L. S. (2016). Social networking, a new online addiction: A review of Facebook and other addiction disorders. *MedicalExpress (São Paulo), 3*(1), M160101. DOI: 10.5935/MedicalExpress.2016.01.01

Guess, A. M., & Munger, K. (2023). Digital literacy and online political behavior. *Political Science Research and Methods, 11*(1), 110–128. DOI: 10.1017/psrm.2022.17

Heller, A. S., & Casey, B. J. (2016). The neurodynamics of emotion: Delineating typical and atypical emotional processes during adolescence. *Developmental Science, 19*(1), 3–18. DOI: 10.1111/desc.12373 PMID: 26548573

Heung, S., Jiang, L., Azenkot, S., & Vashistha, A. (2024, May). "Vulnerable, Victimized, and Objectified": Understanding Ableist Hate and Harassment Experienced by Disabled Content Creators on Social Media. In *Proceedings of the CHI Conference on Human Factors in Computing Systems* (pp. 1-19).

Kuss, D. J., & Griffiths, M. D. (2011). Online Social Networking and Addiction—A Review of the Psychological Literature. *International Journal of Environmental Research and Public Health, 8*(9), 3528–3552. DOI: 10.3390/ijerph8093528 PMID: 22016701

Lebni, J. Y., Toghroli, R., & Abbas, J. (2020). A study of internet addiction and its effects on mental health: A study based on Iranian University Students. *Journal of Education and Health Promotion*, *9*(1), 205. DOI: 10.4103/jehp.jehp_148_20 PMID: 33062738

Lough, E., & Fisher, M. H. (2016). Internet use and online safety in adults with Williams syndrome. *Journal of Intellectual Disability Research*, *60*(10), 1020–1030. DOI: 10.1111/jir.12281 PMID: 27174494

Machado, B., de Faria, P. L., Araújo, I., & Caridade, S. (2024). Cyber interpersonal violence: Adolescent perspectives and digital practices. *International Journal of Environmental Research and Public Health*, *21*(7), 832. DOI: 10.3390/ijerph21070832 PMID: 39063409

Mahendra, Y., Jundi, R., Wulandari, G., & Munawar, A. (2024). The Urgency of Digital Literacy in Shaping Students' Civic Virtue: Challenges and Opportunities in the Technological Era. *ICoCSE Proceedings*, 1, 17-22.

McHugh, B. C., Wisniewski, P., Rosson, M. B., & Carroll, J. M. (2018). When social media traumatizes teens: The roles of online risk exposure, coping, and post-traumatic stress. *Internet Research*, *28*(5), 1169–1188. DOI: 10.1108/IntR-02-2017-0077

Menon, V. A., Prasad, A., Puthur, L. A., K K, S., & Joseph, L. (2023). Social Media Dependency and Facebook Usage among the Older Adults of Kerala. *Studies in Media and Communication*, *11*(4), 202–208. DOI: 10.11114/smc.v11i4.6060

Mooy, M. E., Natalia, M., & Taneo, J. (2023). The Effectiveness of Reality Group Counseling in Reducing Social Media Dependency. *Bulletin of Counseling and Psychotherapy*, *5*(3). Advance online publication. DOI: 10.51214/00202305459000

Mousa, S. E. A. (2023). The effectiveness of cognitive-behavioral therapy in alleviating social media addiction among university youth groups. *Egyptian Journal of Social Work*, *15*(1), 175–200. DOI: 10.21608/ejsw.2023.164679.1163

Nesi, J., & Prinstein, M. J. (2015). Using social media for social comparison and feedback-seeking: Gender and popularity moderate associations with depressive symptoms. *Journal of Abnormal Child Psychology*, *43*(8), 1427–1438. DOI: 10.1007/s10802-015-0020-0 PMID: 25899879

Oberst, U., Wegmann, E., Stodt, B., Brand, M., & Chamarro, A. (2017). Negative consequences from heavy social networking in adolescents: The mediating role of fear of missing out. *Journal of Adolescence*, *55*(1), 51–60. DOI: 10.1016/j.adolescence.2016.12.008 PMID: 28033503

Orosz, G., Faragó, L., Paskuj, B., & Krekó, P. (2024). Strategies to combat misinformation: Enduring effects of a 15-minute online intervention on critical-thinking adolescents. *Computers in Human Behavior*, *159*, 108338. DOI: 10.1016/j.chb.2024.108338

Pew Research Center. (2024, November 13). *Social Media Fact Sheet.*https://www.pewresearch.org/internet/fact-sheet/social-media/

Pradana, P. H., Agustini, K., Dantes, G. R., & Sudatha, I. G. W. (2024). The urgency of digital literacy learning in educational units: Systematic literature review. *Child Education Journal*, *6*(1), 25–33. DOI: 10.33086/cej.v6i1.6100

Primack, B. A., Shensa, A., Sidani, J. E., Whaite, E. O., Lin, L., Rosen, D., Colditz, J. B., Radovic, A., & Miller, E. (2017). Social media use and perceived social isolation among young adults in the US. *American Journal of Preventive Medicine*, *53*(1), 1–8. DOI: 10.1016/j.amepre.2017.01.010 PMID: 28279545

Roberts, A. G., & Lopez-Duran, N. L. (2019). Developmental influences on stress response systems: Implications for psychopathology vulnerability in adolescence. *Comprehensive Psychiatry*, *88*, 9–21. DOI: 10.1016/j.comppsych.2018.10.008 PMID: 30466015

Roberts, T. A., Daniels, E. A., Weaver, J. M., & Zanovitch, L. S. (2022). "Intermission!" A short-term social media fast reduces self-objectification among pre-teen and teen dancers. *Body Image*, *43*, 125–133. DOI: 10.1016/j.bodyim.2022.08.015 PMID: 36152479

Sadagheyani, H. E., & Tatari, F. (2021). Investigating the role of social media on mental health. *Mental Health and Social Inclusion*, *25*(1), 41–51. DOI: 10.1108/MHSI-06-2020-0039

Satici, S. A., Gocet Tekin, E., Deniz, M. E., & Satici, B. (2023). Doomscrolling scale: Its association with personality traits, psychological distress, social media use, and wellbeing. *Applied Research in Quality of Life*, *18*(2), 833–847. DOI: 10.1007/s11482-022-10110-7 PMID: 36275044

Sujarwoto, S., Saputri, R. A. M., & Yumarni, T. (2023). Social media addiction and mental health among university students during the COVID-19 pandemic in Indonesia. *International Journal of Mental Health and Addiction*, *21*(1), 96–110. DOI: 10.1007/s11469-021-00582-3 PMID: 34230820

Sweet, K. S., LeBlanc, J. K., Stough, L. M., & Sweany, N. W. (2020). Community building and knowledge sharing by individuals with disabilities using social media. *Journal of Computer Assisted Learning*, *36*(1), 1–11. DOI: 10.1111/jcal.12377

Tamir, D. I., & Mitchell, J. P. (2012). Disclosing information about the self is intrinsically rewarding. *Proceedings of the National Academy of Sciences of the United States of America, 109*(21), 8038–8043. DOI: 10.1073/pnas.1202129109 PMID: 22566617

Tandoc, E. C.Jr. (2020). Tools of disinformation: How fake news gets to deceive. In *Disinformation and fake news* (pp. 35–46). Springer Singapore.

Tang, C. S. K., & Koh, Y. Y. W. (2017). Online social networking addiction among college students in Singapore: Comorbidity with behavioral addiction and affective disorder. *Asian Journal of Psychiatry, 25*, 175–178. DOI: 10.1016/j.ajp.2016.10.027 PMID: 28262144

Tateno, M., Teo, A. R., Ukai, W., Kanazawa, J., Katsuki, R., Kubo, H., & Kato, T. A. (2019). Internet addiction, smartphone addiction, and Hikikomori trait in Japanese young adult: Social isolation and social network. *Frontiers in Psychiatry, 10*, 455. DOI: 10.3389/fpsyt.2019.00455 PMID: 31354537

Twenge, J. M., Joiner, T. E., Rogers, M. L., & Martin, G. N. (2018). Increases in depressive symptoms, suicide-related outcomes, and suicide rates among US adolescents after 2010 and links to increased new media screen time. *Clinical Psychological Science, 6*(1), 3–17. DOI: 10.1177/2167702617723376

Twenge, J. M., Martin, G. N., & Spitzberg, B. H. (2019). Trends in US Adolescents' media use, 1976–2016: The rise of digital media, the decline of TV, and the (near) demise of print. *Psychology of Popular Media Culture, 8*(4), 329–345. DOI: 10.1037/ppm0000203

Ulfatari, N., Wibowo, M. E., & Japar, M. (2022). The effectiveness of reality group counseling with confrontation techniques to reduce smartphone addiction symptoms in college students. *Jurnal Bimbingan Konseling, 11*(1), 53–59.

Vosoughi, S., Roy, D., & Aral, S. (2018). The spread of true and false news online. *science*, 359(6380), 1146-1151.

Wacks, Y., & Weinstein, A. M. (2021). Excessive smartphone use is associated with health problems in adolescents and young adults. *Frontiers in Psychiatry, 12*, 669042. DOI: 10.3389/fpsyt.2021.669042 PMID: 34140904

Ye, X. L., Zhang, W., & Zhao, F. F. (2023). Depression and internet addiction among adolescents: A meta-analysis. *Psychiatry Research, 326*, 115311. DOI: 10.1016/j.psychres.2023.115311 PMID: 37348449

Zhao, S., Grasmuck, S., & Martin, J. (2008). Identity construction on Facebook: Digital empowerment in anchored relationships. *Computers in Human Behavior*, *24*(5), 1816–1836. DOI: 10.1016/j.chb.2008.02.012

Zhou, X., Rau, P. L. P., Yang, C. L., & Zhou, X. (2021). Cognitive behavioral therapy-based short-term abstinence intervention for problematic social media use: Improved well-being and underlying mechanisms. *The Psychiatric Quarterly*, *92*(2), 761–779. DOI: 10.1007/s11126-020-09852-0 PMID: 32989636

Chapter 4
Gaming Disorder and Its Impact on Adolescents' Mental Health

Gabriela Rangel
https://orcid.org/0009-0007-7554-4407
University of Texas Rio Grande Valley, USA

ABSTRACT

This chapter explores Gaming Disorder (GD) and its impact on adolescents. GD is defined as a condition in which excessive gaming negatively affects various life aspects (American Psychiatric Association, 2023). The chapter identifies key sources for recognizing GD symptoms, which can aid practitioners (American Psychiatric Association, 2023). It examines the prevalence of GD among adolescents, highlighting contributing factors like stress, family dynamics, and mental health conditions such as depression and ADHD (Gao et al., 2022). Emphasizing the importance of therapists understanding the gaming world of adolescents, it discusses how gaming practices can lead to addiction, thus guiding effective treatment (Van der Schyff et al., 2023). The chapter outlines strategies for parents to prevent GD (Young, 2009) and highlights effective counseling techniques for practitioners (Kim & Chun, 2022). Lastly, it promotes healthy gaming practices, helping adolescents engage in gaming more balanced and healthfully (Educational Advancement, 2022).

DOI: 10.4018/979-8-3373-0518-9.ch004

I. INTRODUCTION

Definition of Gaming Disorder (GD)

Gaming disorder (GD) is a condition with significant mental health concerns where individuals lose control over their gaming habits, leading to negative consequences in areas such as self-care, social relationships, school, and work. This condition can occur both during online and offline gaming experiences (American Psychiatric Association, 2023). While video game use has raised concerns, it remains an ambiguous topic within the field (American Psychiatric Association, 2023).

Diagnostic and treatment interventions for GD, particularly those focused on symptom-based criteria, can be restrictive and potentially confusing (American Psychiatric Association, 2023). The purpose of this chapter is not to condemning gaming, but rather to highlight GD as a stage in which an individual's life is substantially affected across multiple domains. While there is a growing body of research indicating the potential benefits of gaming, such as fostering pleasure and well-being (Nguyen et al., 2018), it is essential to recognize that it can also become problematic when taken to excess (Griffiths, 2018).

Diagnosing GD

Gaming disorder has been identified in two primary reference sources for counselors: the *Diagnostic and Statistical Manual of Mental Disorders* (DSM-5-TR) and the *International Classification of Diseases* (ICD-11). The definition of GD is still controversial, and both the DSM-5 and ICD-11, which are authoritative references, offer different interpretations of the disorder, leading to differences in prevalence, etiology, assessment, and intervention (Borges et al., 2021; Ko et al., 2020). Counselors may reference both the DSM-5-TR and ICD-11 when assessing gaming-related concerns, though only the latter provides an official diagnosis.

DSM-5-TR

The first recorded classification of GD appears in DSM-5-TR as a "condition for further study" and a "tentative disorder," with nine criteria for clinical assessment (American Psychiatric Association, 2023). However, GD has not been officially recognized as a formal mental disorder due to insufficient research and lack of consensus regarding its classification as a behavioral addiction (American Psychiatric Association, 2023).

The DSM-5-TR categorizes GD as a potential new diagnosis that can be classified as mild, moderate, or severe, based on the degree of disruption to normal activities. Less severe cases involve fewer symptoms and minimal disruption, while severe cases may result in significant time spent gaming and substantial harm to relationships or career and school opportunities (American Psychiatric Association, 2013). Furthermore, GD may manifest through online gaming, non-internet gaming, or traditional gaming systems. The DSM-5-TR notes that genetic and physiological factors may predispose certain populations, particularly Asian males and adolescents, to GD (American Psychiatric Association, 2013).

ICD-11

A second key reference for GD comes from the *International Classification of Diseases* (ICD-11), published by the World Health Organization (WHO). In 2016, GD was included in the beta draft of the ICD-11 (Aarseth et al., 2016; Pontes & Griffiths, 2019). This inclusion was preceded by significant debate among psychologists, psychiatrists, and clinicians who studied and treated GD. Opinions were divided on whether GD should be formally recognized as an addictive disorder (Griffiths et al., 2017; Pontes & Griffiths, 2019). Some experts advocated for its classification as a mental health disorder, while others, particularly from the field of media psychology, opposed this view, citing insufficient evidence to support GD as a mental disorder (Van Rooij et al., 2018; Pontes & Griffiths, 2019).

Despite these disagreements, WHO officially recognized GD as a mental health disorder in 2019 (Pontes & Griffiths, 2019). The WHO defines GD as "a pattern of gaming behavior characterized by impaired control over gaming, increasing priority given to gaming over other activities, and continuation or escalation of gaming despite negative consequences" (WHO, 2020). According to the WHO, GD symptoms must persist for 12 months and significantly impact key areas of functioning, including personal, familial, social, educational, and occupational domains (WHO, 2020). Based on the effort to have a visualization of both sources, the author summarizes the diagnostic criteria from each source DSM-5-TR (5th ed., text rev.; American Psychiatric Association, 2022) and the ICD-11 (World Health Organization, 2019) in Table 1.

Table 1. Comparison of DSM-5-TR and ICD-11 Diagnostic Criteria for GD.

Category	DSM-5-TR (Proposed)	ICD-11 (Official)
Diagnostic Status	Condition for further study	Official diagnosis
Criteria	At least 5 of 9 symptoms within 12 months	All 3 core criteria within 12 months
Symptoms	1. Preoccupation 2. Withdrawal 3. Tolerance 4. Loss of control 5. Loss of interest 6. Continued use despite problems 7. Deceiving others 8. Gaming to escape 9. Jeopardizing relationships or jobs	1. Impaired control 2. Priority given to gaming 3. Continuation despite negative consequences
Duration	Symptoms present for at least 12 months	Symptoms must be present for 12 months (shorter duration acceptable if symptoms are severe)
Functional Impairment	Required (e.g., social, academic, or occupational)	Required (e.g., personal, family, social, educational, or occupational)

II. GROWING CONCERNS AND PREVALENCE

A 2023 survey conducted by the Pew Research Center with 1,423 U.S. adolescents aged 13 to 17 revealed that 85% of adolescents play video games, with 41% reporting daily gaming. Additionally, 40% of adolescents identify as "gamers" (Gottfried & Sidoti, 2024). Gaming is also seen as a social activity, as 72% of adolescents report spending time with others while playing, and 47% have made online friends through gaming (Gottfried & Sidoti, 2024). Although 50% of adolescents report that gaming has improved their problem-solving skills, 41% note a negative impact on their sleep (Gottfried & Sidoti, 2024). Moreover, gaming has exposed adolescents to bullying, with 80% of them reporting harassment while playing and 41% experiencing offensive name-calling (Gottfried & Sidoti, 2024).

There are also gender and socioeconomic differences in gaming patterns. A greater proportion of male adolescents (62%) identify as gamers compared to female adolescents (17%), and male adolescents also play more frequently (61% vs. 22%) (Gottfried & Sidoti, 2024). Household income also correlates with gaming frequency, with 53% of adolescents from families earning less than $30,000 per year playing daily, compared to 42% of those from households with an income of $30,000 to $74,999 and 39% from households earning $75,000 or more (Gottfried

& Sidoti, 2024). Gaming is more common among Black (17%) and Hispanic (18%) adolescents compared to White adolescents (8%) (Gottfried & Sidoti, 2024).

In terms of motivation, the majority of adolescents play video games to stay entertained (87%), while others play to satisfy social needs (50%) or to learn something new (Gottfried & Sidoti, 2024). Over the past decade, the gaming industry has achieved remarkable financial success, surpassing both Hollywood and the music industry combined. In 2021, global gaming revenues reached $180 billion (Wijman, 2021). Additionally, studies have found that 19% of boys and 7.8% of girls aged 10 to 14 report problematic gaming, with boys more likely to engage in problematic gaming and girls tending to struggle more with social media and mobile phone use (Gordon-Larsen et al., 2000).

III. EVOLUTION OF VIDEO GAMES

Video games have evolved significantly over time, with various genres such as first-person shooters, strategy games, massively multiplayer online role-playing games (MMORPGs), and life simulations (Von et al., 2019). The journey of video games began with the release of *Atari* in 1972, the first video game that offered players an opportunity to engage for extended periods, trying to achieve higher scores and progress through levels (Goethe, 2019). Since then, the gaming industry has seen a shift toward more sophisticated designs, where the inclusion of complex characters and intricate storylines has become commonplace (Saini & Hodgins, 2023). These types of games are especially popular among introverted adolescents who enjoy role-playing as characters with special powers. Online multiplayer features often serve as a preferred alternative to in-person socializing.

At present, GD has gained recognition as a behavior similar to compulsive gambling. Individuals with GD can experience a rush akin to that of winning in gambling (Watkins, 2023). This phenomenon has been compared to substance use disorder (SUD) due to the brain's reward system being activated in similar ways by both.

In 2004, game researchers introduced a concept known as "MDA: A Formal Approach to Game Design and Game Research," which outlined a framework based on three central components: *mechanics*, *dynamics*, and *aesthetics* (Hunicke, 2004).

1. Mechanics are the core systems, rules, and objectives that players must follow to succeed in the game providing structure and competition (Hunicke, 2004).
2. Dynamics refer to the unpredictable outcomes that occur as a result of player choices and the game's rules, contributing to the ongoing flow and excitement of the game (Hunicke, 2004).

3. Aesthetics encompass the emotional and sensory experiences, such as visuals and sound design, that contribute to the player's enjoyment and immersion in the game world (Hunicke, 2004).

This framework provides insight into why video games can captivate players for long stretches of time, making them enjoyable yet, at times, addictive (Andersen & MoldStud Research Team, 2024). Building on this understanding of game mechanics and player engagement, researchers have also explored the psychological factors that influence gaming behaviors and addiction as follows.

IV. NEUROLOGICAL IMPACT OF GD

In 2011, a study examining brain activity and the desire for gaming identified similarities between GD and SUD (Han et al., 2011). Specifically, activation was observed in the prefrontal cortex, orbitofrontal cortex, parahippocampal gyrus, and thalamus in individuals with both conditions (Han et al., 2011). Moreover, the limbic structures appear to play a central role in the reward and addiction circuits in both disorders (Cooper et al., 2017).

Individuals affected by these disorders experience cravings and triggers linked to the dopamine reward system, similar to those associated with substance use and behavioral addiction (Ko et al., 2009; Han et al., 2011). Additionally, research suggests that the dopamine release stimulated by competitive video gaming is comparable to that induced by psychostimulant drugs (Koepp et al., 1998; Yau et al., 2012).

Neurological studies have demonstrated that GD can impair neurocognitive function (Jiang et al., 2020), contribute to executive dysfunction (Lee et al., 2020), and lead to emotional difficulties (Yen et al., 2017). These effects have a holistic impact, influencing physical, mental, and behavioral well-being, particularly among adolescents and young adults (Chen, 2025).

V. EFFECTS OF GD

According to Young (2009), adolescents with GD experience consequences that affect various aspects of their lives, including sleep patterns, nutrition, and real-life interactions, as they prioritize gaming progress over daily responsibilities. Some adolescents engage in gaming sessions lasting 10 to 15 hours or more without taking breaks (Young, 2009). Prolonged gaming can lead to health issues such as back strain, eye strain, carpal tunnel syndrome, and repetitive stress injuries (Ivanova, 2020).

In addition to physical health concerns, excessive gaming negatively impacts academic performance and future aspirations related to education and career development (Gómez-Gonzalvo et al., 2020). Adolescents often struggle to concentrate in class or complete assignments due to their preoccupation with gaming (Johnson, 2023). Furthermore, GD can disrupt social relationships, as individuals may prioritize gaming over spending time with family, friends, or romantic partners, leading to social isolation and a diminished sense of connection (Colwell & Kato, 2003). Building on the broader consequences of GD, it is essential to examine the underlying risk factors that contribute to its development among adolescents.

VI. WHO'S AT RISK FOR GD?

A systematic review and meta-analysis examining the prevalence and potential risk factors of GD among adolescents and young adults identified stress as the most significant contributing factor, followed by the amount of time spent gaming and family-related issues (Gao et al., 2022).

Interpersonal Issues

Interpersonal problems are considered social risk factors for GD, including bullying, being a victim of bullying, and other interpersonal difficulties (Bussone et al., 2020). These interpersonal problems often lead individuals to form emotional connections and commitments during gaming, fostering a social identity within the gaming environment (Lozano-Blasco et al., 2021a). Studies have identified a high level of interpersonal sensitivity among adolescents with GD (Torres-Rodríguez et al., 2018).

Adolescents who experience psychological stress due to maladaptive personality traits are more prone to developing addictive gaming behaviors (Laier et al., 2018). Furthermore, when adolescents exhibit violent tendencies, the prevalence of GD is even higher (Gao et al., 2022). For instance, adolescents who engage in bullying may use violent video games as an outlet for aggression, while those who are victims of bullying may turn to gaming as a means of escaping reality (Vadlin et al., 2016).

Psychological Contributors

Depression, anxiety, emotional distress, and low self-esteem are common factors contributing to the development of GD among adolescents, with depression and anxiety being the most significant (Gao et al., 2022). Anxiety is considered to emerge before depression (Moriarity et al., 2018), and adolescents who experience anxiety during their adolescents age years are more likely to develop depression in adulthood (Johnson et al., 2018). This has been confirmed through longitudinal studies, which have identified that a history of depression and anxiety can predict gaming behavior and the likelihood of developing GD (Teng et al., 2021).

Adolescents who struggle with emotional regulation tend to avoid their emotions, which places them at risk of developing addictive behaviors (Yen et al., 2017), such as excessive gaming, as they seek relief from emotional discomfort (Chang et al., 2020). Those with low self-esteem, particularly those who experience frequent criticism or bullying, may turn to video games as a means of escaping the real world, as they feel safer within the gaming environment (Scerri et al., 2019). Furthermore, studies have shown a negative correlation between self-efficacy and GD, indicating that adolescents with GD perceive themselves as incapable individuals (Jeong & Kim, 2011).

Family Instability

The family environment is a significant risk factor for adolescents, particularly when affected by family issues such as parental separation, poor parent-child relationships, the absence of a parent, or experiences of abandonment (Gao et al., 2022). Family dysfunction can lead adolescents to seek refuge in video games as a means of escaping reality (Park et al., 2008). Engaging in video games may become an unhealthy coping mechanism, allowing adolescents to avoid feelings of sadness or anger resulting from family problems (Schneider et al., 2017).

Academic Performance

The academic performance of adolescents with GD has been identified as being below the passing average, significantly impacting their overall academic achievement (Hawi et al., 2018). Gaming requires time, which limits the availability of adolescents to complete assignments or study (Kuss & Griffiths, 2012). Additionally, poor academic performance influences behavioral outcomes, such as students skipping classes or failing courses (Gao et al., 2022). It is crucial for the school environment to monitor video game usage among adolescents who exhibit these behaviors (Gao et al., 2022).

Males have a higher prevalence of GD than females (Gao et al., 2022) as most popular games consist of role-playing, shooting, battle arenas, and action games (Han et al., 2020). These games share themes of competition, fighting, aggression, and violence, which attract males more significantly than females (Krahé & Möller, 2004). Adolescents addicted to video games may be at a higher risk of developing addictions to other substances later in life, such as drugs or alcohol (Turel & Bechara, 2019). GD has been strongly correlated with various mental health conditions, further complicating the well-being of affected individuals.

VII. GD AND ITS EFFECTS ON MENTAL HEALTH

GD has been linked to several mental health disorders, including depression (González-Bueso et al., 2018; King et al., 2013), anxiety (King et al., 2013), and attention deficit hyperactivity disorder (ADHD) (Rehbein et al., 2015). Individuals with ADHD often struggle with impulse control and attention regulation, these difficulties make them more susceptible to the immediate and intense rewards provided by video games (Rehbein et al., 2015).

Another research published in the Journal of Clinical Child & Adolescent Psychology discovered that adolescents with ADHD who spent more time playing video games displayed more difficulties in controlling themselves and in their decision-making abilities, which are important challenges for people with ADHD (Rehbein et al., 2015).

Studies on neuroanatomy have shown that cortical maturation in individuals with ADHD is delayed (Shaw et al., 2007; Shaw et al., 2012b). This delay affects cognitive processes such as attention and reward evaluation, which may impair an individual's control over addictive behaviors, including substance use, potentially leading to long-term addiction issues (Shaw et al., 2012a). As a result, adolescents with a history of childhood ADHD symptoms may be more susceptible to gaming addiction due to the delayed development of their executive control system (Lee et al., 2017).

Overall, counselors need to be aware of the potential links between ADHD and GD and the potential negative impacts on academic and social functioning (Gao et al., 2022). Despite the growing recognition of gaming disorder, many adolescents face significant stigmas and barriers when seeking support.

VIII. STIGMAS & BARRIERS FOR GD

Many taboos and obstacles surrounding adolescents GD can make it challenging for both adolescents and their parents to get the help they need and even to recognize that a problem exists (Young, 2010). Some people view GD as a sign of weakness or laziness rather than a legitimate mental disorder and the reason is that parents perceive adolescents as just sitting for long periods of time and neglecting other activities, even those they used to enjoy before (Young, 2010).

There are many misconceptions surrounding GD, such as the belief that it only affects boys (APA, 2013). As mentioned in the DSM-5TR adolescent males seem to be at a greater risk of developing GD than girls (APA, 2013) leaving girls who experience GD without proper support. Lastly, parents and caregivers may be concerned that their adolescents spend too much time playing video games; however, they may not recognize it as a complex issue that requires professional help (Mott Poll, 2020).

For certain cultures and their communities, family is prioritized, which may limit individuals in seeking help as they feel compelled to continue supporting the family as a whole and to strengthen familial relationships and unity. This can make it challenging for adolescents to seek help with GD, as they may fear disappointment or burdening their family members (Cauce & Domenech-Rodriguez, 2002). As a result, several countries have introduced regulations aimed at managing and mitigating the negative effects of GD, especially among adolescents.

IX. GOVERNMENT RESPONSES TO GD

The identification of GD varies across countries. In the U.S., there are inconsistencies regarding the sources available for counselors to formally diagnose, despite its prevalence and need for services while other countries have gone as far as developing regulations to prevent and reduce its occurrence (Long et al., 2021).

China has taken direct action to address video game use, particularly among adolescents, who have been the most affected by this issue (Xiao, 2021). By 2009, approximately 10% of China's population, more than 30 million people, had been affected by GD (Young, 2009), with 30% of those identified as children and adolescents (Brooke, 2021).

The impact of GD was observed in poor academic performance, social isolation, and mental health issues such as depression and anxiety (Young, 2009). The situation nearly reached epidemic levels, prompting Chinese authorities to implement strict regulations, including shutting down internet cafes and instituting laws to limit the amount of time adolescents could spend playing online games (Young, 2009).

These restrictions allow gamers to play only during holidays and weekends, with a time limit of one hour, from 8 PM to 9 PM (Brooke, 2021). Additionally, regulations were put in place to ensure that accurate user information, such as name and age, was registered by gaming companies to create a legal record of users (Brooke, 2021). The new rules in China also require gamers to register with a state-run anti-addiction system (Brooke, 2021). While these regulations aim to curb excessive gaming and promote healthier habits, the COVID-19 pandemic has added new challenges to the landscape of GD.

X. COVID-19 AND THE IMPACT OF GD

During the COVID-19 pandemic, isolated children and adolescents reported an increase in gaming hours as a way to cope with psychological distress and avoid social isolation (Han et al., 2022). A growing body of research suggests that these factors may contribute to increased vulnerability to GD (Giardina, 2021). During the COVID-19 pandemic, the prevalence of GD among adolescents intensified (Han et al., 2022). The primary causes were the lack of parental supervision, and the stress adolescents faced due to feelings of loneliness (Han et al., 2022). Additionally, adolescent groups with greater vulnerability during this time were those with a psychiatric history, such as ADHD (Han et al., 2022).

Another important element is that male adolescents were the most affected by GD; however, female adolescents sought out video games as a response to feelings of loneliness (Han et al., 2022). Given these gender differences in the experience of GD, it becomes important to explore how assessments for the disorder are structured. This next section will focus on the tools and methods currently used to evaluate GD and their effectiveness in addressing the unique challenges faced by individuals affected by GD.

XI. ASSESSMENT FOR GD

Currently, there are various assessments for GD, however, it is crucial to examine recent studies and their findings to evaluate the reliability and validity of these instruments. Various assessments for GD have been developed, but consistency in measurement remains a challenge (King et al., 2020).

In a systematic review study, it was identified that out of 32 instruments for measuring GD, none stood out as being superior to the others (King et al., 2020). However, the scales from the Short Version of the Game Addiction Scale for Adolescents GAS-7 (Lemmens et al., 2009), the DSM-5 (American Psychiatric Association, 2013), the 9-Item Internet Gaming Disorder Scale-Short Form IGDS9-SF, (Pontes & Griffiths, 2015), YDQ, and the Internet Gaming Disorder Scale IGDS (Lemmens et al., 2015) received the most support in terms of their psychometric properties (Gao et al., 2022).

It is important to note that these scales are merely screening tools with no diagnostic value, and the results should be interpreted with caution (Gao et al., 2022). The next section will explore the approaches mental health professionals can implement to support clients struggling with GD, offering effective strategies for intervention and treatment.

XII. UNDERSTANDING GD IN CLINICAL PRACTICE

One of the primary goals when working with adolescents in counseling is to establish a strong therapeutic alliance, as this connection significantly influences engagement, retention, and overall treatment outcomes (Flack, 2020). However, it is common for adolescents to demonstrate resistance and limited rapport in the early stages of therapy (Raymer, 2021).

An effective way to develop rapport and build trust, particularly with resistant clients, the counselor sharing their own experiences related to video games. Finding common ground through shared interests can help create a more open and collaborative therapeutic environment (Raymer, 2021).

Unlike the treatment of SUD, the primary goal in addressing GD is not necessarily complete abstinence from gaming. Instead, the focus is on managing and reducing gaming time to normalize behavior in a way that does not negatively impact key areas of an adolescent's life, including their physical and mental health (Raymer, 2021).

To provide effective support, it is also essential for counselors to understand the types of video games adolescents are engaging with (van der Schyff et al., 2023). Furthermore, staying informed about gaming trends enables professionals to remain relevant and responsive, thereby promoting adolescents' overall well-being and assisting them in navigating challenges associated with excessive gaming (Anderson, 2017).

XIII. STRATEGIES FOR COUNSELORS WORKING WITH ADOLESCENTS WITH GD

When working with adolescents, it is important for counselors to consider how to approach them, as many adolescents may not even be aware of their addiction problem (Young, 2009). Therefore, it is suggested that counselors take the following elements into consideration.

The Therapeutic Alliance

The establishment of a therapeutic relationship is the first step in building rapport with adolescents. Without trust, adolescents may not feel comfortable sharing personal information or discussing the challenges they are facing (My People Patterns, 2023). In a study focused on group therapy for adolescents with GD, it was emphasized that counselors were strictly required to possess experience and knowledge related to computer games in order to effectively respond to the participants' dynamics and engagement (Wendt et al., 2021).

Identification of Triggers and Underlying Issues

For some adolescents, GD serves as a way to escape their real-life problems, and the activity acts as a coping mechanism that allows them to forget about the stress or difficulties they face. This behavior is similar to individuals with SUD, who use drugs or alcohol to escape problems they are unable to confront. Similarly, individuals with GD use video games to avoid dealing with challenging situations (Young, 2009). Counselors can support adolescents by helping them identify what motivates or triggers excessive gaming, uncovering underlying issues that may contribute to addiction, such as anxiety, depression, or stress (Newport Academy, 2024).

Developing Coping Strategies

Counselors can also work with adolescents to help them learn healthy coping strategies to manage the triggers and cravings associated with gaming. Some of these strategies include the practice of mindfulness, engaging in physical activities such as sports, or finding alternative activities to gaming as identifying and practicing a new hobby (Sharma et al., 2021).

Psychoeducation

It is important for adolescents to have conversations where they can learn about the benefits but also the effect of GD physically and mentally. While gaming is a common activity among adolescents, the consequences of excessive gaming, particularly GD, are rarely discussed (Wendt et al., 2021).

Family involvement

Involving the adolescents' family in the treatment process can significantly support the adolescent's recovery (Horigian et al., 2016). Counselors can collaborate with the family to establish boundaries around gaming, improve communication, and address any family-related issues that may contribute to the addiction (Horigian et al., 2016).

Referral

There may come a point where counselors feel they are not adequately equipped to support an adolescent struggling with gaming issues (Raymer, 2021). However, it is crucial to establish a rapport to understand how the individual is being affected by addiction and to what extent gaming is impacting their life and environment (Raymer, 2021). If the counselor does not feel sufficiently prepared to assist the client, it is important to consider referring the client to a therapist who is trained to provide the necessary support (Raymer, 2021).

After exploring various strategies to support adolescents with GD, it is crucial for counselors to be equipped with specific resources, including counseling techniques, to best support their clients. \

XIV. TREATMENT APPROACHES FOR GD

The following techniques can provide valuable tools for counselors, ensuring that adolescents with GD receive the most effective support possible.

Motivational Interview (MI)

An evidence-based approach to address addictions as GD in adolescents is MI (Miller & Rollnick, 2023; Lindenberg et al., 2022). The primary goal of MI is to help individuals clarify ambivalence and motivate them to change behaviors that negatively impact their health (Miller & Rollnick, 2023). Initially, MI was developed specifically for the treatment of addictions (Galbraith et al., 2022). A published article highlighted the successful application of MI in the case of an adolescent with GD. The following case study is presented to help counselors gain a practical understanding of how to implement this approach effectively (Verma, 2019).

Case Study. A 15-year-old male student enrolled in the 10th grade was referred for counseling due to escalating online gaming behaviors and associated functional impairments over the past year. In recent weeks, his parents reported increased irritability, social withdrawal, disrupted sleep patterns, skipped meals, and neglect of personal hygiene. He regularly spent 14 to 15 hours per day engaged in online multiplayer gaming. Socially, the adolescent had become increasingly isolated. He expressed disinterest in academics and recently stated his intent to discontinue school to pursue a career as a professional gamer.

According to his parents, the adolescent began engaging with online games in 7th grade, after persistent requests, they purchased a gaming computer. Since then, his gaming hours have progressively increased, while his ability to manage time and meet responsibilities has declined. Given the adolescent's resistance to traditional therapy and reluctance to acknowledge the behavioral impact of his gaming, MI was selected as the primary intervention framework. The initial sessions were introduced as career counseling, aligning with the adolescent's expressed interest in professional gaming. This approach facilitated rapport-building and helped avoid early resistance or confrontation (Verma, 2019).

Table 2 summarizes MI-based strategies outlined by Verma (2019) that counselors can use when working with adolescents exhibiting similar behavioral patterns.

Table 2. Applying MI in GD.

Therapeutic Target	MI Strategy or Technique
Initial Engagement	Frame sessions around the adolescent's own goals (e.g., becoming a professional gamer).
Resistance to Change	Avoid confrontation; explore ambivalence and reinforce autonomy through open dialogue.
Behavioral Framing	Approach excessive gaming as a behavioral addiction, similar to substance use interventions.
MI Core Principles (RULE)	- **R**esist the righting reflex - **U**nderstand motivation - **L**isten with empathy - **E**mpower the client

continued on following page

Table 2. Continued

Therapeutic Target	MI Strategy or Technique
MI Communication Tools (OARS)	- **O**pen-ended questions - **A**ffirmations - **R**eflective listening - **S**ummaries
Change Process Support	Facilitate movement through the stages of change (precontemplation, contemplation, preparation, action and maintenance), focusing on readiness and self-directed goals.

Cognitive Behavioral Therapy (CBT)

CBT is a well-established therapeutic approach that helps individuals recognize and restructure maladaptive beliefs, thoughts, emotions, and behaviors. According to Han et al. (2020), CBT significantly improved symptoms of GD, as well as associated issues such as anxiety, impulsivity, and social avoidance, when compared to problematic gamers who received supportive therapy. CBT enables individuals struggling with GD to better understand their behavioral patterns and reduce the risk of relapse (El-Sherbini & Abdou, 2020; Mestre-Bach et al., 2022). As noted by Tambunan et al. (2023), CBT aims to transform negative thinking patterns into more adaptive ones; in adolescents, this often involves challenging immature or distorted beliefs about the consequences of excessive gaming.

CBT is widely recognized as an effective treatment for various mental health conditions, including SUD, gambling disorder, and eating disorders, due to its foundation in the cognitive-behavioral model. This model posits that thoughts influence both emotions and behaviors; therefore, modifying maladaptive thought patterns can result in meaningful behavioral change (Young, 2007). In a neuroimaging study involving adolescent participants with GD, symptoms were shown to decrease following CBT interventions (Han et al., 2018).

CBT emphasizes the role of cognition in gaming use (Davis, 2001). CBT can be divided into three distinct stages (Ding & Li, 2023). Each stage addresses a specific aspect of the behavior, ranging from reducing excessive use to targeting underlying cognitive and functional challenges. Table 3 outlines these stages along with their corresponding therapeutic goals (Young, 2004; Young, 2011; Malinauskas & Malinauskiene, 2019; Ding & Li, 2023).

Table 3. Three-Stage CBT Approach for GD

Stage	Focus	Therapeutic Goals
1. Behavioral Modification	Gradual reduction of online/gaming hours; building healthy offline routines.	- Reduce time spent online - Introduce structured daily schedules
2. Cognitive Reconstruction & Rationalization	Identifying and challenging distorted thoughts or justifications for excessive use.	- Recognize excessive use and internal triggers - Correct maladaptive beliefs - Improve self-regulation
3. Functional Restoration & Relapse Prevention	Addressing underlying emotional, social, and academic problems linked to gaming.	- Maintain recovery - Prevent relapse

Other Counseling Techniques

When adolescents are dealing with underlying issues such as anxiety, depression, or stress that have not been addressed, they can be taught coping strategies through psychoeducation and mindfulness exercises to help them relax and alleviate the exacerbated symptoms (Mayo Clinic, 2022). Other counseling techniques include Solution-Focused Therapy (Kaptsis et al., 2016), and Person-Centered Therapy (Torres-Rodriguez et al., 2018).

Building on these counseling techniques, it is equally important to involve the family in the treatment process. Parental support plays a crucial role in helping adolescents manage and overcome GD as they can be essential to the support of the stages of change during the treatment (Verma, 2019). Therefore, the next section focuses on strategies for parents to effectively support their children with GD.

XV. PARENTAL STRATEGIES FOR GD SUPPORT

Parents need to receive education about GD, its signs and symptoms, and the potential risks and consequences (Kim & Chun, 2022). Adolescents need the support and encouragement from their parents more than extremes actions that can hazard the trust and communication between them (Kim & Chun, 2022).

The use of boundaries imposed by parents or guardians are suggested for video game use, such as limiting screen time, setting specific days and times for gaming, taking breaks, and doing other activities to rest (Young. 2009). Parents and caregivers need to agree to the expected rules and have a plan when those rules are not followed (Young. 2009). Counselors can support the parents and adolescents in finding alternative activities to gaming, such as sports, hobbies, or other social activities (Young. 2009).

Adolescents learn by observing the people around them, and parents and guardians exert considerable influence on adolescents (Raising Children Network, 2024). Therefore, it is important for parents to understand the concept of modeling and how their behavior can be observed and mirrored by their adolescents (Raising Children Network, 2024). Instead of spending excessive time in front of the screen, parents can encourage activities such as reading a book or engaging in exercise (Color Bliss, 2024).

The primary recommendation when discussing these issues, whether socially or within the community, is to always advise seeking professional help (Cleveland Clinic, 2022). Mental health professionals must be prepared to assist adolescents or refer them to professionals who can help identify GD and support adolescents in their recovery treatment (Griffiths & Meredith, 2009). As we are near the conclusion of this chapter, which discussed the importance of professional support, it is critical to consider strategies for the healthy use of video games. Achieving a balance between hobbies, activities, and responsibilities is essential for adolescents. The following section presents ways to promote healthy gaming practices.

XVI. PLAYING VIDEO GAMES IN A HEALTHY WAY

In the United States, approximately two out of every three students play video games as a form of distraction, recreation, or even as an organized competitive activity in schools. While gaming can serve as a hobby or social outlet, extended playtime has been associated with potential health consequences. A growing debate in the mental health field centers on whether adolescents should adopt an abstinence-based approach or follow a harm reduction model when addressing problematic gaming behaviors (Grinspoon, 2020).

One recognized benefit of gaming is its capacity to connect individuals virtually, fostering the development of online communities. This was particularly evident during the COVID-19 pandemic, when in-person interactions were restricted. During that time, video games played a significant role in facilitating global social connections across all age groups (Grinspoon, 2020).

A 2022 study published by the National Institutes of Health examined 2,000 children and reported that those who played video games for three or more hours per day demonstrated stronger cognitive skills, including impulse control and working memory, compared to children who had never played. However, in 2023, the same publication issued a retraction and replacement, clarifying that children who engaged in three or more hours of daily gaming showed significantly higher levels of attention problems, depressive symptoms, and ADHD-related behaviors than those who did not play video games (National Institutes of Health, 2023).

These mixed findings indicate that video games can pose both benefits and risks for adolescents. As a result, two main approaches have been proposed to manage gaming behaviors. The first is abstinence, which may be necessary when gaming leads to serious problems that negatively affect an adolescent's overall well-being, making complete cessation the most appropriate response (Evans et al., 2018). The second is harm reduction, which encourages adolescents to engage in gaming in a healthier manner without requiring them to stop completely (King et al., 2017b). The decision between these approaches depends on the severity of gaming's impact on the adolescent's life.

Abstinence

A study examined gaming abstinence in different areas such as withdrawal, affect, and distress in adolescent habitual gamers (Evans et al., 2018). Participants were adolescents identified as at-risk gamers, a term used to describe individuals whose gaming behaviors may lead to adverse outcomes, such as daily gaming, difficulty maintaining a balanced routine, and concerns from others about excessive play. The findings suggested that recommending breaks and fostering critical thinking about gaming may be a more effective means of promoting behavioral change than more authoritarian or punitive approaches (Schneider et al., 2017).

Additionally in the same study, some adolescents reported feelings of boredom during periods of abstinence due to the disruption of their regular gaming routines. However, many were able to redirect their time toward alternative activities, such as spending time with family or engaging in outdoor physical exercise (Shin et al., 2015).

Harm Reduction

Harm reduction has been linked to cognitive and behavioral approaches in adolescents with GD, as discussed earlier in this chapter. The therapeutic goal of this strategy is to support adolescents in managing their video game use through targeted interventions, rather than requiring them to quit gaming entirely (King et al., 2017b).

One way to assist adolescents with GD is by negotiating a personalized and adaptive gaming schedule. This strategy is particularly useful because maintaining designated gaming periods can prevent negative attitudes toward gaming restrictions, which might otherwise lead to resistance or increased desire to play as a form of rebellion.

Evans et al. (2018) recommend developing a schedule in which adolescents avoid gaming on certain days a strategy grounded in harm reduction principles. These breaks are intended not to eliminate gaming entirely, but to create space for self-reflection. By stepping away periodically, adolescents may better identify their motivations for playing and evaluate the potential costs and benefits of their gaming behavior.

While playing video games can be a fun and engaging activity, it is essential for adolescents to do so in a balanced and healthy manner. Several harm reduction strategies have been identified to support this goal and help adolescents maintain healthier gaming habits (Young, 2009; Educational Advancement, 2022). These strategies are outlined in Table 4.

Table 4. Harm Reduction Strategies

Strategy	Description
Setting Limits	Establishing clear boundaries on gaming time
Engaging in Other Activities	Encouraging participation in alternative activities, including physical exercise, new hobbies, promoting a more balanced lifestyle.
Taking Breaks	Taking short breaks approximately every 20 minutes while gaming.
Maintaining Balance	Ensuring that gaming does not interfere with school, relationships, or physical health.

CHAPTER SUMMARY

This chapter focused on GD and its impact on adolescents. It discussed the definition of GD as a condition where excessive gaming leads to significant negative consequences in various aspects of life, such as social relationships, school performance, and mental well-being. Adolescents are particularly vulnerable to GD due to factors like stress, family dynamics, and underlying mental health conditions, such as depression, anxiety, and ADHD. The chapter emphasized the importance of counselors understanding adolescents' gaming habits and experiences to provide effective support and treatment. It also highlights strategies for parents, such as setting gaming limits and encouraging alternative activities, to help prevent GD. By promoting healthy gaming practices, such as balancing gaming with other activities and ensuring breaks during play, adolescents can engage in gaming in a more balanced and healthy manner.

REFERENCES

Aarseth, E., Bean, A. M., Boonen, H., Colder Carras, M., Coulson, M., Das, D., Deleuze, J., Dunkels, E., Edman, J., Ferguson, C. J., Haagsma, M. C., Helmersson Bergmark, K., Hussain, Z., Jansz, J., Kardefelt-Winther, D., Kutner, L., Markey, P., Nielsen, R. K. L., Prause, N., & Van Rooij, A. J. (2017). Scholars' open debate paper on the World Health Organization ICD-11 Gaming Disorder proposal. *Journal of Behavioral Addictions*, *6*(3), 267–270. DOI: 10.1556/2006.5.2016.088 PMID: 28033714

American Psychiatric Association. (2013). *Diagnostic and statistical manual of mental disorders* (5th ed.). American Psychiatric Publishing.

American Psychiatric Association. (2023, January). Internet gaming. *James Sherer, M.D.*https://www.psychiatry.org/patients-families/internet-gaming

Anderson, R. (2017). Understanding video game mechanics as a tool in creating a sustainable relationship with digital media. In J. Christenson & A. Merritts (Eds.), *Family therapy with adolescents in residential treatment* (pp. 49□70). Springer, Cham. https://doi.org/DOI: 10.1007/978-3-319-51747-6_4

Bickham, D. S., Vandewater, E. A., Huston, A. C., Lee, J. H., Caplovitz, A. G., & Wright, J. C. (2003). Predictors of children's electronic media use: An examination of three ethnic groups. *Media Psychology*, *5*(2), 107–137. DOI: 10.1207/S1532785XMEP0502_1

Bliss, C. (2024, January 22). Beyond the screens: Discover engaging activities with screen time management tips. *Color Bliss*. https://colorbliss.com/blog/beyond-the-screens-discover-engaging-activities-with-screen-time-management-tips

Borges, G., Orozco, R., Benjet, C., Martínez, K., Contreras, E. V., Pérez, A., Cedrés, A., Uribe, P., Couder, M., Gutiérrez-García, R., Chávez, G., Albor, Y., Méndez, E., Medina-Mora, M. E., Mortier, P., & Ayuso-Mateos, J. (2021). (Internet) Gaming disorder in DSM-5 and ICD-11: A case of the glass half empty or half full. *Canadian Journal of Psychiatry*, *66*(5), 477–484. DOI: 10.1177/0706743720948431 PMID: 32806957

Brooke, S. (2021, November 16). What to make of the new regulations in China's gaming industry. *China Briefing*. https://www.china-briefing.com/news/what-to-make-of-the-new-regulations-in-china-online-gaming-industry/

Bussone, S., Trentini, C., Tambelli, R., & Carola, V. (2020). Early-life interpersonal and affective risk factors for pathological gaming. *Frontiers in Psychiatry*, *11*, 423. DOI: 10.3389/fpsyt.2020.00423 PMID: 32499728

Carson, N., Lê Cook, B., Chen, C. N., & Alegria, M. (2012). Racial/ethnic differences in video game and Internet use among US adolescents with mental health and educational difficulties. *Journal of Children and Media*, *6*(4), 450–468. DOI: 10.1080/17482798.2012.724592 PMID: 29167696

Cauce, A. M., & Domenech-Rodriguez, M. (2002). Latino families: Myths and realities. *Latino children and families in the United States: Current research and future directions*, 3-25.

Chang, Y. H., Chang, K. C., Hou, W. L., Lin, C. Y., & Griffiths, M. D. (2021). Internet gaming as a coping method among schizophrenic patients facing psychological distress. *Journal of Behavioral Addictions*, *9*(4), 1022–1031. DOI: 10.1556/2006.2020.00081 PMID: 33128519

Chen, Z., Ge, J., Gan, Q., Fu, Y., & Chen, Z. (2025). Protocol for a Randomized Controlled Trial to Enhance Executive Function via Brief Mindfulness Training in Individuals with Internet Gaming Disorder. *PLoS One*, *20*(4), e0320305. DOI: 10.1371/journal.pone.0320305 PMID: 40168432

China Legal Experts. (2024, July 9). China gaming laws. *China Legal Experts*. https://www.chinalegalexperts.com/news/china-gaming-laws

Cillero, I. H., & Jago, R. (2010). Systematic review of correlates of screen-viewing among young children. *Preventive Medicine*, *51*(1), 3–10. DOI: 10.1016/j.ypmed.2010.04.012 PMID: 20417227

Cleveland Clinic. (2022, May 27). Video game addiction. *Cleveland Clinic*. https://my.clevelandclinic.org/health/diseases/23124-video-game-addiction

Colwell, J., & Kato, M. (2003). Investigation of the relationship between social isolation, self-esteem, aggression and computer game play in Japanese adolescents. *Asian Journal of Social Psychology*, *6*(2), 149–158. DOI: 10.1111/1467-839X.t01-1-00017

Cooper, S., Robison, A. J., & Mazei-Robison, M. S. (2017). Reward circuitry in addiction. *Neurotherapeutics; the Journal of the American Society for Experimental NeuroTherapeutics*, *14*(3), 687–697. DOI: 10.1007/s13311-017-0525-z PMID: 28324454

Davis, R. A. (2001). A cognitive-behavioral model of pathological Internet use. *Computers in Human Behavior*, *17*(2), 187–195. DOI: 10.1016/S0747-5632(00)00041-8

Ding, K., & Li, H. (2023). Digital addiction intervention for children and adolescents: A scoping review. *International Journal of Environmental Research and Public Health*, *20*(6), 4777. DOI: 10.3390/ijerph20064777 PMID: 36981687

Dong, G., Zheng, H., Liu, X., Wang, Y., Du, X., & Potenza, M. N. (2018). Gender-related differences in cue-elicited cravings in Internet gaming disorder: The effects of deprivation. *Journal of Behavioral Addictions*, *7*(4), 953–964. DOI: 10.1556/2006.7.2018.118 PMID: 30556781

Educational Advancement. (2022, May 21). The good and the bad effects of video games on children. *Educational Advancement*. https://educationaladvancement.org/blog-the-good-and-the-bad-effects-of-video-games-on-children/#:~:text=Discourage%20children%20to%20do%20well,detrimental%20to%20your%20child's%20development

El-Sherbini, H. H., & Abdou, R. A. (2020). Effect of Cognitive Behavioral Therapy on Internet Gaming Disorder and Quality of Life Among Preparatory School Students in Alexandria. *Assiut Scientific Nursing Journal*, *8*(23), 22–38. DOI: 10.21608/asnj.2020.46217.1057

Evans, C., King, D. L., & Delfabbro, P. H. (2018). Effect of brief gaming abstinence on withdrawal in adolescent at-risk daily gamers: A randomized controlled study. *Computers in Human Behavior*, *88*, 70–77. DOI: 10.1016/j.chb.2018.06.024

Flack, D. (2020, May). Engaging avoidant teens. https://www.counseling.org/publications/counseling-today-magazine/article archive/article/legacy/engaging-avoidant-teens

Galbraith, N., Rose, C., & Rose, P. (2022). The roles of motivational interviewing and self-efficacy on outcomes and cost-effectiveness of a community-based exercise intervention for inactive middle-older aged adults. *Health & Social Care in the Community*, *30*(4), e1048–e1060. DOI: 10.1111/hsc.13510 PMID: 34260782

Gao, Y. X., Wang, J. Y., & Dong, G. H. (2022). The prevalence and possible risk factors of internet gaming disorder among adolescents and young adults: Systematic reviews and meta-analyses. *Journal of Psychiatric Research*, *154*, 35–43. DOI: 10.1016/j.jpsychires.2022.06.049 PMID: 35926424

Giardina, A., Di Blasi, M., Schimmenti, A., King, D. L., Starcevic, V., & Billieux, J. (2021). Online gaming and prolonged self-isolation: Evidence from Italian gamers during the COVID-19 outbreak. *Clinical Neuropsychiatry*, *18*(1), 65. PMID: 34909021

Goethe, O. (2019). Visual aesthetics in games and gamification. In *Gamification Mindset* (pp. 85–92). Springer., DOI: 10.1007/978-3-030-11078-9_8

Gómez-Gonzalvo, F., Devís-Devís, J., & Molina-Alventosa, P. (2020). Video game usage time in adolescents' academic performance. *Comunicar: Media Education Research Journal*, *28*(65), 87–96. DOI: 10.3916/C65-2020-08

González-Bueso, V., Santamaría, J. J., Fernández, D., Merino, L., Montero, E., & Ribas, J. (2018). Association between internet gaming disorder or pathological video-game use and comorbid psychopathology: A comprehensive review. *International Journal of Environmental Research and Public Health, 15*(4), 668. DOI: 10.3390/ijerph15040668 PMID: 29614059

Gordon-Larsen, P., McMurray, R. G., & Popkin, B. M. (2000). Determinants of adolescent physical activity and inactivity patterns. *Pediatrics, 105*(6), e83–e83. DOI: 10.1542/peds.105.6.e83 PMID: 10835096

Gottfried, J., & Sidoti, O. (2024, May 9). Adolescentss and video games today. *Pew Research Center*. https://www.pewresearch.org/internet/2024/05/09/adolescentss -and-video- gamestoday/#fnref-165467-1

Griffiths, M. D. (2018). The therapeutic and health benefits of playing video games.

Griffiths, M. D., & Meredith, A. (2009). Videogame addiction and its treatment. *Journal of Contemporary Psychotherapy, 39*(4), 247–253. DOI: 10.1007/s10879-009-9118-4

Grinspoon, P. (2020, December 22). *The health effects of too much gaming*. Harvard Health. https://www.health.harvard.edu/blog/the-health-effects-of-too-much -gaming-2020122221645

Han, D. H., Bolo, N., Daniels, M. A., Arenella, L., Lyoo, I. K., & Renshaw, P. F. (2011). Brain activity and desire for Internet video game play. *Comprehensive Psychiatry, 52*(1), 88–95. DOI: 10.1016/j.comppsych.2010.04.004 PMID: 21220070

Han, H., Jeong, H., Jo, S. J., Son, H. J., & Yim, H. W. (2020). Relationship between the experience of online game genre and high risk of Internet gaming disorder in Korean adolescents. *Epidemiology and Health, 42*, e2020016. Advance online publication. DOI: 10.4178/epih.e2020016 PMID: 32272007

Han, J., Seo, Y., Hwang, H., Kim, S. M., & Han, D. H. (2020). Efficacy of cognitive behavioral therapy for internet gaming disorder. *Clinical Psychology & Psychotherapy, 27*(2), 203–213. DOI: 10.1002/cpp.2419 PMID: 31881100

Han, T. S., Cho, H., Sung, D., & Park, M. H. (2022). A systematic review of the impact of COVID-19 on the game addiction of children and adolescents. *Frontiers in Psychiatry, 13*, 976601. DOI: 10.3389/fpsyt.2022.976601 PMID: 36061296

Han, X., Wang, Y., Jiang, W., Bao, X., Sun, Y., Ding, W., Cao, M., Wu, X., Du, Y., & Zhou, Y. (2018). Resting-state activity of prefrontal-striatal circuits in internet gaming disorder: Changes with cognitive behavior therapy and predictors of treatment response. *Frontiers in Psychiatry*, *9*, 341. DOI: 10.3389/fpsyt.2018.00341 PMID: 30123144

Hawi, N. S., Samaha, M., & Griffiths, M. D. (2018). Internet gaming disorder in Lebanon: Relationships with age, sleep habits, and academic achievement. *Journal of Behavioral Addictions*, *7*(1), 70–78. DOI: 10.1556/2006.7.2018.16 PMID: 29486571

Hill, J. P., & Lynch, M. E. (1983). The intensification of gender-related role expectations during early adolescence. In *Girls at Puberty: Biological and Psychosocial Perspectives* (pp. 201-228). Springer US. DOI: 10.1007/978-1-4899-0354-9_10

Horigian, V. E., Anderson, A. R., & Szapocznik, J. (2016). Family-based treatments for adolescent substance use. *Child and Adolescent Psychiatric Clinics of North America*, *25*(4), 603–628. DOI: 10.1016/j.chc.2016.06.001 PMID: 27613341

Hunicke, R., LeBlanc, M., & Zubek, R. (2004, July). MDA: A formal approach to game design and game research. In *Proceedings of the AAAI Workshop on Challenges in Game AI* (Vol. 4, No. 1, p. 1722).

Ivanova, V. (2020). Carpal tunnel syndrome symptoms in esports players. *Journal of Clinical Rehabilitation*, *34*(3), 115–123.

Jeong, E. J., & Kim, D. H. (2011). Social activities, self-efficacy, game attitudes, and game addiction. *Cyberpsychology, Behavior, and Social Networking*, *14*(4), 213–221. DOI: 10.1089/cyber.2009.0289 PMID: 21067285

Jiang, C., Li, C., Zhou, H., & Zhou, Z. (2020). Individuals with internet gaming disorder have similar neurocognitive impairments and social cognitive dysfunctions as methamphetamine-dependent patients. Adicciones, 1342(10.20882).

Johnson, D., Dupuis, G., Piche, J., Clayborne, Z., & Colman, I. (2018). Adult mental health outcomes of adolescent depression: A systematic review. *Depression and Anxiety*, *35*(8), 700–716. DOI: 10.1002/da.22777 PMID: 29878410

Johnson, K. (2023, February 13). Kids and video games: The good and the bad. *Akron Children's Hospital*. https://www.akronchildrens.org/inside/2023/02/13/kids-and-video-games-the-good-and-the-bad/#:~:text=Studies%20show%20playing%20video%20games,been%20linked%20with%20developing%20obesity

Kaptsis, D., King, D. L., Delfabbro, P. H., & Gradisar, M. (2016). Withdrawal symptoms in internet gaming disorder: A systematic review. *Clinical Psychology Review*, *43*, 58–66. DOI: 10.1016/j.cpr.2015.11.006 PMID: 26704173

Khang, H., Kim, J. K., & Kim, Y. (2013). Self-traits and motivations as antecedents of digital media flow and addiction: The Internet, mobile phones, and video games. *Computers in Human Behavior*, *29*(6), 2416–2424. DOI: 10.1016/j.chb.2013.05.027

Kim, S., & Chun, J. (2022). The impact of parental and peer attachment on gaming addiction among out-of-school adolescents in South Korea: The mediating role of social stigma. *International Journal of Environmental Research and Public Health*, *20*(1), 72. DOI: 10.3390/ijerph20010072 PMID: 36612398

Kim, S. M., Han, D. H., Lee, Y. S., & Renshaw, P. F. (2012). Combined cognitive behavioral therapy and bupropion for the treatment of problematic online game play in adolescents with major depressive disorder. *Computers in Human Behavior*, *28*(5), 1954–1959. DOI: 10.1016/j.chb.2012.05.015

King, D. L., Chamberlain, S. R., Carragher, N., Billieux, J., Stein, D., Mueller, K., Potenza, M. N., Rumpf, H. J., Saunders, J., Starcevic, V., Demetrovics, Z., Brand, M., Lee, H. K., Spada, M., Lindenberg, K., Wu, A. M. S., Lemenager, T., Pallesen, S., Achab, S., & Delfabbro, P. H. (2020). Screening and assessment tools for gaming disorder: A comprehensive systematic review. *Clinical Psychology Review*, *77*, 101831. DOI: 10.1016/j.cpr.2020.101831 PMID: 32143109

King, D. L., Delfabbro, P. H., Doh, Y. Y., Wu, A. M., Kuss, D. J., Pallesen, S., Mentzoni, R., Carragher, N., & Sakuma, H. (2018). Policy and prevention approaches for disordered and hazardous gaming and Internet use: An international perspective. *Prevention Science*, *19*(2), 233–249. DOI: 10.1007/s11121-017-0813-1 PMID: 28677089

King, D. L., Haagsma, M. C., Delfabbro, P. H., Gradisar, M., & Griffiths, M. D. (2013). Toward a consensus definition of pathological video-gaming: A systematic review of psychometric assessment tools. *Clinical Psychology Review*, *33*(3), 331–342. DOI: 10.1016/j.cpr.2013.01.002 PMID: 23396015

Ko, C. H., Kiraly, O., Demetrovics, Z., Chang, Y. M., & Yen, J. Y. (2020). Identifying individuals in need of help for their uncontrolled gaming: A narrative review of concerns and comments regarding gaming disorder diagnostic criteria. *Journal of Behavioral Addictions*, *9*(3), 572–588. DOI: 10.1556/2006.2020.00058 PMID: 33011711

Ko, C. H., Liu, G. C., Hsiao, S., Yen, J. Y., Yang, M. J., Lin, W. C., Yen, C.-F., & Chen, C. S. (2009). Brain activities associated with gaming urge of online gaming addiction. *Journal of Psychiatric Research*, *43*(7), 739–747. DOI: 10.1016/j.jpsychires.2008.09.012 PMID: 18996542

Koepp, M. J., Gunn, R. N., Lawrence, A. D., Cunningham, V. J., Dagher, A., Jones, T., Brooks, D. J., Bench, C. J., & Grasby, P. M. (1998). Evidence for striatal dopamine release during a video game. *Nature*, *393*(6682), 266–268. DOI: 10.1038/30498 PMID: 9607763

Krahé, B., & Möller, I. (2004). Playing violent electronic games, hostile attributional style, and aggression-related norms in German adolescents. *Journal of Adolescence*, *27*(1), 53–69. DOI: 10.1016/j.adolescence.2003.10.006 PMID: 15013260

Kuss, D. J., & Griffiths, M. D. (2012). Online gaming addiction in children and adolescents: A review of empirical research. *Journal of Behavioral Addictions*, *1*(1), 3–22. DOI: 10.1556/JBA.1.2012.1.1 PMID: 26166826

Laier, C., Wegmann, E., & Brand, M. (2018). Personality and cognition in gamers: Avoidance expectancies mediate the relationship between maladaptive personality traits and symptoms of Internet-gaming disorder. *Frontiers in Psychiatry*, *9*, 304. DOI: 10.3389/fpsyt.2018.00304 PMID: 30042702

Lee, D., Lee, J., Lee, J. E., & Jung, Y. C. (2017). Altered functional connectivity in the default mode network in Internet gaming disorder: Influence of childhood ADHD. *Progress in Neuro-Psychopharmacology & Biological Psychiatry*, *75*, 135–141. DOI: 10.1016/j.pnpbp.2017.02.005 PMID: 28174127

Lemmens, J. S., Valkenburg, P. M., & Peter, J. (2009). Development and validation of a game addiction scale for adolescents. *Media Psychology*, *12*(1), 77–95. DOI: 10.1080/15213260802669458

Leonhardt, M., & Overå, S. (2021). Are there differences in video gaming and use of social media among boys and girls?—A mixed methods approach. *International Journal of Environmental Research and Public Health*, *18*(11), 6085. DOI: 10.3390/ijerph18116085 PMID: 34200039

Lindenberg, K., Kindt, S., & Szász-Janocha, C. (2022). Effectiveness of cognitive behavioral therapy–based intervention in preventing gaming disorder and unspecified internet use disorder in adolescents: A cluster randomized clinical trial. *JAMA Network Open*, *5*(2), e2148995–e2148995. DOI: 10.1001/jamanetworkopen.2021.48995 PMID: 35179587

Lischer, S., Jeannot, E., Brülisauer, L., Weber, N., Khazaal, Y., Bendahan, S., & Simon, O. (2022). Response to the regulation of video games under the Youth Media Protection Act: A public health perspective. *International Journal of Environmental Research and Public Health*, *19*(15), 9320. DOI: 10.3390/ijerph19159320 PMID: 35954678

Long, J., Bhad, R., Potenza, M. N., Orsolini, L., Phan, V., Kanabar, M., & Achab, S. (2022). Public health approaches and policy changes after the inclusion of gaming disorder in ICD-11: Global needs. *BJPsych International*, *19*(3), 63–66. DOI: 10.1192/bji.2021.57 PMID: 36287819

Lozano-Blasco, R., Latorre-Martínez, M. P., & Cortes-Pascual, A. (2021). Analyzing adolescents: An analysis from the perspective of gamers on YouTube. *Sustainability (Basel)*, *13*(20), 11391. DOI: 10.3390/su132011391

Mayo Foundation for Medical Education and Research. (2023, April 11). *Psychotherapy*. Mayo Clinic. https://www.mayoclinic.org/tests-procedures/psychotherapy/about/pac-20384616

McDaniel, C. C., Kavookjian, J., & Whitley, H. P. (2022). Telehealth delivery of motivational interviewing for diabetes management: A systematic review of randomized controlled trials. *Patient Education and Counseling*, *105*(4), 805–820. DOI: 10.1016/j.pec.2021.07.036 PMID: 34366228

Mestre-Bach, G., Fernandez-Aranda, F., & Jiménez-Murcia, S. (2022). Exploring Internet gaming disorder: An updated perspective of empirical evidence (from 2016 to 2021). *Comprehensive Psychiatry*, *116*, 152319. DOI: 10.1016/j.comppsych.2022.152319 PMID: 35526417

Miller, W. R., & Rollnick, S. (2012). *Motivational interviewing: Helping people change*. Guilford Press.

Moriarity, D. P., McArthur, B. A., Ellman, L. M., Coe, C. L., Abramson, L. Y., & Alloy, L. B. (2018). Immunocognitive model of depression secondary to anxiety in adolescents. *Journal of Youth and Adolescence*, *47*(12), 2625–2636. DOI: 10.1007/s10964-018-0905-7 PMID: 30088131

My People Patterns. (2023, February 1). *Building rapport with teens so they talk in therapy*. Building Rapport With Teens So They Talk In Therapy. https://www.mypeoplepatterns.com/blog/rapport

Nagata, J. M., Ganson, K. T., Iyer, P., Chu, J., Baker, F. C., Gabriel, K. P., & Bibbins-Domingo, K. (2022). Sociodemographic correlates of contemporary screen time use among 9- and 10-year-old children. *The Journal of Pediatrics*, *240*, 213–220. DOI: 10.1016/j.jpeds.2021.08.077 PMID: 34481807

National Institutes of Health. (2022). *Video gaming may be associated with better cognitive performance in children*. National Institutes of Health.

New York Times. (2022, February 8). Parents and adolescentss: Finding balance when it comes to screen time. https://www.nytimes.com/guides/well/family/screen-time

Nguyen, H. V., Huang, H. C., Wong, M. K., Yang, Y. H., Huang, T. L., & Teng, C. I. (2018). Moderator roles of optimism and weight control on the impact of playing exergames on happiness: The perspective of social cognitive theory using a randomized controlled trial. *Games for Health Journal, 7*(4), 246–252. DOI: 10.1089/g4h.2017.0165 PMID: 29708775

Park, S. K., Kim, J. Y., & Cho, C. B. (2008). Prevalence of Internet addiction and correlations with family factors among South Korean adolescents. *Adolescence, 43*(172). PMID: 19149152

Poll, M. (2020, January 20). Game on: Adolescentss and video games (Vol. 35, Issue 4). Mott Poll. https://mottpoll.org/reports/game-adolescentss-and-video-games

Pontes, H. M., & Griffiths, M. D. (2015). Measuring DSM-5 internet gaming disorder: Development and validation of a short psychometric scale. *Computers in Human Behavior, 45*, 137–143. DOI: 10.1016/j.chb.2014.12.006

Pontes, H. M., & Griffiths, M. D. (2019). A new era for gaming disorder research: Time to shift from consensus to consistency. *Addictive Behaviors*. PMID: 31473045

Priyono, D., & Fradianto, I. (2022). Coping strategies in adolescents with online games addiction. *International Journal of Progressive Sciences and Technologies, 34*(1), 20. DOI: 10.52155/ijpsat.v34.1.4534

Raising Children Network. (2024, February 8). Parents as role models for pre-adolescents and adolescents. Raising Children Network.

Raymer, D. L., Jr. (2021, September). Internet gaming disorder: A real mental health issue on the rise in adolescents and young adults. *Counseling Today*. https://www.counseling.org/publications/counseling-today-magazine/article-archive/article/legacy/internet-gaming-disorder--a-real-mental-health-issue-on-the-rise-in-adolescents-and-young-adults#:~:text=It%20is%20important%20to%20establish,time%20spent%20playing%20video%20games

Rehbein, F., Mößle, T., Rumpf, H. J., Bischof, G., & Bischof, A. (2015). Lebenszeit-und 12-Monatsprävalenz der Internet Gaming Disorder in der deutschen Erwachsenenbevölkerung: Wie sich das Spielverhalten Betroffener von unauffälligen Spielern unterscheidet. *Suchttherapie, 16*(S 01), S_07_02.

Scerri, M., Anderson, A., Stavropoulos, V., & Hu, E. (2019). Need fulfilment and internet gaming disorder: A preliminary integrative model. *Addictive Behaviors Reports, 9*, 100144. DOI: 10.1016/j.abrep.2018.100144 PMID: 31193898

Schneider, L. A., King, D. L., & Delfabbro, P. H. (2017). Family factors in adolescent problematic Internet gaming: A systematic review. *Journal of Behavioral Addictions*, *6*(3), 321–333. DOI: 10.1556/2006.6.2017.035 PMID: 28762279

Sharma, M. K., Bhargav, H., Kumar, A., Digambhar, V., & Mani, T. A. (2021). Mindfulness-based interventions: Potentials for management of internet gaming disorder. *International Journal of Yoga*, *14*(3), 244–247. DOI: 10.4103/ijoy.ijoy_46_21 PMID: 35017867

Shaw, P., Eckstrand, K., Sharp, W., Blumenthal, J., Lerch, J. P., Greenstein, D. E. E. A., Clasen, L., Evans, A., Giedd, J., & Rapoport, J. L. (2007). Attention-deficit/hyperactivity disorder is characterized by a delay in cortical maturation. *Proceedings of the National Academy of Sciences of the United States of America*, *104*(49), 19649–19654. DOI: 10.1073/pnas.0707741104 PMID: 18024590

Shaw, P., Malek, M., Watson, B., Sharp, W., Evans, A., & Greenstein, D. (2012). Development of cortical surface area and gyrification in attention-deficit/hyperactivity disorder. *Biological Psychiatry*, *72*(3), 191–197. DOI: 10.1016/j.biopsych.2012.01.031 PMID: 22418014

Shin, S. M., Ryu, S. J., Kim, B. J., Lee, D., & Chung, Y. (2015). The development and effectiveness of MI group counseling program for adolescents internet-addiction. *Sangdamhag Yeon'gu*, *16*(4), 89–109. DOI: 10.15703/kjc.16.4.201508.89

Staff, N. A. (2024, June 19). Teens & Video Games: New Research on Teenage Video Game Addiction. https://www.newportacademy.com/resources/treatment/teenage-video-game- addiction/

Tambunan, H. R., Kumboyono, K., & Lestari, R. (2023). Cognitive Behaviour Therapy (CBT) lowers online game addiction rates in adolescents. *Jurnal Aisyah: Jurnal Ilmu Kesehatan*, *8*(S1), 361–368. DOI: 10.30604/jika.v8iS1.1665

Teng, Z., Pontes, H. M., Nie, Q., Griffiths, M. D., & Guo, C. (2021). Depression and anxiety symptoms associated with internet gaming disorder before and during the COVID-19 pandemic: A longitudinal study. *Journal of Behavioral Addictions*, *10*(1), 169–180. DOI: 10.1556/2006.2021.00016 PMID: 33704085

Torres-Rodríguez, A., Griffiths, M. D., Carbonell, X., & Oberst, U. (2018). Internet gaming disorder in adolescence: Psychological characteristics of a clinical sample. *Journal of Behavioral Addictions*, *7*(3), 707–718. DOI: 10.1556/2006.7.2018.75 PMID: 30264606

Turel, O., & Bechara, A. (2019). Little video-gaming in adolescents can be protective, but too much is associated with increased substance use. *Substance Use & Misuse*, *54*(3), 384–395. DOI: 10.1080/10826084.2018.1496455 PMID: 30654698

Vadlin, S., Åslund, C., Hellström, C., & Nilsson, K. W. (2016). Associations between problematic gaming and psychiatric symptoms among adolescents in two samples. *Addictive Behaviors*, *61*, 8–15. DOI: 10.1016/j.addbeh.2016.05.001 PMID: 27203825

Van Brunt, B. (2014). *Treating video game addiction: Three brief sessions*. American Counseling Association.

van der Schyff, E. L., Forsyth, R., Amon, K. L., Ridout, B., & Campbell, A. J. (2023). Increasing access to mental health services: Videogame players' perspectives. *International Journal of Environmental Research and Public Health*, *20*(6), 4772. DOI: 10.3390/ijerph20064772 PMID: 36981681

Van Rooij, A. J., Ferguson, C. J., Colder Carras, M., Kardefelt-Winther, D., Shi, J., Aarseth, E., Bean, A. M., Bergmark, K. H., Brus, A., Coulson, M., Deleuze, J., Dullur, P., Dunkels, E., Edman, J., Elson, M., Etchells, P. J., Fiskaali, A., Granic, I., Jansz, J., & Przybylski, A. K. (2018). A weak scientific basis for gaming disorder: Let us err on the side of caution. *Journal of Behavioral Addictions*, *7*(1), 1–9. DOI: 10.1556/2006.7.2018.19 PMID: 29529886

Verma, T.el. (2019). Managing online video gaming-related addictive behaviors through motivational interviewing. *Indian Journal of Social Psychiatry*, *35*(3), 217–219. DOI: 10.4103/ijsp.ijsp_113_18

Von der Heiden, J. M., Braun, B., Müller, K. W., & Egloff, B. (2019). The association between video gaming and psychological functioning. *Frontiers in Psychology*, *10*, 1731. DOI: 10.3389/fpsyg.2019.01731 PMID: 31402891

Watkins, M. (Ed.). (2024, November 29). Video game addiction symptoms and treatment. American Addiction Centers. https://americanaddictioncenters.org/behavioral-addictions/video-gaming-addiction

Wendt, L. M., Austermann, M. I., Rumpf, H. J., Thomasius, R., & Paschke, K. (2021). Requirements of a group intervention for adolescents with internet gaming disorder in a clinical setting: A qualitative interview study. *International Journal of Environmental Research and Public Health*, *18*(15), 7813. DOI: 10.3390/ijerph18157813 PMID: 34360106

Wijman, T. (2021, December 22). *The games market and beyond in 2021: The Year in numbers | newzoo*. The Games Market and Beyond in 2021: The Year in Numbers. https://newzoo.com/resources/blog/the-games-market-in-2021-the-year-in-numbers- esports-cloud-gaming

World Health Organization. (2020, October 22). Addictive behaviours: Gaming disorder. https://www.who.int/news-room/questions-and-answers/item/addictive-behaviours-gaming-disorder

Xiao, L. Y. (2021). People's Republic of China legal update: The notice on further strictly regulating and effectively preventing online video gaming addiction in minors (published August 30, 2021, effective september 1, 2021). *Gaming Law Review*, *25*(9), 379–382. DOI: 10.1089/glr2.2021.0026

Yau, Y. H., Crowley, M. J., Mayes, L. C., & Potenza, M. N. (2012). Are Internet use and video- game-playing addictive behaviors? Biological, clinical and public health implications for youths and adults. *Minerva Psichiatrica*, *53*(3), 153. PMID: 24288435

Yen, J.-Y., Lin, P.-C., Wu, H.-C., & Ko, C.-H. (2022). The withdrawal-related affective, gaming urge, and anhedonia symptoms of internet gaming disorder during abstinence. *Journal of Behavioral Addictions*. Advance online publication. DOI: 10.1556/2006.2022.00008 PMID: 35338772

Yen, J. Y., Yeh, Y. C., Wang, P. W., Liu, T. L., Chen, Y. Y., & Ko, C. H. (2018). Emotional regulation in young adults with internet gaming disorder. *International Journal of Environmental Research and Public Health*, *15*(1), 30. DOI: 10.3390/ijerph15010030 PMID: 29295597

Young, K. (2009). Understanding online gaming addiction and treatment issues for adolescents. *The American Journal of Family Therapy*, *37*(5), 355–372. DOI: 10.1080/01926180902942191

Young, K. S. (2004). Internet addiction: A new clinical phenomenon and its consequences. *The American Behavioral Scientist*, *48*(4), 402–415. DOI: 10.1177/0002764204270278

Young, K. S. (2007). Cognitive behavior therapy with Internet addicts: Treatment outcomes and implications. *Cyberpsychology & Behavior*, *10*(5), 671–679. DOI: 10.1089/cpb.2007.9971 PMID: 17927535

Young, K. S. (2010). When gaming becomes an obsession: Help for parents and their children to treat online gaming addiction. *Retrieved October, 17*, 2013.

Chapter 5 Intra–Interpersonal Consequences of Pornographic Addiction in Youth

Ayush Dwivedi
https://orcid.org/0009-0001-2103-7342
Graphic Era University, Dehradun, India

Ravindra Singh
https://orcid.org/0000-0003-3062-1812
Magadh University, Bodh Gaya, India

Aditya Ratna Tripathi
https://orcid.org/0009-0001-7011-7242
Graphic Era University, Dehradun, India

ABSTRACT

Addiction is not having control over doing something to the extent that it is harmful to an individual. Recent studies show pornographic addiction can also lead to such compulsivity in behavior. The technological advancements and long quarantine period of the COVID-19 pandemic have caused a significant increase in the user base of pornographic materials. It is estimated that about 74% of men and 41% of women watch porn. The purpose of this study is to examine the consequences of pornographic addiction on the life of an individual. This is a systematic review paper and it is based on data collected from Research Papers Existing literature on pornographic addictions shows that it can lead to impairments in the psychological well-being (Feelings of loneliness, frustration, guilt,t, etc.) of an individual. Additionally, it can

DOI: 10.4018/979-8-3373-0518-9.ch005

lead to depression, stress disorders, mood disorders, etc. Pornographic addiction also hampers one's ability to sustain good social relationships. Moreover, it was also reported by previous studies that pornography hurts the sexual life of an individual.

1. INTRODUCTION

The concern about intra- and interpersonal consequences of Pornographic addiction among youth and adolescents has become a growing concern in contemporary society. This book chapter attempts to explore the psychological, emotional, and social ramifications of excessive pornography consumption. Additionally, it is also keen to understand how pornography affects the various cognitive phenomena (e.g., self-perception, emotional regulation, cognitive functioning, and relationship dynamics). High Pornography content consumption has been normalized in the modern digital era. The excessive engagement with Pornography material can lead to detrimental consequences, particularly among impressionable youth. The accessibility, accessibility, affordability, and anonymity of online pornography content force compulsive consumption patterns and foster a cycle of addiction.

Addiction is not having control over doing something to an extent that it is harmful to an individual. Addiction can be substance-related (drugs and alcohol) and also to primary needs like food and sex. The DSM-5-TR heavily associates addiction with substance abuse with non-substance-based addictions being limited to gambling addiction. However, pornography addiction is a recent diagnostic label that helps define patients with a propensity and tendency to frequently view pornography. Alongside, these patients show signs of distress when not allowed access to pornographic images and videos (Ley et al., 2014). Products that are used commercially to encourage or induce sexual pleasure and are fictitious in nature are termed *pornography* (Kumbhare, 2022). Pornography has mainly two kinds, hard- core porn and soft- core porn (George et al., 2019). Modern technological developments are the key reason for the widespread availability of pornography among the young generation. As, current digitalization process has made the internet so effortless, it has inflated the exposure of pornographic content all around the world (Astuti & Winarti, 2022). Considering the appearance of pornography on the internet, its affordability, anonymity, and accessibility (AAA) have attracted millions of users (Kühn & Gallinat, 2014). Although it is difficult to measure the rate of consumption of pornography. A study by Rich (2001) has evaluated that a capital of 10 to 14 billion dollars is generated from pornography. Which is mostly from pay-per-view movies on satellites and cable, in room hotel movies, internet websites, porn networks, sex toys and magazines, phone sex etc. (Rich, 2001). It was estimated that nowadays pornography has become a bigger business than professional baseball, football, and basketball combined (Rich, 2001). Also, it was pointed out that people are paying more for pornography in America than they do for buying movie tickets and watching performing arts put together (Rich, 2001).

Furthermore, pornography these days tends to be more powerful and immediate because of its more interactive and consumer-driven nature (for e.g. individuals can easily select what and who they want to see, also can interact with them via video camera) (Keilty, 2018). Thus, a major proportion of the population, especially adults, have reported exposure to various explicit sexual material (Paolucci et al., 1997).

Burtăverde et al. (2021) have done empirical research, which states that men usually engage in more pornographic content than women. They have suggested four factors that lead to watching pornography in both genders. First factor is increased sex drive which comprises feeling of pleasure while watching porn. The second factor is enhancing sexual performance, which includes learning about sex and exploring their own sexuality. The third factor is social and instrumental reasons, which comprise non-sexual reasons like peer pressure. The fourth factor is a lack of relational and emotional skills, which includes feelings of loneliness and mood regulation (for instance, getting rid of stressful thoughts due to a lack of any romantic relationship). Furthermore, children and adolescents are the most vulnerable viewers to pornographic material. As (1) they have limited physiological, emotional, and cognitive abilities to process the obscene material encountered involuntarily and voluntarily. (2) They usually develop unrealistic expectations due to fantasy-based videos on their future sexual relationships. (3) They can be easily persuaded to consume pornography or convinced into the production of it. (4) Can easily be addicted to it, same like adults. Furthermore, fake and traumatic messages spread about sexuality and relationships can negatively impact their social and sexual development (Manning, 2006).

Although pornography is the source of entertainment for most people but for some it can result in seeking treatment for out-of-control behavior (Gola et al., 2016). The prolonged exposure to pornographic content has caused negative consequences on the development of individuals (Astuti & Winarti, 2022). Pornographic material (especially via the internet) is often consumed privately by a household member. Nevertheless, its effects are observed in entire family systems and then in communities. Marital relationship specifically is dealing with its consequences as it is the foundational familial and social unit (Attwood, 2004). People depend on pornography in order to stimulate their sexual excitement (Love et al., 2015). The individuals who are actively consuming pornography on a daily basis give increased importance to sexual relations without emotional involvement. It was also commonly found with pornography users that they started objectification of their partner rather than continuing a meaningful interaction (Attwood, 2004).

The consequences of pornographic addiction are a matter of debate that is going on for a long time. Many people who are addicted to pornography material have more behavioral problems. They display a greater number of depressive symptoms, less emotional bonding, and a lower level of social integration (Mc-Bride, 2019). Additionally, such individuals also feel loneliness, anxiety, and self-blame, and seek mental health support. (George et al., 2019). Furthermore, pornography has a destructive effect on the public health of our society. Overconsumption of pornography material can cause sexual aggression which is usually from males to females (Foubert, 2017). Thus, pornographic content available must be monitored, filtered, and some should be banned. This included showing sadomasochism, bestiality, aggression, etc. (Chawla & Kar, 2021).

1.1 Key consequences of pornography:

1.2 Psychological Distress

Prior research highlights a significant gender-based disparity in the impact of pornographic addiction. Studies report that males are more likely to develop compulsive consumption patterns. On the flip side, females tend to experience more severe emotional distress and a moderate level of compulsiveness due to pornography use (Setyawati et al., 2020). Additionally, female adolescents who consume pornography frequently report higher levels of body dissatisfaction and distorted self-image (Mattebo et al., 2013.). Studies indicate a correlation between excessive pornography consumption and increased anxiety, depression, and low self-esteem in adolescents struggling with pornographic addiction. It may involve cognitive dissonance, social isolation, and feelings of guilt (Grubbs & Kraus, 2015). Excessive pornography use has been linked to symptoms of low self-worth. Adolescents often develop unrealistic sexual expectations, leading to dissatisfaction with real-life experiences (Laier et al., 2013).

1.3 Emotional Dysregulation

Excessive pornography consumption can be associated with heightened emotional instability (George et al., 2019). Pornographic addiction has been linked to emotional instability, mood swings, and increased impulsivity. This dysregulation can contribute to emotional distress and decreased overall life satisfaction (Privara & Bob, 2023). Pornographic addiction is linked to emotional instability, including heightened anxiety, depression, and stress (George et al., 2019). Research indicates that frequent exposure to pornography may lead to maladaptive coping mechanisms, reducing the ability to manage negative emotions effectively (Bancroft et al., 2003).

1.4 Cognitive Changes

The systematic exposure to pornographic material is linked to impaired cognitive functions contributing to compulsive behavior and difficulty in managing stress and emotion. A study also indicate that pornography can alter perceptions of normal sexual relationships and objectify sexual partners (Lim et al., 2016). Neurological studies on pornography indicate that compulsive pornography use alters brain reward pathways. It reduces impulse control and increases dependence. Research suggests that prolonged exposure to explicit material affects the brain's reward system, leading to an increased threshold for pleasure and emotional desensitization. The reward system of the human brain experiences changes due to constant dopamine surges in several regions, contributing to a dependency tendency (Di Chiara et al., 2004). On the other hand, the absence of such a stimulus leads to withdrawal symptoms when access to pornography is restricted (Gustirini & Putri., 2019). Further, it decreases motivation for real-world achievements due to reliance on instant gratification. Adolescents develop unrealistic self-expectations regarding body image and sexual performance, leading to dissatisfaction and self-doubt. Adolescents struggling with pornography addiction often experience body image issues and diminished self-confidence. Feelings of shame and guilt contribute to secrecy and further psychological distress (Setyawati et al., 2020).

1.5 Neurological Implications

Neuroscientific studies highlight that excessive pornography consumption affects the brain's reward system, particularly the dopaminergic pathways (Di Chiara et al., 2004). This leads to increased impulsivity, diminished executive control, and a heightened need for novel stimuli, reinforcing addictive behavior (De Sousa & Lodha, 2017). Research suggests that prolonged pornography consumption alters brain structures associated with addiction, including the prefrontal cortex, which is responsible for impulse control, and the reward pathway (Di Chiara et al., 2004). These neurological changes mimic those found in substance abuse disorders, reinforcing compulsive behaviors and reducing an individual's ability to regulate consumption. Research in neuropsychology suggests that compulsive pornography use alters neural pathways, particularly in the prefrontal cortex and reward system. Overstimulation of dopamine receptors due to repeated exposure can lead to addictive behaviors similar to substance dependence (Di Chiara et al., 2004).

1.6 Distorted Sexual Expectations and Objectification

Exposure to unrealistic portrayals of sexuality contributes to distorted perceptions of consent, gender roles, and relationship dynamics, influencing risky sexual behaviors (Love et al., 2015). Pornography often portrays exaggerated and unrealistic sexual encounters, which can distort a young individual's expectations of real-life intimacy. This misrepresentation may contribute to issues such as reduced empathy toward partners, objectification of individuals, and unrealistic performance anxiety in sexual relationships (Love et al., 2015).

1.7 Diminished Self-Esteem and Declining Academic Performance

Research highlights a negative correlation between frequent pornography use and self-esteem (Peter & Valkenburg, 2016). Adolescents may compare themselves unfavorably to unrealistic portrayals of sexual performance, leading to feelings of inadequacy and self-doubt (Bridges et al., 2010). Persistent engagement with pornographic content can lead to decreased focus, reduced academic motivation, and impaired executive functioning (Che Nozid et al., 2023).

1.8 Relationship and Social Impact

Pornographic addiction can distort adolescents' understanding of healthy sexual relationships (Peter & Valkenburg, 2008). Research indicates that habitual exposure to explicit content contributes to unrealistic expectations regarding physical appearance, sexual performance, and relational dynamics (Minarcik et al., 2016). Adolescents with compulsive pornography habits often struggle with real-life interpersonal relationships. Findings suggest that excessive consumption fosters avoidance behaviors, leading to reduced interest in social interactions and potential romantic partnerships (Minarcik et al., 2016). Previous literature also associates pornographic addiction with an increased likelihood of engaging in unsafe sexual practices. These include early sexual initiation, multiple sexual partners, and reduced use of contraceptives, which elevate the risk of sexually transmitted infections and unintended pregnancies (Pathmendra et al., 2023). Youth and adolescents exposed to excessive pornography often develop unrealistic expectations about sex, leading to dissatisfaction and impaired bonding in real-life relationships (Bridges et al., 2010; Peter & Valkenburg, 2008).

2. RESEARCH METHODOLOGY

This systematic review consists of secondary data. The data is collected from various online databases like Google Scholar, PubMed, Science Direct, and Research Gate. The content for this study is collected from Empirical studies, Meta-analytical papers, Systematic reviews, Books, etc. Papers only in the English language are included for this study. Furthermore, various keywords like impact of pornography on behavior, social impacts of pornography, negative consequences of pornography, inter- and intra-personal consequences of pornographic addiction, pornography impact on adolescents, pornographic addiction and cognition, psychological impacts of pornographic addiction, psychosocial impacts of pornographic addiction, pornography and sexual aggression, pornography and sexual violence, public harms of pornography, causes of pornographic addiction, pornography in modern era, treatment of pornography, pornography, compulsive sexual behavior disorder (CBSD) in ICD-11, Public harms of pornography, Internet and pornography, neurobiology of pornography, neuroscience perspective on pornography, dopamine imbalance in pornography etc. were used to collect data for this review paper.

2.1 Inclusion criteria:

A total of 88 research studies were selected during the search process, however, only 50 of them got included in this paper. The selection was based on the relevance and correlation of the papers with this review. Only those papers were included which tell (a) what is pornographic addiction and its causes, (b) why pornographic addiction is developing more in modern day generation and also in adults, (c) intra and interpersonal consequences of pornographic addiction or other consequences which are in relation with them, (d) how pornography can lead to more sexual aggression and violence (mainly towards female), (e) how pornography is effecting modern societies and changes that should be brought to solve it, (f) concerns about more studies in future for better knowledge and diagnosis of this problem. An in-depth investigation was done by the authors for a good selection of papers. Furthermore, for more information, references and citations of other research were included for a more informative review. Then, all the information was compiled effectively by the authors, which contains all the information about the issue and also about the steps that should be followed in the future in order to solve the problem.

3. REVIEW OF LITERATURE:

Pornography has adverse effect on individuals. Additionally, it has more negative consequences when the pornographic content is consumed by adolescents. As youth is a foundational period in the life of an individual, it is a stage in which the development of beliefs, attitudes, values, habits, and worldviews happens (De Alarcón et al., 2019). Preventing experiences like addiction to pornography, which can hamper the overall development and ability to maintain long-term family and marital relationships, must be a top priority for educators, parents, and policymakers (De Alarcón et al., 2019). Furthermore, due to these reasons, it is illegal to consume pornography by minors. Yet the widespread availability and accessibility of the internet have slowed down the process and destabilized the progression to stop this illegal activity at the global level. Hence, this has indirectly and directly caused negative consequences in the child's world and family processes (Manning, 2006). Therefore, the following study has shown some intra- and interpersonal consequences that a pornographic addict faces.

3.1 Intra-Personal Consequences:

Various intrapersonal psychological impairments of watching excessive pornographic content include forms of guilt, irritability, stress, frustration, difficulty concentrating, difficulty sleeping, feelings of depression, and other psychosomatic symptoms (Astuti & Winarti, 2022). Additionally, similar studies have also shown that excessive sexual behavior due to pornography can deteriorate an individual's mental health, which can cause depression or depressive mood and anxiety (Bancroft et al., 2003; Laier et al., 2013; Peter and Valkenburg, 2011; Ross et al., 2012). Furthermore, research also shows that pornography addicts also face difficulty in emotional regulation and mind control strategies. Thus, it also causes frustration, guilt, and irritation to an individual (Molla et al., 2018). Also, pornography addicts have problems with work functioning and daily life activities (Souza & Lodha, 2017). Consuming excessive pornographic content can cause sexual compulsivity, impairment in academic or professional performance, distress, etc. (Cooper et al.,1999). Pornographic addicts also face numerous problems related to focus or concentration. They are constantly thinking of sexual fantasies and intercourse scenes. Furthermore, individuals who continuously watch pornographic content are more vulnerable to having sexual urges regularly (Gustirini & Putri, 2019).

A significant number of researchers advocate that one of the factors that causes more problematic pornography is essentially more associated with interpretations of the use rather than the use itself. Religion can be a similar cause for the same. It is observed that religiously based moral disapproval is one of the causes for self-reported addiction to pornography. This clearly suggests that moral incongruence can complicate the diagnosis of CBSD. This was also supported by the fact that many authors on diagnostic criteria for CBSD claimed that moral distress over sexual behavior is not alone sufficient for the diagnosis of CBSD (Grubbs & Kraus, 2021). Furthermore, much research has also shown that culture and religiosity, highlighting sexual purity, can lead to feelings of guilt and negative emotions in an individual (Grubbs et al., 2015).

Increasing internet access to individuals can lead to loss of self-control, which can cause vulnerability to watch internet pornography (Block, 2008; Daneback et al., 2006, 2012; Ross et al., 2012). Furthermore, it has been found in research that pornography addicts face immersion. Immersion is simply a feeling of preoccupation with pornographic content (Griffiths et al., 2016). It was observed that addicts find it difficult to get rid of pornographic videos revolving in their minds. Also, they face relapse, which is a condition when an individual re-accesses pornographic content after trying to hold back (Camilleri et al., 2021). Thus, there are many factors causing individuals to consume pornography, which also includes curiosity, loneliness, and sexual satisfaction etc. Loneliness is the main factor why adolescent engages in online sexual behavior (Habibi & Kurniawan, 2021).

3.2 Interpersonal Consequences:

The addiction to Pornographic content among youth and adolescents has profound intra- and interpersonal consequences. Such a serious kind of addiction hinders the emotional and social development of children and adolescents and makes interpersonal relationships fragile. Addressing the issue requires a multi-level approach involving various stakeholders from different streams like education, counseling, and policy interventions. Cognitive-behavioral therapy (CBT) and mindfulness-based approaches have shown promise in helping individuals regain control over their consumption patterns (Nasser, 2021). Previous research; highlight significant negative consequences, such as decreased emotional well-being, impaired social skills, and distorted perceptions of relationships and sexuality (Habibi & Kurniawan, 2021).

Various social effects of pornographic addiction include withdrawal from social circumstances, difficulty in establishing interpersonal relationships with other people, preferring to remain silent, and feeling distant from society (Astuti & Winarti, 2022). Thus, pornographic addiction can cause disturbance in the social identity of a person. Also, today's pornographic material is enormously different from what was available in the past. The limitless supply of novel images that can be clicked through in seconds has deviated the concepts of sex and violence in the developing brain of today's young generation. It was found in research that 88% of scenes in these movies are totally based on physical and verbal aggression, which is usually towards females (Foubert, 2017). Furthermore, various studies have shown that excessive pornographic use can cause greater sexual objectification of partners (mainly women), risk of sexual aggression, casual sexual behaviour, and more stereotypical beliefs about gender roles (Peter & Valkenburg, 2016). Furthermore, studies also suggest that pornography provides unrealistic stimuli which have no relation with actual psychosocial contacts and interpersonal relations, leading to abnormal emotional response (Burtăverde et al., 2021; Laier et al., 2013; Mauer-Vakil and Bahji, 2020; Ross et al., 2012; Štulhofer et al., 2016). It has been proposed that pornographic addiction that certain themes of aggression, impulse gratification, and objectification in pornography can severely deviate one's attitude and behaviour (Paolucci et al., 1997). With the context of social learning theory, an individual viewing pornography may interpret it as the portrayal of reality. With that expectation they may engage in behaviour which is not socially acceptable or morally sound (Paolucci et al., 1997) Also, findings from major researches show that 95% of the time during sexual violence in pornography (usually from male to female), the female shows a liking to the violent behaviour without any objections. This can cause deviance in sexual attitude and behaviour of the viewer, as they can think it to be normal. (Bridges et al., 2010).

Furthermore, a general theoretical model, (HCM) hierarchical confluence model of sexual aggression interprets the consequences of pornography with relation to individual differences and personality types, which correlates to sexual aggressive attitudes (Hald et al., 2014). A study using a representative sample of young Danish adults and a randomized experimental design. It was found that both women and men with lower agreeableness, excessive past pornography consumption significantly predict a higher level of ASV (attitude promoting sexual violence against women) (Hald & Malamuth, 2014). In order to have an impact on solving or ending the issue of sexual violence against women, one must tackle the problem of pornographic addiction (Foubert, 2017). Furthermore, excessive pornography use can negatively affect the enjoyment of sexual intimate behavior with a partner as it causes distraction by sexual thoughts, sexual boredom in a relationship, and frequent masturbation. Additionally, pornographic addiction can cause tolerance to natural sexual intercourse, which causes lesser level of excitement (Sun et al., 2014; Peter & Valkenburg, 2008; Carvalheira et al., 2015). These difficulties are more common in couples with one partner regularly engages in pornographic material, which results in a loss of interest in sexual intimacy (Schneider, 2000).

Thus, pornography has a negative effect on inmate relationships (Deloy, 2007). Furthermore, research also show that excessive pornography use can adversely affect the sexual health of individuals. For example, cases of erectile dysfunction (ED) are skyrocketing, which is directly related to excessive use of pornography content. Recent data showed that a man is 60% more likely to have ED if he is addicted to pornography (Foubert,2017). All these men have ED when they are actually with a partner not when they are consuming porn (Landripet & Štulhofer, 2015; Negash et al., 2015). Similarly, Norwegian and Croatian samples, respectively, were found to be using pornography several times a week. About 14.2%-28.3% of the participants reported erectile dysfunction, 16.3%-37.4% reported hypoactive sexual dysfunction, and 6.2%-19.9% had delayed ejaculation (Landripet & Štulhofer, 2015; Negash et al., 2015). Furthermore, pornographic addiction can cause certain changes in neural processes that are similar to substance addiction (De Sousa & Lodha, 2017). Additionally, pornographic addiction causes changes in the Mesolimbic Dopamine Pathway (DP). This circuitry is responsible for reward seeking, reinforcement, pleasure, and impulsivity (Di Chiara et al., 2004). It has been shown by research that when somebody chronically watches pornography. There is excessive release of dopamine to the reward system, which stimulates a neuroplastic change that reinforces the experience. These changes build brain maps for sexual arousal (Love et al., 2015). Now these maps cause individuals to watch more pornographic content to maintain high sexual excitement, which can't be matched with normal sexuality (Hilton, 2015).

Individuals perceive fantasies shown in pornography as reality, which results in a negative attitude and faulty sexual behavior, especially when sexual information is limited (Lim et al., 2016). Many recent studies showed that people are looking for pornography for sexual relaxation and a feeling of satisfaction through masturbation (Ross et al., 2012; Mauer-Vakil & Bahji, 2020). These changes cause changes in the normal sexual functioning of an individual from a partner relationship to compulsively watching pornographic content.

Furthermore, the following table shows data from studies in the last decade, which shows the psychological and social impact of pornography on the lives of individuals.

Summery table of the major finding of the previous article. (Table 1.)

Table 1.

S. No.	Author(S)	Type of research	Main Objective	Major Findings
1.	Setyawati et al., (2020)	Empirical research	To study the psychological impacts of internet pornography addictions	Impacts of pornographic addiction involves obsession with pornographic content, find difficulty in sleep and focus on regular activities, withdrawal from social setting and, inability to form interpersonal relationships.
2.	George et al., (2019)	Review paper	To examine psychosocial consequences of pornographic addiction	Pornographic addicts have thoughts of sex revolving in their mind, sexual compulsivity, problems with social integration etc. Hence, it's important to design pornography addiction education program in order to educate students
3.	Camilleri et al., (2021)	Empirical research	Investigate the relationship between pornography use and mental health among university students	Pornography addiction causes impaired control (like preoccupation, dependence etc.), problem with social integration and various psychological problems like depression, stress, frustration etc. Which have a negative impact on mental health of an individual
4.	Deloy, (2006)	Empirical research	To study effect of sexually explicit material (SEM) or pornography on males who are involved in romantic relationship	Males who actively use SEM have a significant decrease in relationship satisfaction
5.	Bridges et al., (2010)	Content analysis	Examine the depiction of aggression and similar variables in popular pornographic videos	There is significant reinforcement to verbal and non-verbal aggression during sexual intercourse in popular pornographic videos
6.	Foubert, (2017)	Review paper	Map the public health hazards of internet Pornography.	It was found that internet pornography consumption leads to sexual objectification of women in brain of male consumers, skyrocketed the cases of erectile dysfunction (ED) and a cause of sexual violence against women
7.	Hald & Malamuth, (2014)	Empirical research	Investigate the effects of personality traits and past pornographic consumption on attitude supporting violence against women (ASV)	Pornographic consumption may increase ASV on individuals who have lower level of Agreeableness (personality dimension)
8.	Minarcik et al., (2016)	Empirical research	Impact of Sexually explicit materials (SEM) on relationship dynamics.	Investment in SEM usage by it's users is the determinant of its negative consequences in relationships

continued on following page

Table 1. Continued

S. No.	Author(S)	Type of research	Main Objective	Major Findings
9.	Sun et al., (2014)	Empirical research	Impact of pornography on real world sexual encounters between man and women.	Men who frequently watch pornography are more likely to rely on pornography to become sexually excited and integrate pornography on sexual activities hence have diminished enjoyment of sexually inmate behaviour
10.	Peter & Valkenburg, (2011)	Empirical research	To investigate whether sexually explicit internet material (SEIM) have effect on sexual risk behaviour of adults and adolescent.	SEIM can cause sexual risk behaviour on adults but not in adolescents
11.	Grubbs et al., (2015)	Empirical research	Role of moral disapproval and religious belief on self-perceived addiction to internet pornography.	Religiosity leads to moral disapproval to pornography use; therefore, these moral attitudes lead to self-perceived addiction to internet pornography
12.	Astuti & Winarti, (2022)	Review paper	Impact of pornographic addition on adolescents.	Pornographic addiction has three major effects i.e. psychological (guilt, frustration etc.), social (disturbing interpersonal relationship etc.), and medical (decreasing cognitive functions).
13.	Che Nozid et al., (2023)	Empirical research	Psychological impacts of pornographic consumption on university students in Kuantan.	Pornographic addiction can be the cause of anxiety and depression, which would lead to lower academic performance in students
14.	Burtăverde et al., (2021)	Empirical research	To map the reasons for pornography consumption in individuals.	There are four factors due to which people watch pornography i.e. increase sex drive, enhancing sexual performance, social and instrumental motives (like learning from peers), lack of emotional and relational skills
15.	Molla et al., (2018)	Empirical research	Examine the role of thought control strategies and emotional regulation on pornographic use.	Pornography use was positively influenced by difficulties in emotion regulation and negatively influenced with social control and distraction
16.	De Souza & Lodha, (2017)	Review paper	Clinical orientation of neurobiology of pornographic addiction.	Pornographic addiction causes a surge of dopamine in reward system of brain which reinforces the addiction. Also changes in limbic system due to excessive pornographic use is similar to drug addiction
17.	Gola et al., (2016)	Empirical research	To investigate whether people seek treatment for problematic pornographic use (PU) due to quantity of pornographic content or due to severe negative symptoms attached to it.	Treatment of Problematic pornography must be focussed on impact of pornography (like negative behavioural consequences) in an individual's life rather than it's mere frequency (quantity)

continued on following page

Table 1. Continued

S. No.	Author(S)	Type of research	Main Objective	Major Findings
18.	Later et al., (2013)	Empirical research	To discuss development and maintenance factors of cybersex addiction.	Positive reinforcement like sexual arousal and craving (sexual gratification) is the key for maintenance of cybersex addiction
19.	De Alarcon et al., (2019)	Systematic review	Summarize existing knowledge on problematic internet pornography use as a pathological entity.	Excessively watching pornographic content can lead to addiction and have adverse effects like sexual dysfunction and psychosexual dissatisfaction
20.	Nasser, (2021)	Empirical research	Identify pornographic addiction in teenagers and middle school students.	Males are more often addicted to pornography in comparison with females and search pornographic content on internet to satisfy their sexual instinct and obtain pleasure

4. DISCUSSION

Pornography addiction is a feeling of an urge to watch pornographic materials compulsively despite facing its consequences. Its maladaptive nature causes hindrance in various domains of life of an individual. Furthermore, it has a serious impact on the well-being of a person, their family, and hence on communities. An individual usually watches pornographic material through magazines, DVDs, erotic books, the internet (blogs, videos, photos, live calls, chats, and video calls), etc. Moreover, sources of pornography materials have changed over the course of time. Earlier, pornographic material had certain limits to its accessibility because people had to actually go out to buy such stuff. But nowadays pornography has become more anonymous, accessible, and affordable because of improving technology and the internet. This means any individual can watch pornography anytime in their own personal space without any interference from other people. This has caused an enormous increase in viewership of pornography (especially online). Additionally, in 2012, it was estimated that 37 million Google hits contained the phrase "porn movies", and 506 million searches included the word "sex" (Kar, 2016). Also, online pornography is evolving day by day; the introduction of various new themes of porn has attracted millions of viewers and also caused them to revisit these sites. This has triggered more vulnerability to develop this addiction in the present generation, which can cause immediate disturbances in their personal and social lives.

Talking about the various effects of pornography, this review consists of various inter- and intrapersonal consequences of pornography. Intrapersonal consequences of pornography include various psychological impairments, including forms of guilt, irritability, stress, frustration, difficulty concentrating, difficulty sleeping, feelings of depression, and psychosomatic symptoms. Furthermore, thoughts of pornography continuously revolve in the mind of a pornographic addict, which causes disturbances in the ability of an individual to successfully complete daily tasks and activities. Also, pornography (mainly through the internet) shows such acts and fantasies which are very unrealistic (such as hard-core anal porn, verbal or physical aggression in various scenes, etc.). This can lead to certain expectations in the minds of viewers that are not morally and ethically sound and affect their sexual attitudes and behavior. Now coming to various interpersonal consequences of pornographic addiction, which include difficulty in maintaining a healthy sexual relationship with a partner, preferring to remain in isolation, not actively participating in social interaction with other people, etc. Hence, pornographic addicts face a lower level of excitement during natural sexual intercourse with their partner, as they are habituated to feeling orgasms to pornographic material, which leads to a negative effect on intimate relationships. It is also found that excessive pornography can lead to sexual objectification of the partner, which may lead to the sexual violence, sexual aggression, and casual sexual behavior.

This systematic review provides knowledge of the consequences of pornographic addiction as mentioned above. However, we also recommend a more in-depth analysis of this issue in future research for better understanding and to create a better diagnosis to solve this problem. More empirical studies should be done in this area to have concrete evidence for its impact on individuals and also to quantify and map the causes of problematic pornography use. Furthermore, we also suggest spreading awareness of this issue to parents, teachers, and especially to teenagers and children, as they are more vulnerable to its negative effects. As childhood is the period of life where the development of personality, attitude, etc. happens at its peak, so in order to ensure their healthy development, it's important to guide them through this period of their lives.

5. CONCLUSION:

Pornography (especially through the internet) is a massive business these days. Since, technological advancements and limitless internet connectivity have boosted its availability several times than it was before. As of now, the content can be consumed by anyone at any age, including Adolescents. Furthermore, excessive use of pornography is a problem of today, and with growing technological advancements, this issue is getting more disastrous. Additionally, there is certain negligence given to the topic in research and diagnosis criteria. Most of the addictive behaviors mentioned in the latest edition of the Diagnostic and Statistical Manual of Mental

Health (DSM-5-TR) are related to substances. The only non-substance-related disorder mentioned there is gambling. Pornography is under CBSD (compulsive sexual behavior disorder) in ICD-11. Even so, where and how it should be classified must be a matter of debate in future studies (Lew-Starowicz & Coleman, 2022). Also, there is no clinical diagnosis of withdrawal symptoms of pornographic addiction in the eleventh version of the International Classification of Diseases (ICD-11).

Pornography addiction has a multi-level negative impacts on an individual's life. Where, an addict may suffer from irritability, anxiety, guilt, frustration and depression with difficulty in sleeping and concentrating. A concerning effect of excessive pornography are sexual aggression, casual sexual behavior, partner's objectification etc. Furthermore, they may also face social withdrawal, avoid interaction with others, feeling of loneliness etc. Furthermore, we need domain-specific research on this topic for in-depth knowledge and better diagnosis in the future. Additionally, we also need funding agencies to support research related to pornography, specifically if it is related to treatment-seeking attitudes of individuals to problematic pornography or any other CBSD-related behavior.

6. INTERVENTION STRATEGIES

To counter the pornographic addiction in youth, Cognitive-behavioral therapy (CBT) has shown significant benefit in treating pornography addiction. Research suggests that CBT interventions effectively help adolescents develop healthier coping mechanisms. It reduces cognitive distortions and emotional distress to reduce maladaptive behaviors in youth. Moreover, Mindfulness-based interventions also help in improving emotion regulation. Additionally, comprehensive targeted sex education programs on pornography and its effects can promote awareness. Family-based interventions can also offer significant reinforcement to reduce compulsive pornography behaviors. Further, encouraging open discussions about online pornographic content can mitigate exposure to explicit material. Official representatives should consider age restrictions, digital literacy programs, and stricter regulations on explicit content accessibility to protect vulnerable populations.

7. FUTURE SCOPE AND LIMITATION

Pornography use is a behavior that intersects with many other research domains and influences outcomes, which has been previously studied by psychologists. Thus, pornography should be studied as a separate and specific domain, however, it is treated as a subdivision of other research areas. It has been concluded that pornography as a research domain is in need of continued empirical studies from several domains of psychology. That too should focus on a variety of behaviors, ranging from positive to negative effects (Grubbs & Kraus, 2021). Also, it is very crucial to introduce specifically designed pornography addiction education programs in order to educate students about the adverse impacts of pornography. Also, direct treatment programs for pornography abuse, sexual addiction, and sexual abuse must be presented for the individuals who need support (George et al., 2019). There is also a need for encouraging researchers who are already studying this topic to implement more specific methodologies, such as experimental methods, ecological momentary assessments, and longitudinal dyadic studies (Grubbs & Kraus, 2021). Future research must focus on the recognition of various types and subtypes in the given heterogeneity of the issue. Furthermore, research must be done on clinical assessment, better instrumentation, and examining fundamental entities within the population (Lew-Starowicz & Coleman, 2022). Studies in the future should also focus on employing robust research designs (e.g., longitudinal cohort design, nationally representative sample, etc.) while investigating the relationship between psychological well-being and pornography use (Grubbs & Kraus, 2021).

REFERENCES

Astuti, S. A. T., & Winarti, Y. (2022). A scoping review: the impact of pornography addiction on adolescents. *Proceeding of Muhammadiyah International Public Health and Medicine Conference (MIPHMC), 2*(1), 366-381. DOI: 10.61811/miphmp.v1i2.265

Attwood, F. (2004). Pornography and objectification. *Feminist Media Studies, 4*(1), 7–19. DOI: 10.1080/1468077041001674617

Bancroft, J., Janssen, E., Strong, D., Carnes, L., Vukadinovic, Z., & Long, J. S. (2003). The relation between mood and sexuality in heterosexual men. *Archives of Sexual Behavior, 32*(3), 217–230. DOI: 10.1023/A:1023409516739 PMID: 12807294

Block, J. J. (2008). Issues for dsm-v: Internet addiction. *The American Journal of Psychiatry, 165*(3), 306–307. DOI: 10.1176/appi.ajp.2007.07101556 PMID: 18316427

Bridges, A. J., Wosnitzer, R., Scharrer, E., Sun, C., & Liberman, R. (2010). Aggression and sexual behavior in best-selling pornography videos: A content analysis update. *Violence Against Women, 16*(10), 1065–1085. DOI: 10.1177/1077801210382866 PMID: 20980228

Burtăverde, V., Jonason, P. K., Giosan, C., & Ene, C. (2021). Why do people watch porn? An evolutionary perspective on the reasons for pornography consumption. *Evolutionary Psychology, 19*(2). Doi.org .DOI: 10.1177/14747049211028798

Camilleri, C., Perry, J. T., & Sammut, S. (2021). Compulsive Internet Pornography Use and Mental Health: A Cross-Sectional Study in a Sample of University Students in the United States. *Frontiers in Psychology, 11*, 613244. Doi.org/10./fpsyg.2020.613244. DOI: 10.3389/fpsyg.2020.613244 PMID: 33510691

Carvalheira, A., Træen, B., & Stulhofer, A. (2015). Masturbation and pornography use among coupled heterosexual men with decreased sexual desire: How many roles of masturbation? *Journal of Sex & Marital Therapy, 41*(6), 626–635. DOI: 10.1080/0092623X.2014.958790 PMID: 25189834

. Chawla, K., & Sujita, K. K. (2021). Pornography addiction and its influence on sexual behavior, intimate relationship and other life domains. *Indian journal of health, sexuality & culture, 7* (1), 80-83. Doi.org/10.5281/zenodo.5151912.

. Che Nozid, N. R., Rostam, M. A., & Uzir, B. F. (2023). Psychological impacts of pornography exposure among university students in pahang. *International journal of allied health sciences, 7*(2), 2909–2916. https://doi.org/DOI: 10.31436/ijahs.v7i2.780

Cooper, A., Putnam, D., Planchon, L., & Boies, S. (1999). Online sexual compulsivity: Getting tangled in the net. *Sexual Addiction & Compulsivity*, *6*(2), 79–104. DOI: 10.1080/10720169908400182

Daneback, K., Månsson, S. A., Ross, M. W., & Markham, C. M. (2012). The internet as a source of information about sexuality. *Sex Education*, *12*(5), 583–598. DOI: 10.1080/14681811.2011.627739

Daneback, K., Ross, M. W., & Månsson, S. A. (2006). Characteristics and behaviors of sexual compulsives who use the internet for sexual purposes. *Sexual Addiction & Compulsivity*, *13*(1), 53–67. DOI: 10.1080/10720160500529276

De Alarcón, R., de la Iglesia, J. I., Casado, N. M., & Montejo, A. L. (2019). Online Porn Addiction: What We Know and What We Don't-A Systematic Review. *Journal of Clinical Medicine*, *8*(1), 91. Doi.org/10.3390/jcm8010091. DOI: 10.3390/jcm8010091 PMID: 30650522

De Sousa, A., & Lodha, P. (2017). Neurobiology of pornography addiction – a clinical review. *Telangana Journal of Psychiatry*, *3*(2), 66–67. DOI: 10.18231/2455-8559.2017.0016

Deloy, J. (2006). Patterns of relationship satisfaction and sexual behavior as a function of pornography use among college men. *Theses and Dissertations*. 2532. https://commons.und.edu/theses/2532

Di Chiara, G., Bassareo, V., Fenu, S., De Luca, M. A., Spina, L., Cadoni, C., Acquas, E., Carboni, E., Valentini, V., & Lecca, D. (2004). Dopamine and drug addiction: The nucleus accumbens shell connection. *Neuropharmacology*, *47*(1), 227–241. DOI: 10.1016/j.neuropharm.2004.06.032 PMID: 15464140

. Foubert, J. D. (2017). The public health harms of pornography: the brain, erectile dysfunction and sexual violence. *Dignity: A journal on sexual exploitation and Violence, 2*(3). DOI: 10.23860/dignity.2017.02.03.06

George, M., Maheshwari, S., Chandran, S., & Rao, T. S. S. (2019). Psychosocial aspects of pornography. *Journal of Psychosexual Health*, *1*(1), 44–47. DOI: 10.1177/2631831818821535

Gola, M., Lewczuk, K., & Skorko, M. (2016). What matters: Quantity or quality of pornography use? Psychological and behavioral factors of treatment-seeking for problematic pornography use. *Journal of Sexual Medicine*, *13*(5), 815–824. DOI: 10.1016/j.jsxm.2016.02.169 PMID: 27012817

Griffiths, M. D., Kuss, D. J., Billieux, J., & Pontes, H. M. (2016). The evolution of internet addiction: A global Perspective. *Addictive Behaviors*, *53*, 193–195. DOI: 10.1016/j.addbeh.2015.11.001 PMID: 26562678

Grubbs, J. B., Exline, J. J., Pargament, K. I., Hook, J. N., & Carlisle, R. D. (2015). Transgression as addiction: Religiosity and moral disapproval as predictors of perceived addiction to pornography. *Archives of Sexual Behavior*, *44*(1), 125–136. DOI: 10.1007/s10508-013-0257-z PMID: 24519108

Grubbs, J. B., & Kraus, S. W. (2021). Pornography use and psychological science: A call for consideration. *Current Directions in Psychological Science*, *30*(1), 68–75. DOI: 10.1177/0963721420979594

Gustirini, R., & Putri, A. (2020). Peningkatan pengetahuan remaja tentang dampak negatif paparan pornografi di sma negeri 14 palembang. *Khidmah*, *2*(1), 96–101. DOI: 10.52523/khidmah.v2i1.308

Habibi, L. A. N., & Kurniawan, A. (2021). Loneliness relationship with cybersex behaviour in emerging adult. [BRPKM]. *Psychology and Mental Health Research Bulletin*, *1*(1), 722–733. DOI: 10.20473/brpkm.v1i1.26863

Hald, G. M., Seaman, C., & Linz, D. (2014). Sexuality and pornography. In D. L. Tolman, L. M. Diamond, J. A. Bauermeister, W. H. George, J. G. Pfaus, & L. M. Ward (Eds.), *APA handbook of sexuality and psychology, Vol. 2. Contextual approaches* (pp. 3–35). American Psychological Association. DOI: 10.1037/14194-001

Hald, M. G., & Malamuth, N. N. (2014). Experimental effects of exposure to pornography: The moderating effect of personality and mediating effect of sexual arousal. *Archives of Sexual Behavior*, *44*(1), 99–109. DOI: 10.1007/s10508-014-0291-5 PMID: 24729134

Hilton, D. L.Jr. (2013). Pornography addiction – a supranormal stimulus considered in the context of neuroplasticity. *Socioaffective Neuroscience & Psychology*, *3*(1), 20767. DOI: 10.3402/snp.v3i0.20767 PMID: 24693354

Kar, S. K. (2016). Lost online, then lust online. *New Journal of Psychiatric Nursing*, *5*(3), 117–119. DOI: 10.21088/jpn.2277.9035.5316.4

Keilty, P. (2018). Desire by design: Pornography as technology industry. *Porn Studies*, *1–5*(3), 338–342. Advance online publication. DOI: 10.1080/23268743.2018.1483208

Kühn, S., & Gallinat, J. (2014). Brain Structure and Functional Connectivity Associated With Pornography Consumption. *JAMA Psychiatry*, *71*(7), 827. DOI: 10.1001/jamapsychiatry.2014.93 PMID: 24871202

Kumbhare, K. (2022). Effect Pornography has on an Individual's Personality. *International Journal of Indian Psychology, 10*(3). Doi.org/10.25215/1003.156

Laier, C., Pawlikowski, M., Pekal, J., Schulte, F. P., & Brand, M. (2013). Cybersex addiction: Experienced sexual arousal when watching pornography and not real-life sexual contacts makes the difference. *Journal of Behavioral Addictions, 2*(2), 100–107. DOI: 10.1556/JBA.2.2013.002 PMID: 26165929

Landripet, I., & Štulhofer, A. (2015). Is Pornography Use Associated with Sexual Difficulties and Dysfunctions among Younger Heterosexual Men? *Journal of Sexual Medicine, 12*(5), 1136–1139. DOI: 10.1111/jsm.12853 PMID: 25816904

Lew-Starowicz, M., & Coleman, E. (2022). Mental and sexual health perspectives of the international classification of diseases (icd-11) compulsive sexual behavior disorder •. *Journal of Behavioral Addictions, 11*(2), 226–229. DOI: 10.1556/2006.2022.00032 PMID: 35895453

Ley, D., Prause, N., & Finn, P. (2014). The emperor has no clothes: A review of the 'pornography addiction' model. *Current Sexual Health Reports, 6*(2), 94–105. DOI: 10.1007/s11930-014-0016-8

Lim, M. S., Carrotte, E. R., & Hellard, M. E. (2016). The impact of pornography on gender-based violence, sexual health and well-being: What do we know? *Journal of Epidemiology and Community Health, 70*(1), 3–5. DOI: 10.1136/jech-2015-205453 PMID: 26022057

Love, T., Laier, C., Brand, M., Hatch, L., & Hajela, R. (2015). Neuroscience of internet pornography addiction: A review and update. *Behavioral Sciences (Basel, Switzerland), 5*(3), 388–433. DOI: 10.3390/bs5030388 PMID: 26393658

Manning, J. C. (2006). The impact of internet pornography on marriage and the family: A review of the research. *Sexual Addiction & Compulsivity, 13*(2–3), 131–165. DOI: 10.1080/10720160600870711

Mattebo, M., Larsson, M., Tydén, T., & Häggström-Nordin, E. (2013). Professionals' perceptions of the effect of pornography on Swedish adolescents. *Public Health Nursing (Boston, Mass.), 31*(3), 196–205. DOI: 10.1111/phn.12058 PMID: 24720654

Mauer-Vakil, D., & Bahji, A. (2020). The addictive nature of compulsive sexual behaviours and problematic online pornography consumption: A review. *The Canadian Journal of Addiction, 11*(3), 42–51. DOI: 10.1097/CXA.0000000000000091

Mc-Bride, J. F. (2019). Addiction and mindfulness; pornography addiction and mindfulness-based therapy act. *Sexual Addiction & Compulsivity, 26*(1–2), 42–53. DOI: 10.1080/10720162.2019.1576560

Minarcik, J., Wetterneck, C. T., & Short, M. B. (2016). The effects of sexually explicit material use on romantic relationship dynamics. *Journal of Behavioral Addictions, 5*(4), 700–707. DOI: 10.1556/2006.5.2016.078 PMID: 27784182

Molla, M. D., Shirazi, M., & Nikmanesh, Z. (2018). The role of difficulties in emotion regulation and thought control strategies on pornography use. *Practice in Clinical Psychology, 6*(2), 119–128. DOI: 10.29252/nirp.jpcp.6.2.119

Nasser, A. S. (2021). Teenagers' Addiction to Pornography. *Psychology (Savannah, Ga.), 58*(2), 979–993. Doi.org/10.17762/pae.v58i1.847. DOI: 10.17762/pae.v58i1.847

Negash, S., Sheppard, N. V., Lambert, N. M., & Fincham, F. D. (2016). Trading later rewards for current pleasure: Pornography consumption and delay discounting. *Journal of Sex Research, 53*(6), 689–700. DOI: 10.1080/00224499.2015.1025123 PMID: 26305628

Paolucci, E. O., Genuis, M., & Violato, C. (1997). *A meta-analysis of the published research on the effects of pornography. The Changing Family and Child Development.* Ashgate Publishing Ltd.

Pathmendra, P., Raggatt, M., Lim, M. S., Marino, J. L., & Skinner, S. R. (2023). Exposure to pornography and adolescent sexual behavior: Systematic review. *Journal of Medical Internet Research, 25*, e43116. DOI: 10.2196/43116 PMID: 36853749

Peter, J., & Valkenburg, P. M. (2008). Adolescents' exposure to sexually explicit internet material and sexual preoccupancy: A three-wave panel study. *Media Psychology, 11*(2), 207–234. DOI: 10.1080/15213260801994238

Peter, J., & Valkenburg, P. M. (2011). The influence of sexually explicit internet material on sexual risk behavior: A comparison of adolescents and adults. *Journal of Health Communication, 16*(7), 750–765. DOI: 10.1080/10810730.2011.551996 PMID: 21476164

Peter, J., & Valkenburg, P. M. (2016). Adolescents and pornography: A review of 20 years of research. *Journal of Sex Research, 53*(4-5), 509–531. DOI: 10.1080/00224499.2016.1143441 PMID: 27105446

Privara, M., & Bob, P. (2023). Pornography consumption and cognitive-affective distress. *The Journal of Nervous and Mental Disease, 211*(8), 641–646. DOI: 10.1097/NMD.0000000000001669 PMID: 37505898

Rich, F. (2001). Naked capitalists. In Stombler, M., Burgess, E. O., Donnelly, D., & Simonds, W. (Eds.), *Sex matters: The sexuality and society reader* (pp. 462–466). Pearson Education Inc.

Ross, M. W., Månsson, S. A., & Daneback, K. (2012). Prevalence, severity, and correlates of problematic sexual internet use in swedish men and women. *Archives of Sexual Behavior*, *41*(2), 459–466. DOI: 10.1007/s10508-011-9762-0 PMID: 21562915

Schneider, J. P. (2000). Effects of cybersex addiction on the family: Results of a survey. *Sexual Addiction & Compulsivity*, *7*(1), 31–58. DOI: 10.1080/10720160008400206

Setyawati, R., Hartini, N., & Suryanto, S. (2020). The psychological impacts of internet pornography addiction on adolescents. *Humaniora*, *11*(3), 235–244. DOI: 10.21512/humaniora.v11i3.6682

Štulhofer, A., Jurin, T., & Briken, P. (2016). Is high sexual desire a facet of male hypersexuality? Results from an online study. *Journal of Sex & Marital Therapy*, *42*(8), 665–680. DOI: 10.1080/0092623X.2015.1113585 PMID: 26569650

Sun, C., Bridges, A., Johnason, J., & Ezzell, M. (2014). Pornography and the male sexual script: An analysis of consumption and sexual relations. *Archives of Sexual Behavior*, *45*(4), 983–994. Doi.org/10.1007/s10508-014-0391-2. DOI: 10.1007/s10508-014-0391-2 PMID: 25466233

Chapter 6
Unraveling Compulsive Buying Disorder:
A Comprehensive Review of the Causes, Impact, and Treatment of Compulsive Buying Disorder

Fathima Yusaira
https://orcid.org/0000-0002-0334-3960
St. Francis de Sales College, Bangalore, India

Lakshmi Balakrishnan
https://orcid.org/0009-0004-9001-7064
St. Francis de Sales College, Bangalore, India

Papia Saraf
St. Francis de Sales College, Bangalore, India

Benita Raj Prince
St. Francis de Sales College, Bangalore, India

Dakshina U. Kanthy
https://orcid.org/0000-0002-2901-6167
St. Francis de Sales College, Bangalore, India

Diliya Joseph
St. Francis de Sales College, Bangalore, India

ABSTRACT

This chapter examines Compulsive Buying Disorder (CBD), a behavioral addiction characterized by uncontrollable purchasing despite adverse consequences. Prevalence rates (2-8%) highlight disproportionate impacts on women and youth, driven by impulsivity, digital retail access, and emotional dysregulation. Neurobiological mechanisms link CBD to striatal hyperactivity and dopaminergic dysfunction, paralleling substance addiction. Diagnostic challenges stem from exclusion in DSM-5/ICD-11 and overlaps with OCD/impulse-control disorders. Evidence-based treatments prioritize cognitive-behavioral therapy and pharmacotherapy, though

DOI: 10.4018/979-8-3373-0518-9.ch006

relapse remains common. Sociocultural drivers, including materialism and digital marketing, underscore the need for holistic interventions. The chapter advocates standardized diagnostic criteria and integrated approaches to address CBD's multifactorial etiology.

INTRODUCTION

In the modern era, shopping has evolved far beyond its utilitarian roots. Fueled by advances in technology, the global expansion of consumer culture, and shifting psychological norms, it has become embedded in everyday life as a recreational activity, a form of identity expression, and, for some individuals, a means of emotional escape. This cultural transformation has coincided with increasing reliance on mobile devices and social media, exposing users to relentless digital marketing tactics. As a result, many people—especially younger demographics—are drawn into compulsive purchasing behaviors, which can strain both their mental well-being and financial stability.

Compulsive Buying Disorder (CBD), also known as shopping addiction or oniomania, is a behavioral condition marked by an irresistible drive to make purchases, often in disregard of actual need or financial limitations. Despite its widespread impact, CBD often remains under-recognized due to societal norms that glorify consumption and material success. Similar to other behavioral addictions, CBD is typified by a cycle of impulsivity, loss of control, temporary psychological relief, and subsequent guilt or distress, which often reinforces the compulsion. The emergence of online retail platforms has amplified this behavior, offering 24/7 access to shopping opportunities. Research suggests that CBD disproportionately affects women, a pattern possibly linked to social expectations, emotional engagement with consumption, and media-driven standards of appearance and lifestyle (Sathya et al., 2023).

Defining Compulsive Buying Disorder

Historically, compulsive buying was identified as a form of pathological impulse—grouped with conditions like kleptomania and pyromania (Bleuler, 1930). Benson (2000) coined the term "Spendaholism" to capture the compulsive nature of this behavior and its ties to self-concept and personal identity. While CBD is not formally recognized as a distinct diagnosis in the DSM-5 (5th ed.; DSM-5; American Psychiatric Association, 2013), it is commonly understood as a behavioral addiction with serious consequences across emotional, social, occupational, and financial domains.

Scholars have debated its classification, associating CBD variously with addiction models (Krych, 1989), obsessive-compulsive tendencies (Hollander, 1993), and affective disorders (Lejoyeux et al., 1996). Though excluded from DSM-IV, it had previously been listed in DSM-III-R under "impulse control disorder not otherwise specified." Efforts by McElroy and colleagues (1994) focused on developing criteria that reflect the cognitive and behavioral underpinnings of the disorder. Some critics argue that pathologizing CBD contributes to the medicalization of lifestyle behaviors (Lee, 2004). However, dismissing the disorder in this way ignores substantial evidence pointing to the debilitating effects CBD can have on affected individuals and undermines legitimate efforts to understand and treat it.

Core Features of Compulsive Buying Disorder

Compulsive Buying Disorder (CBD) manifests through persistent and overwhelming urges to shop, which significantly impair an individual's functioning and emotional well-being. Lifetime prevalence estimates range from 2% to 8% globally, with the condition occurring more frequently in women (Black, 2001; Black, 2007; Filomensky & Tavares, 2021; Aboujaoude, 2014). Gender-based prevalence may be influenced by cultural narratives that place heightened importance on appearance and consumption among women (Tavares et al., 2008; Narayanan et al., 2025). Young adults, especially university students, appear to be particularly susceptible, likely due to their increased exposure to digital retail environments and social peer pressures (Amin et al., 2022).

The consequences of CBD are not merely psychological; individuals often face chronic debt, strained relationships, and legal complications arising from their uncontrolled spending behaviors (Weinstein et al., 2016; Müller & Zwaan, 2010). Although cognitive-behavioral therapy (CBT) has shown promising outcomes, pharmacological options have yet to demonstrate consistent effectiveness (Black, 2001; Filomensky & Tavares, 2021). Shopping is frequently used by individuals with CBD as a maladaptive emotional regulation strategy, offering temporary relief from negative affect but often worsening financial hardship over time (Weinstein et al., 2016).

Psychological Dynamics and Personality Correlates

The psychological profile of CBD is multifaceted. Core features include diminished self-esteem, chronic stress, and impulsivity, often compounded by co-occurring psychiatric conditions such as depression, anxiety, and other impulse-control disorders

(Vasiliu & Vasile, 2017; González-Fuente & Jiménez, 2024; Filomensky & Tavares, 2021). The interplay between emotional dysregulation and compulsive urges highlights the disorder's complexity. Affected individuals frequently report high stress levels, with shopping acting as an emotional release mechanism (Leftwich, 2022).

Impulsivity plays a critical role in compulsive buying behaviors. Research shows that individuals with elevated impulsivity are more prone to making spontaneous, irrational purchases (González-Fuente & Jiménez, 2024). Depressive symptoms are also prevalent, suggesting that some individuals may turn to consumption to alleviate emotional discomfort (Leite & Silva, 2014). While CBD spans all age groups, it is particularly prominent in youth populations—possibly due to their greater interaction with digital marketing and reduced emotional regulation skills (González-Fuente & Jiménez, 2024).

Qureshi et al. (2024) explored the influence of personality traits using the HEXACO model, uncovering important distinctions. For example, lower conscientiousness predicted greater cognitive impulsivity, while higher emotionality was linked to emotionally driven purchases. These insights underscore the need for individualized intervention strategies that account for personality-driven vulnerabilities. Supporting this, Rachubińska et al. (2024) found that women at risk for CBD scored lower in agreeableness and conscientiousness, and a significant portion also showed tendencies toward workaholism—pointing to an intricate overlap between personality dimensions and compulsive behaviors.

Sociocultural Dimensions of Compulsive Buying

The influence of culture and societal norms on consumer behavior cannot be overstated. In many societies, especially those with collectivist or masculine cultural traits, shopping behaviors are shaped by the desire to achieve social validation. Purchasing high-status or luxury items is often used as a means of signaling social worth (Strizhak & Mancheva, 2022). Belk (1988) posited that material goods act as extensions of the self, serving as tools for constructing identity and signaling social belonging.

Consumer decisions are also influenced by perceived social expectations. People often measure their self-worth based on how their purchases are perceived by others (Ordabayeva et al., 2022). When combined with personality traits such as neuroticism or extraversion, these sociocultural pressures can amplify compulsive tendencies (Tarka & Harnish, 2023). Moreover, studies indicate that those vulnerable to CBD often experience dissatisfaction with their social lives and resort to shopping as a compensatory strategy to cope with emotional or psychological voids.

Signs and Symptoms of Compulsive Buying Disorder

Compulsive Buying Disorder presents through a distinct set of behavioral and emotional symptoms. Individuals often report an overwhelming preoccupation with shopping, alongside frequent urges to make purchases that feel difficult or impossible to resist (Müller et al., 2021). These buying episodes are typically unplanned and impulsive, leading to temporary gratification but followed by intense guilt, regret, or psychological discomfort (Darrat et al., 2022; Müller et al., 2020).

Financial strain is a common consequence, as excessive spending habits often outpace income, resulting in debt accumulation and potential legal troubles (Ünübol et al., 2022). The compulsive nature of the disorder not only jeopardizes financial stability but also contributes to relationship difficulties, as affected individuals may conceal purchases or lie about spending. Emotional responses such as shame, anxiety, and low self-worth are closely linked to these behaviors, creating a vicious cycle in which distress fuels further compulsive shopping (Darrat et al., 2022).

The pattern of repeated spending, followed by negative emotional fallout, distinguishes CBD from normative consumer behavior. As a result, clinical interventions must focus not only on behavior management but also on addressing the emotional and psychological underpinnings of the disorder.

HISTORICAL BACKGROUND OF COMPULSIVE BUYING DISORDER

This section will focus on the historical background of compulsive buying disorder backed with theories of compulsive buying. Compulsive Buying Disorder (CBD) was first described clinically by Emil Kraepelin and Eugen Bleuler in their textbooks early in the 20th century. Kraepelin described this disorder as ' buying mania' characterized by compulsive shopping and called them 'Oniomaniacs': 'Onio' in Greek meant 'for sale' and 'mania' meant 'insanity'. He described it as a pathological condition, whereby the individual is addicted to buying things and services and spending leisure time shopping (Jose, 2023). Eugen Bleuler elaborated the concept further in 1924 categorising it as 'reactive impulse' alongside pyromania and kleptomania (Jose, 2023; Tavaeres et al., 2008). Throughout the twentieth century, compulsive buying disorder received limited attention after its initial description,except for among consumer behaviorists and psychoanalysts. In the early nineteenth and twentieth century, compulsive buying started to be identified as a psychiatric illness. While some researchers considered CBD as an addictive disorder, others considered it as a part of obsessive compulsive disorder and mood disorder (Tavares et al., 2008). A resurgence of compulsive buying occurred in the early 1990s with three independent clinical case series involving 90 subjects published, reviving academic and clinical interest in the disorder (Tavares et al.,2018; Black, 2007).

THEORIES OF COMPULSIVE BUYING

Disease theory and biological factors have identified the underlying genetic predisposition of CBD, suggesting that compulsive buying runs in families and that within these families, mood, anxiety, and substance use disorders are excessively prevalent (Workman & Paper, 2010). Neurobiological explanations suggest the neural circuits of compulsive buying to be similar to that of other addictions like gambling and that such behaviours are maintained by the brain's reward system (Lejoyeux & Weinstein, 2010). Neurobiological theories explain disturbances in the serotonergic, dopaminergic, and opioid transmission networks to be the reason for compulsive buying. Research says that the dopaminergic system that regulates pleasure and reward tends to be hyperactive in compulsive buyers, leading to heightened sensitivity to positive reinforcement of shopping (Black, 2007). This is similar to other addictive behaviours like gambling. Sociocultural theories have explained compulsive buying as a sociocultural phenomenon facilitated by contemporary marketing strategies. Cultural mechanisms essential for compulsive buying to develop included the presence of a market-based economy, availability of a wide variety of goods, disposable income and significant leisure time (Tavares et al.,2008). Social learning theories have examined the role of feedback in compulsive buying. These theorists argue that compulsive buyers are less likely to reduce or stop their excessive shopping behaviors if they remain isolated, depressed, separated from non-compulsive consumers, or surrounded by other compulsive buyers. Additionally, when compulsive buyers receive predominantly positive reinforcement for their excessive shopping habits, they may feel psychologically validated or enabled, further encouraging their behavior. Consequently, many compulsive buyers align with the personality, disease, sociocultural, and social learning theoretical models previously discussed (Workman & Paper, 2010).

NEUROLOGICAL AND BIOLOGICAL UNDERPINNINGS

Brain Regions Involved in Compulsive Buying Disorder

Ventral Striatum (Nucleus Accumbens)

The ventral striatum, particularly the nucleus accumbens (NAcc), is central to reward anticipation and craving in CBD. Raab et al. (2011) demonstrated that compulsive buyers exhibit heightened NAcc activation during product presentation compared to non-compulsive buyers, correlating with increased purchasing propensity. This aligns with Trotzke et al. (2021), who found that ventral striatum activity in individuals with CBD is positively associated with symptom severity, suggesting its role in encoding the hedonic value of shopping-related cues. These findings mirror mechanisms observed in substance-use disorders, where the NAcc drives reward-seeking behavior through dopaminergic signaling (Raab et al., 2011; Trotzke et al., 2021).

Dorsal Striatum

The dorsal striatum, critical for habit formation and compulsive behaviors, shows heightened activation in CBD during cue-exposure. Trotzke et al. (2021) reported increased dorsal striatum (caudate nucleus) activity in CBD individuals when exposed to shopping cues, consistent with the transition from goal-directed to habitual behavior in later addiction stages. This shift may explain the persistent, uncontrollable urges to shop despite negative consequences, as the dorsal striatum mediates habitual "wanting" rather than conscious reward evaluation (Trotzke et al., 2021).

Insula

The insula, involved in processing negative arousal and loss aversion, exhibits reduced activity in CBD during price evaluation. Raab et al. (2011) found that compulsive buyers show diminished insular activation when confronted with product prices, impairing their sensitivity to financial loss. This hypoactivity may diminish the "pain of paying," facilitating impulsive purchases. In contrast, non-compulsive buyers display stronger insula engagement, reflecting heightened aversion to monetary costs (Raab et al., 2011).

Anterior Cingulate Cortex (ACC)

The ACC, implicated in conflict monitoring and emotional regulation, demonstrates altered function in CBD. Raab et al. (2011) observed heightened ACC activity in compulsive buyers during purchasing decisions, potentially linked to comorbid depression or decision-related conflict. This hyperactivity may reflect inefficient resolution of competing motivations (e.g., desire to buy vs. financial consequences), contributing to maladaptive decision-making (Raab et al., 2011).

Dopaminergic Pathways

Dopamine, a key neurotransmitter in reward processing, underpins striatal dysregulation in CBD. Trotzke et al. (2021) posit that dorsal striatum hyperactivity in CBD aligns with dopaminergic modulation of habitual behaviors, while ventral striatum engagement reflects residual reward anticipation. Raab et al. (2011) similarly associate NAcc activation with dopaminergic signaling, mirroring patterns in substance addiction where cues elicit dopamine release, reinforcing compulsive behaviors. These findings suggest that dopaminergic pathways mediate both the initial reward-driven phase and the later compulsive phase of CBD (Trotzke et al., 2021; Raab et al., 2011).

Clinical and Policy Implications

Understanding CBD's neural substrates informs therapeutic strategies. Trotzke et al. (2021) emphasize targeting cue-reactivity and craving through exposure therapy or mindfulness-based interventions to modulate striatal hyperactivity. Raab et al. (2011) highlight the need for policies recognizing CBD as a neuropsychiatric disorder, advocating for consumer protections (e.g., stricter credit regulations) to mitigate triggers. Delving deep into the neurological underpinnings underscore the importance of integrating neurobiological insights into psychotherapy to enhance inhibitory control and decision-making (Trotzke et al., 2021; Raab et al., 2011).

CBD is rooted in dysfunctions of the ventral and dorsal striatum, insula, and ACC, driven by dopaminergic reward pathways. These neural abnormalities parallel those in substance addiction, supporting CBD's classification as a behavioral addiction. Future research should explore longitudinal changes in striatal activity and dopaminergic modulation to refine therapeutic approaches.

PSYCHOLOGICAL AND COGNITIVE FACTORS

Cognitive Processes Associated with Addiction

Impulsivity: A Core Driver of CBD

Impulsivity, defined as a predisposition toward rapid, unplanned actions without regard for consequences, is a hallmark of CBD. Individuals with CBD exhibit elevated levels of trait impulsivity across multiple dimensions, including motor impulsivity (acting without thinking), attentional impulsivity (difficulty focusing), and non-planning impulsivity (lack of forethought) (Black et al., 2012). The Barratt Impulsiveness Scale (BIS) reveals that CBD patients score significantly higher than controls, particularly in motor impulsivity, which reflects immediate behavioral disinhibition (Black et al., 2012). This impulsivity fosters spontaneous purchasing, as individuals struggle to resist urges triggered by environmental cues (e.g., retail environments or online advertisements).

Impulsivity also mediates the relationship between personality traits and CBD. For instance, neuroticism and openness to experience indirectly influence compulsive buying through heightened impulsive tendencies (Shehzadi et al., 2016). Impulsive acts provide temporary relief from negative emotions, reinforcing the cycle of compulsive shopping (Black et al., 2012). Over time, chronic impulsivity escalates into compulsive patterns, as individuals increasingly rely on shopping to regulate emotional states (Shehzadi et al., 2016).

CBD patients exhibit elevated ADHD symptoms, particularly inattention and hyperactivity, which correlate with impulsivity. The ADHD Rating Scale reveals higher scores in CBD patients for items like “difficulty waiting turn” and “loses things” (Black et al., 2012). These symptoms suggest executive dysfunction, such as impaired inhibitory control and working memory, which may exacerbate impulsive buying. Notably, ADHD symptoms in CBD patients decline with treatment, indicating a bidirectional relationship where CBD and ADHD symptoms mutually reinforce maladaptive behaviors (Black et al., 2012).

Compulsivity: Persistence Despite Negative Consequences

Compulsivity in CBD manifests as repetitive shopping behaviors persisted despite adverse outcomes (e.g., financial debt, interpersonal conflict). While CBD shares features with obsessive-compulsive spectrum disorders (OCSD), neuropsychological studies reveal no significant deficits in executive function (e.g., cognitive flexibility, decision-making) in CBD patients, distinguishing it from traditional compulsivity seen in OCD (Black et al., 2012). Instead, compulsivity in CBD may stem from maladaptive coping mechanisms, where shopping serves as an escape from distress (Vasiliu, 2022). Functional MRI studies highlight heightened activation in the nucleus accumbens—a brain region associated with reward processing—during shopping episodes, suggesting that compulsive buying is reinforced by dopamine-driven pleasure responses (Black et al., 2012). This neurobiological overlap with behavioral addictions (e.g., gambling disorder) underscores the role of reward-seeking rather than cognitive control deficits in CBD compulsivity.

Cognitive Distortions: Skewed Thinking Patterns

Cognitive distortions perpetuate CBD by rationalizing excessive spending. Common distortions include:

- Denial: Minimizing the severity of financial or social consequences (e.g., "I can stop anytime").
- Justification: Framing purchases as necessary or deserved (e.g., "I work hard, so I deserve this").
- Emotional Reasoning: Associating shopping with emotional relief (e.g., "Buying this will make me feel better") (Shehzadi et al., 2016).

Cognitive-behavioral therapy (CBT) interventions target these distortions by challenging irrational beliefs and promoting adaptive coping strategies (Vasiliu, 2022). For example, restructuring thoughts like "I need this item to be happy" reduces the emotional dependency on shopping. Studies using the Yale-Brown Obsessive-Compulsive Scale-Shopping Version (YBOCS-SV) demonstrate that addressing such distortions significantly lowers CBD severity (Black et al., 2012).

Visual Perception and Product Involvement

CBD patients perform better on visual perception tasks (e.g., the WASI Picture Completion subtest), suggesting heightened attention to product (Black et al., 2012). This cognitive strength may increase susceptibility to marketing cues, as individuals fixate on aesthetic or sensory features of products, amplifying cravings.

Personality Traits Linked to CBD

Neuroticism: Emotional Instability as a Risk Factor

Neuroticism, characterized by emotional instability, anxiety, and susceptibility to stress, is strongly associated with CBD. Individuals high in neuroticism use shopping to alleviate negative affective states, such as sadness or loneliness (Shehzadi et al., 2016). The Temperament and Character Inventory (TCI) reveals that CBD patients score higher in novelty seeking and harm avoidance, traits linked to emotional dysregulation (Black et al., 2012). Neuroticism also correlates with comorbid mood and anxiety disorders, which exacerbate compulsive buying tendencies (Vasiliu, 2022). For instance, depressive symptoms may drive "retail therapy" as a short-term mood enhancer, perpetuating the cycle of CBD.

Sensation Seeking and Novelty Seeking

Novelty seeking, a dimension of Cloninger's psychobiological model, reflects a desire for new experiences and stimulation. CBD patients exhibit elevated novelty seeking, which is theorized to stem from low basal dopamine activity (Black et al., 2012). This trait drives individuals to seek excitement through shopping, as acquiring new items provides transient dopamine-mediated pleasure. Functional imaging studies corroborate this, showing heightened nucleus accumbens activation in CBD patients when exposed to desirable products (Black et al., 2012). Additionally, openness to experience—a Big Five trait encompassing curiosity and creativity—mediates impulsive buying, as individuals explore novel products without restraint (Shehzadi et al., 2016).

Conscientiousness as a Protective Factor

Conscientiousness, characterized by self-discipline and goal-directed behavior, is negatively correlated with CBD (Black et al., 2012). Highly conscientious individuals plan purchases, avoid debt, and resist impulsive urges, reducing CBD risk (Shehzadi et al., 2016).

Comorbidities and Psychological Vulnerabilities

CBD patients frequently present with psychiatric comorbidities:

- Mood Disorders: 62% of CBD patients have lifetime major depression (Black et al., 2012).

- Anxiety Disorders: 50% exhibit generalized anxiety or social phobia (Black et al., 2012).
- Impulse Control Disorders: 69% report co-occurring disorders like pathological gambling (Black et al., 2012).

These comorbidities exacerbate CBD by amplifying emotional distress and impairing self-regulation. For instance, depressive symptoms may drive shopping as a form of emotional escape, while anxiety increases susceptibility to impulsive purchases (Vasiliu, 2022).

SOCIAL AND ENVIRONMENTAL FACTORS

Family Dynamics: The Foundational Influence

Family environment plays a pivotal role in shaping compulsive buying tendencies, particularly through parenting styles, communication patterns, and emotional support.

Parental Behavior and Modeling

Parental behavior significantly impacts adolescents' susceptibility to CBD. Roberts et al. (2003) found that parental yielding—giving in to children's demands—increases the likelihood of compulsive buying. This permissive parenting style fails to instill self-regulation, leading to impulsive consumption as a coping mechanism (Gwin et al., 2004). Similarly, socio-oriented communication patterns, which prioritize social harmony over critical thinking, correlate with higher CBD rates. Families emphasizing obedience and conformity over autonomy may inadvertently foster dependency on material goods for emotional validation (Gwin et al., 2004; Singh & Nayak, 2016).

Family Cohesion vs. Conflict

Family cohesion, characterized by emotional bonding, mutual support, and effective conflict resolution, mitigates compulsive buying disorder (CBD) risk by fostering adolescents' self-esteem, which buffers against maladaptive coping mechanisms like compulsive shopping (Singh & Nayak, 2016; Grougiou et al., 2015). Cohesive families provide a secure environment that reduces stress and diminishes reliance on impulsive consumption. In contrast, families marked by low cohesion or conflict—such as unresolved arguments, emotional distance, or harsh disciplinary practices—undermine self-esteem and heighten stress, driving adolescents to seek validation through material possessions (Singh & Nayak, 2016). This dynamic is particularly evident in disrupted family structures (e.g., divorce or single-parent households), where reduced parental supervision and emotional support increase susceptibility to peer influence and impulsive behaviors (Grougiou et al., 2015). Critically, self-esteem fully mediates the relationship between familial discord and CBD, as individuals often turn to shopping to alleviate negative emotions rooted in childhood experiences or to compensate for diminished self-worth (Khorrami et al., 2015; Gwin et al., 2004). Together, these findings underscore the dual role of familial environments: cohesive bonds serve as protective factors, while conflict or emotional neglect perpetuates cycles of distress and compensatory consumption.

Tangible vs. Intangible Family Resources

Family resources also shape CBD trajectories. While intangible resources (e.g., love, attention) reduce compulsivity by fostering resilience, excessive tangible resources (e.g., spending money) paradoxically increase risk. Gwin et al. (2004) noted that adolescents with greater financial access often lack fiscal responsibility, normalizing impulsive purchases. This dichotomy underscores the need for balanced parenting that combines emotional support with financial literacy.

Lower SES exacerbates compulsive tendencies due to limited access to intangible resources like parental attention and emotional guidance. Grougiou et al. (2015) found that adolescents from low-SES families often adopt socio-oriented communication styles, where parents emphasize obedience over autonomy. This stifles cognitive development and encourages emotionally driven behaviors, including impulsive purchases. Conversely, higher-SES families promote concept-oriented communication, fostering critical thinking and reducing reliance on compulsive consumption for emotional relief.

Social Dynamics: Interpersonal Relationships and Communication

Social interactions outside the family unit further influence CBD, particularly through word-of-mouth (WOM) and societal expectations.

Peer Communication About Consumption

Adolescents who frequently discuss consumption matters with peers are more likely to internalize materialistic norms, viewing compulsive buying as a socially desirable behavior (Grougiou et al., 2015). For example, peer groups that glorify brand ownership or frequent shopping trips create environments where compulsive buying is normalized. However, paradoxically, adolescents from disrupted families may avoid such discussions to conceal socio-economic vulnerabilities, yet still engage in covert compulsive behaviors as a form of emotional escapism (Grougiou et al., 2015).

Word-of-Mouth and Social Validation

Khorrami et al. (2015) identified WOM as a critical driver of impulse buying, which escalates into CBD. Recommendations from peers or influencers validate purchasing decisions, creating a feedback loop where social approval becomes tied to consumption. This is exacerbated in cultures where materialism is synonymous with social status, compelling individuals to "keep up" with trends (Singh & Nayak, 2016).

Communication Styles and Social Connectedness

Communication styles within social networks also matter. Socio-oriented individuals, trained to prioritize others' opinions, are more prone to CBD due to fear of social exclusion (Gwin et al., 2004). Conversely, concept-oriented communication, which encourages independent decision-making, correlates with lower compulsivity. However, such communication is rare in environments where communal conformity dominates (Singh & Nayak, 2016).

Cultural and Societal Norms: Materialism and Gender Roles

Cultural values, particularly materialism and gender expectations, institutionalize compulsive buying behaviors.

Materialism as a Cultural Value

Materialistic societies equate self-worth with possessions, normalizing excessive consumption. Khorrami et al. (2015) found that available money directly fuels impulse buying, especially in cultures where wealth signals success. Similarly, Singh and Nayak (2016) linked low self-esteem—often stemming from societal pressure to conform—to higher CBD rates, as individuals use shopping to project an idealized self-image.

Gender Disparities

Gender roles further shape CBD prevalence. Women are disproportionately affected, partly due to socialization that frames shopping as a leisure activity or emotional outlet (Gwin et al., 2004). In patriarchal cultures, women may lack autonomy, leading to repressed emotions that manifest in compulsive buying (Singh & Nayak, 2016). Conversely, men are socialized toward alternative coping mechanisms, such as substance use, reducing their CBD likelihood (Gwin et al., 2004).

Role of Media and Internet Proliferation

The proliferation of digital media and internet technologies has profoundly influenced the emergence and perpetuation of compulsive buying-shopping disorder (CBSD). These platforms leverage psychological mechanisms to amplify consumption behaviors, often blurring the lines between adaptive and maladaptive purchasing patterns.

Mere Exposure Effect and Cognitive Prioritization

The mere exposure effect, which posits that repeated exposure to stimuli increases familiarity and preference, is central to understanding how digital environments foster CBSD. Social media platforms and online marketplaces inundate users with advertisements, product recommendations, and influencer endorsements, creating a continuous loop of exposure to consumer goods. Over time, this repeated exposure elevates the cognitive prioritization of shopping-related cues, making purchasing behaviors more automatic and less deliberative (Müller et al., 2021; Jameel et al., 2024). For instance, constant visibility of "idealized lifestyles" on social networking sites (SNS) triggers upward social comparisons, where individuals perceive material possessions as essential for social validation (Sharif & Yeoh, 2018; Jameel et al., 2024). This dynamic is exacerbated by platforms like Instagram and Facebook, where users curate aspirational content that normalizes excessive consumption (Müller et al., 2021).

Personalized Algorithms and Behavioral Reinforcement

Personalized algorithms play a critical role in shaping compulsive buying tendencies. E-commerce platforms and SNS employ machine learning to tailor content based on users' browsing histories, preferences, and purchasing patterns. These algorithms create "filter bubbles" that prioritize shopping opportunities, making it easier for individuals to encounter products aligned with their interests (Müller et al., 2021; Jameel et al., 2024). For example, targeted ads on social media exploit users' materialistic values by promoting products as solutions to identity confusion or low self-esteem (Sharif & Yeoh, 2018; Jameel et al., 2024). Such personalization not only increases the salience of shopping but also reduces the cognitive effort required to make purchases, fostering impulsive decision-making (Müller et al., 2021).

Coping Mechanisms and Emotional Relief

For many individuals, compulsive buying serves as a distraction-oriented coping strategy to escape negative emotions such as anxiety, loneliness, or stress. The anonymity and convenience of online shopping provide immediate—albeit temporary—emotional relief, reinforcing the behavior through operant conditioning (Müller et al., 2021; Jameel et al., 2024). Studies highlight that individuals with CBSD often experience cravings triggered by emotional distress, leading to cycles of "retail therapy" (Müller et al., 2021). Social media exacerbates this by offering a curated escape from reality, where shopping becomes a means to compensate for unmet psychological needs (Sharif & Yeoh, 2018). For instance, excessive SNS users report higher levels of money anxiety and power-prestige motives, driving them to seek gratification through compulsive purchases (Sharif & Yeoh, 2018).

Economic and Environmental Stressors

Compulsive buying is not only a psychological concern but also a socioeconomic and environmental issue. The financial and ecological consequences of CBSD create feedback loops that perpetuate individual and collective harm.

Debt Accumulation and Financial Instability

The ease of accessing credit systems and "buy now, pay later" schemes has intensified debt accumulation among compulsive buyers. Individuals with CBSD often exhibit poor impulse control, leading to unrestrained spending despite financial constraints (Müller et al., 2021; Jameel et al., 2024). For example, Malaysian youths with excessive SNS use reported higher credit card debts, as materialistic aspirations overshadowed fiscal responsibility (Sharif & Yeoh, 2018). Over time, this behavior results in financial insecurity, limiting long-term savings and exacerbating stress—a factor that paradoxically fuels further compulsive buying (Jameel et al., 2024).

Environmental Impact of Materialism

The environmental ramifications of CBSD are linked to hedonic consumption patterns and a culture of disposability. Materialistic values prioritize short-term gratification over sustainability, leading to frequent purchases of non-essential items (Jameel et al., 2024). This "fast fashion" mentality contributes to waste accumulation, as products are quickly discarded to make room for new acquisitions. While direct references to landfill deposits or resource depletion are limited in the literature, the environmental toll is implicit in studies linking materialism to overconsumption (Jameel et al., 2024). For instance, Saudi Arabian youths' compulsive buying behaviors, driven by social media and TV advertisements, reflect a broader trend of prioritizing status symbols over ecological mindfulness (Jameel et al., 2024).

DIAGNOSTIC CRITERIA OF CBD

Compulsive Buying Disorder (CBD) is a behavioral addiction characterized by chronic and repetitive purchasing triggered by emotional distress and followed by significant negative consequences. The diagnostic criteria was first proposed in 1994 and was later refined (Lejoyeux & Weinstein, 2010). These criteria define CBD as persistent preoccupations with buying or shopping, alongside an inability to resist the impulse, leading to purchases that exceed financial means or are unnecessary. This behavior causes distress, consumes significant time, and interferes with social, financial, or occupational functioning. Notably, CBD occurs independently of manic or hypomanic episodes, distinguishing it from bipolar-related spending behaviors. However, CBD is not officially enlisted as an independent mental disorder in the Diagnostic and Statistical Manual (DSM) 5 or International Classification of Diseases (ICD) 11 (Lejoyeux & Weinstein, 2010; Muller et al.,2021). Also, excessive buying has been considered as an important symptom of hoarding disorder in ICD -11 and as one form of excessive acquisition within the hoarding disorder in DSM -V (Muller et al.,2021). However, it is essential that a diagnostic criteria be developed for CBD to enable advancements in research in this area.

Muller and a group of researchers (2021) developed a diagnostic criteria for CBD using Delphi technique. The proposed draft diagnostic criteria for compulsive buying-shopping disorder given by them is as follows:

A. Persistent and/or recurrent dysfunctional buying/shopping-related behaviors, thoughts and related phenomena, as indicated by the following characteristics:

1. Intrusive and/or irresistible urges and/or impulses and/or cravings and/or preoccupations for buying/shopping as evidenced by:

a. Repetitive impulses to buy/shop
b. Strong desire or irresistible urge to engage in buying/shopping activities
c. Preoccupations with buying/shopping
d. Craving for the high or for relief while buying/shopping
e. Repetitive intrusive thoughts about buying/shopping

2. Diminished control over buying/shopping as evidenced by:
   a. Buying many more things or spending more than necessarily needed/intended
   b. Purchasing many more things than can be afforded
   c. Spending much more time buying/shopping than intended
   d. Repeated unsuccessful efforts to reduce or control buying/shopping activities
   e. Repeated unsuccessful efforts to stop thinking about buying/shopping
   f. Buying/shopping something "on the spur of the moment"
3. Excessive purchasing of items without utilizing them for their intended purposes
4. Use of buying/shopping to regulate internal states, e.g.,
   a. Generate or chase positive mood (e.g., pleasure, excitement, "high" while buying/shopping)
   b. Relieve negative mood (e.g., nervousness, tension, negative feelings and thoughts, discomfort, boredom)
5. Persistent and recurrent dysfunctional buying/shopping symptoms result in negative consequences and impairment in important areas of functioning, e.g.,
   a. Impairment in social life (e.g., familial discord, jeopardizing relationships)
   b. Clinically significant distress
   c. Negative feelings (e.g., shame, guilt, embarrassment, regret)
   d. Financial difficulties including indebtedness and bankruptcy
   e. Loss of interest or impairment in other important areas of functioning, e.g. everyday activities and hobbies, daily responsibilities
   f. Lying to others about buying/shopping (e.g., buying/shopping in secret, hiding bought things)
   g. Impairment in occupational functioning (e.g., risking career opportunities)
6. Reduction or cessation of excessive buying/shopping results in
   a. Negative emotional states (e.g., anxiety, restlessness, agitation, impatience, sadness, irritability, dysphoria, uncertainty, insecurity, anger, sustained tension) and/or
   b. Cognitive symptoms (e.g., worries, rumination, distractibility, cognitive constriction on buying/shopping)

B. Maintenance or escalation of dysfunctional buying/shopping behaviors despite negative consequences

C. The pattern of buying/shopping does not occur exclusively during a period of mania/hypomania

D. The pattern of buying/shopping is not better explained by the symptoms of another mental disorder (e.g., psychosis) or attributable to a medical condition (e.g., organic psycho syndrome)

Specifier: With vs. without excessive hoarding of purchased item.

Individuals with CBD often experience intrusive thoughts and urges related to shopping, resulting in a loss of control over buying behaviour. This causes excessive purchasing of unnecessary items, ultimately resulting in financial loss and interpersonal problems. Impulsivity is a hallmark of compulsive buyers because they struggle to control the urge to purchase, despite negative consequences. Emotional instability with heightened levels of anxiety and depression is common among compulsive buyers (Müller et al.2015). All these behaviours are often used as maladaptive cooing mechanisms to manage negative emotions or unsatisfactory social situations, further perpetuating the cycle of compulsive buying (Rachubińska et al., 2024). CBD is frequently associated with psychiatric comorbidities, notably mood disorders, anxiety, and obsessive-compulsive disorder (OCD). Depression often co-occurs, with studies showing increased prevalence of CBD in individuals experiencing recurrent depressive episodes. Additionally, compulsive buyers commonly report impulse control issues, such as kleptomania or bulimia, and higher rates of borderline and avoidant personality disorders. Materialism, desire for uniqueness and lack of self-control were also found to be positively correlated with compulsive buying (Rana & Malik, 2023). Though some similarities with OCD exist, compulsive buyers exhibit higher impulsivity and quicker decision-making, separating them diagnostically.

Screening and Diagnostic tools

Researchers have developed screening and diagnostic tools to identify CBD. These include the Compulsive Buying Scale, the Yale-Brown Obsessive Compulsive Scale-Shopping Version, the Questionnaire of Addicting Buying Behavior and the Bergen Shopping Addiction Scale (BSAS).

The Compulsive Buying Scale (Faber & O'Guinn, 1992) is a seven-item screening instrument developed to measure compulsive buying. Taking inspiration from this scale, Edwards (1993) developed Edwards Compulsive Buying Scale to assess how compulsive the individual is in their buying behaviour. The Questionnaire of Addictive Buying Behaviour (QABB) is a 19 item scale representing major items of buying behaviour (Lejoyeux & Ades, 1994). Monahan et al. (1996) adapted the Yale-Brown Obsessive Compulsive Scale (Y-BOCS) to assess compulsive shopping behavior, measuring symptom severity, distress, and functional impairment. The Bergen Shopping Addiction Scale was developed by Andreassen et al. (2015) to assess shopping addiction. The scale consisted of 7 items chosen based on the diagnostic criteria for pathological gambling, the Game Addiction Scale and a literature review of common symptoms associated with shopping and buying addiction. The respondents were asked to rate their agreement or disagreement regarding their shopping behaviour (Andreassen et al., 2015). The other screening tools include Canadian Compulsive Buying Measurement Scale, Minnesota Impulsive Buying Disorder Interview and Ridgway's Compulsive Buying Scale (Christenson et al., 1994; Ridgway et al., 2008; Valence et al., 1988). Although these instruments assess the severity of symptoms, preoccupations, urges, and the social or occupational disruptions caused by compulsive shopping, clinical evaluations remain essential, requiring detailed inquiries into buying attitudes, triggers, and consequences (Christenson et al., 1994; Ridgway et al., 2008; Valence et al., 1988).

Clinical challenges in diagnosing CBD

Conceptualizing compulsive buying disorder is a challenge considering the overlap with obsessive-compulsive disorders, addictive disorders and impulsive disorders (Grant & Chamberlain, 2024). There seems to be a significant symptomatic and diagnostic overlap between these disorders and hence differential diagnosis becomes challenging. This emphasizes the importance of a thorough clinical screening to understand frequently overlooked comorbidities and provide individualized treatment. Additionally, there is a critical need for high-quality clinical trials focused on compulsive buying disorder and large-scale longitudinal studies to better understand its presentation over time (Grant & Chamberlain, 2024). Literature says that normal buying should also be ruled out. Shopping is the main time pass of many women, particularly in the US and other developed countries, but this essentially does not qualify for evidence in support of CBD (Black, 2007). During special occasions, normal buying may sometimes take on a compulsive quality. Although research has not identified gender specific patterns of buying, men showed more interest in electronic devices, automotive and hardware, while women were keen on clothing, shoes and compact discs (Black, 2007).

Compulsive buying has a highly complex pathology that encompasses aspects of behavioral addictions, the obsessive-compulsive disorder spectrum, and impulse control disorders. Some individuals may align more closely with behavioural addictions, while others may exhibit stronger impulsivity, and some may present features associated with the OCD spectrum. Additionally, various combinations of these dimensions within a single patient are also theoretically possible. Hence, differential diagnosis is challenging (Vasiliu, 2022). In conclusion, CBD is a distinct behavioral addiction requiring specific diagnostic criteria and tools to differentiate it from related disorders. Comprehensive assessments and clinical insights are vital for effective diagnosis and management.

TREATMENT AND INTERVENTION APPROACHES FOR COMPULSIVE BUYING DISORDER

Compulsive Buying Disorder (CBD) is characterized by excessive, uncontrollable purchasing behaviors that lead to psychological distress and financial harm. Effective interventions often integrate psychotherapeutic, pharmacological, and adjunctive strategies. This chapter synthesizes evidence-based approaches from current research, focusing on major therapeutic modalities, pharmacotherapy, and treatment challenges.

Major Psychotherapeutic Approaches

Cognitive Behavioral Therapy (CBT) and Group CBT

Cognitive Behavioral Therapy (CBT) is the most empirically supported intervention for CBD. Structured protocols typically span 12 weekly sessions, targeting maladaptive thoughts, emotional triggers, and behaviors. Key components include psychoeducation, cognitive restructuring, financial management (e.g., discarding credit cards), exposure with response prevention, and relapse prevention (Mitchell et al., 2006; Mueller et al., 2008). Group CBT enhances accountability and social support, with studies showing significant reductions in compulsive buying symptoms post-treatment and sustained improvements at six-month follow-ups (Mueller et al., 2008). For instance, a randomized trial demonstrated that group CBT reduced Yale-Brown Obsessive-Compulsive Scale-Shopping Version (YBOCS-SV) scores significantly compared to waitlist controls (Mueller et al., 2008).

Motivational Interviewing and Imaginal Desensitization

Motivational interviewing (MI) fosters intrinsic behavioral change by resolving ambivalence, while imaginal desensitization uses guided visualization to reduce urges. A case study combining MI with imaginal desensitization and naltrexone reported reduced compulsive buying behaviors, with effects maintained at six months (Donahue et al., 2011). These techniques help patients confront triggers in a controlled manner, promoting healthier coping strategies.

Acceptance and Commitment Therapy (ACT)

ACT emphasizes psychological flexibility through mindfulness, value-driven actions, and acceptance of distressing emotions. A study on women with CBD found that an 8-session ACT protocol significantly improved emotional self-control, flexibility, and valued living compared to controls (Danesh-Mirkohan et al., 2021). By aligning behaviors with personal values (e.g., financial stability), ACT reduces the reliance on shopping for emotional regulation.

Group Therapy: Stopping Overshopping Model

Structured group interventions, such as the 12-session Stopping Overshopping model, integrate CBT principles with skill-building (e.g., stress management, social skills). Participants learn to replace compulsive behaviors with adaptive alternatives, supported by peer accountability (Mitchell et al., 2006).

Psychopharmacological Treatments

Antidepressants

Selective serotonin reuptake inhibitors (SSRIs), such as fluvoxamine and citalopram, are commonly prescribed. Fluvoxamine (100–200 mg/day) combined with CBT led to symptom remission in case studies (Marcinko & Karlovi, 2005). Similarly, open-label trials report reductions in CBD symptoms with citalopram, though evidence remains limited (McElroy et al., 1994).

Naltrexone

The opioid antagonist naltrexone (50–90 mg/day) has shown promise in curbing craving-driven behaviors. A case study pairing naltrexone with MI and imaginal desensitization highlighted its potential in reducing purchase urges (Donahue et al., 2011).

Other Approaches

Support Groups and Debtors Anonymous

Peer-led support groups, such as Debtors Anonymous, provide accountability and practical strategies for financial recovery. A case study noted improved outcomes when behavioral therapy was supplemented with group participation (Fong et al., 2012).

Challenges in Treatment

Relapse Rates

While CBT and pharmacotherapy yield short-term improvements, relapse remains common. Follow-up studies indicate that 50–60% of patients maintain abstinence at six months, underscoring the need for long-term support (Mueller et al., 2008).

Comorbidities

CBD frequently coexists with mood, anxiety, and impulse-control disorders, complicating treatment. For example, 80% of patients in one sample had comorbid Axis I diagnoses (Mueller et al., 2007). Tailored interventions addressing dual diagnoses are critical.

Diagnosis Challenges

The absence of CBD in the DSM-5 contributes to underdiagnosis and delayed treatment. Clinicians often rely on criteria proposed by McElroy et al. (1994), which emphasize preoccupation with buying, financial harm, and impaired functioning.

CONCLUSION

Effective CBD management requires a multimodal approach, combining CBT, ACT, and pharmacotherapy. Group interventions and support networks enhance sustainability, while addressing comorbidities and relapse risks improves long-term outcomes. Future research should standardize diagnostic criteria and explore novel interventions, such as neuromodulation, to address unresolved challenges.

REFERENCES

Aboujaoude, E. (2014). Compulsive buying disorder: A review and update. *Current Pharmaceutical Design*, *20*(25), 4021–4025. DOI: 10.2174/13816128113199990618 PMID: 24001296

American Psychiatric Association. (2013). *Diagnostic and statistical manual of mental disorders* (5th ed.)., DOI: 10.1176/appi.books.9780890425596

Amin, H. S., Nagshabandi, K., & Alhammad, S. (2022). Compulsive buying disorder (CBD) among medical students in colleges of medicine, dentistry and pharmacy at King Saud University in Riyadh. *Journal of Family Medicine and Primary Care*, *11*(11), 6876–6884. DOI: 10.4103/jfmpc.jfmpc_769_22 PMID: 36993053

Andreassen, C. S., Griffiths, M. D., Pallesen, S., Bilder, R. M., Torsheim, T., & Aboujaoude, E. (2015). The Bergen Shopping Addiction Scale: Reliability and validity of a brief screening test. *Frontiers in Psychology*, *6*, 1374. DOI: 10.3389/fpsyg.2015.01374 PMID: 26441749

Belk, R. W. (1988). Possessions and the extended self. *The Journal of Consumer Research*, *15*(2), 139–168. DOI: 10.1086/209154

Benson, A. L. (Ed.). (2000). *I shop, therefore I am: Compulsive buying and the search for self*. Jason Aronson.

Blac, K. D. W. (2007). A review of compulsive buying disorder. *World Psychiatry; Official Journal of the World Psychiatric Association (WPA)*, *6*(1), 14–18. PMID: 17342214

Black, D. W. (2001). Compulsive buying disorder: Definition, assessment, epidemiology and clinical management. *CNS Drugs*, *15*(1), 17–27. DOI: 10.2165/00023210-200115010-00003 PMID: 11465011

Black, D. W. (2007). Compulsive buying disorder: A review of the evidence. *CNS Spectrums*, *12*(2), 124–132. DOI: 10.1017/S1092852900020630 PMID: 17277712

Black, D. W., Shaw, M., McCormick, B., Bayless, J. D., & Allen, J. (2012). Neuropsychological performance, impulsivity, ADHD symptoms, and novelty seeking in compulsive buying disorder. *Psychiatry Research*, *200*(2-3), 581–587. DOI: 10.1016/j.psychres.2012.06.003 PMID: 22766012

Bleuler, E. (1930). *Textbook of psychiatry*. Macmillan.

Christenson, G. A., Faber, R. J., De Zwaan, M., Raymond, N. C., Specker, S. M., Ekern, M. D., & Eckert, E. D. (1994). Compulsive buying: Descriptive characteristics and psychiatric comorbidity. *The Journal of Clinical Psychiatry*, *55*(1), 5–11. PMID: 8294395

Danesh, M. R. A., Taklavi, S., & Kazemi, R. (2021). The Effectiveness of Acceptance and Commitment Therapy on Emotional Self-Control, Emotional Flexibility, and the Valued Living among Women with Compulsive Buying Disorder.

Darrat, A. A., Darrat, M., & Darrat, M. A. (2022). Does wanting more lead to losing control? Examining the psychological drivers of compulsive buying. *Young Consumers*, *24*(1), 56–73. DOI: 10.1108/YC-01-2022-1453

Donahue, C. B., Odlaug, B. L., & Grant, J. E. (2011). Compulsive buying treated with motivational interviewing and imaginal desensitization. *Annals of Clinical Psychiatry*, *23*, 226–227. PMID: 21808756

Edwards, E. A. (1993). Edwards Compulsive Buying Scale. *Financial Counseling and Planning*.

Faber, R. J., & O'guinn, T. C. (1992). A clinical screener for compulsive buying. *The Journal of Consumer Research*, *19*(3), 459–469. DOI: 10.1086/209315

Filomensky, T. Z., & Tavares, H. (2021). *Compulsive buying disorder*. Springer., DOI: 10.1007/978-3-030-36391-8_69

Fong, T. W., Reid, R. C., & Parhami, I. (2012). Behavioral Addictions Where to Draw the Lines? *The Psychiatric Clinics of North America*, *35*(2), 279–296. DOI: 10.1016/j.psc.2012.03.001 PMID: 22640756

González-Fuente, B., & de la Villa Moral Jiménez, M. (2024). Compra compulsiva online y offline y su relación con la ansiedad estado-rasgo y la impulsividad. *Behavioral Psychology–Psicologia Conductual,* 249–267. https://doi.org/DOI: 10.51668/bp.8324202s

Grant, J. E., & Chamberlain, S. R. (2024). Compulsive buying disorder: Conceptualization based on addictive, impulsive, and obsessive-compulsive features and comorbidity. *Psychiatry Research Communications*, *4*(4), 100199. DOI: 10.1016/j.psycom.2024.100199

Grougiou, V., Moschis, G., & Kapoutsis, I. (2015). Compulsive buying: The role of earlier-in-life events and experiences. *Journal of Consumer Marketing*, *32*(4), 278–289. DOI: 10.1108/JCM-01-2015-1283

Gwin, C. F., Roberts, J. A., & Martínez, C. R. (2004). Nature vs. Nurture: The Role of Family in Compulsive Buying. *Nature*.

Hollander, E. (Ed.). (1993). *Obsessive-compulsive related disorders*. American Psychiatric Press.

Jameel, A., Khan, S., Alonazi, W. B., & Khan, A. A. (2024). Exploring the Impact of Social Media Sites on Compulsive Shopping Behavior: The Mediating Role of Materialism. *Psychology Research and Behavior Management*, *17*, 171–185. DOI: 10.2147/PRBM.S442193 PMID: 38250636

Jose, A. (2023). A study on the effects of compulsive buying behavior and shopping addiction on the self-esteem of college-going female students. *International Journal of Indian Psychology*, *11*(4), 585–592. DOI: 10.25215/1104.052

Khorrami, M. S., Esfidani, M. R., & Delavari, S. (2015). The effect of situational factors on impulse buying and compulsive buying: Clothing. International Journal of Management. *Accounting and Economics*, *2*(8), 823–837.

Krych, R. (1989). Abnormal consumer behavior: A model of addictive behaviors. *Advances in Consumer Research. Association for Consumer Research (U. S.)*, *16*, 745–748.

Lee, S., & Mysyk, A. (2004). The medicalization of compulsive buying. *Social Science & Medicine*, *58*(9), 1709–1718. DOI: 10.1016/S0277-9536(03)00340-X PMID: 14990372

Leftwich, B. M. (2022). Compulsive buying behavior and its association with emotional distress, depression, and impulsivity in general population: An online survey. 1–15. https://doi.org/DOI: 10.1017/S1092852922001109

Leite, P. L., Pereira, V. M., Nardi, A. E., & Silva, A. C. (2014). Psychotherapy for compulsive buying disorder: A systematic review. *Psychiatry Research*, *219*(3), 411–419. DOI: 10.1016/j.psychres.2014.05.037 PMID: 25023363

Lejoyeux, M., & Ades, J. (1994). Les achats pathologiques: Une addiction comportementale. *Neuro-Psy*, *9*(1), 25–32.

Lejoyeux, M., Andes, J., & Tassian, V.. (1996). Phenomenology and psychopathology of uncontrolled buying. *The American Journal of Psychiatry*, *152*, 1524–1529. PMID: 8942446

Lejoyeux, M., & Weinstein, A. (2010). Compulsive Buying. *The American Journal of Drug and Alcohol Abuse*, *36*(5), 248–253. DOI: 10.3109/00952990.2010.493590 PMID: 20560822

Marcinko, D., & Karlovi, D. (2005). Oniomania—successful treatment with fluvoxamine and cognitive-behavioral psychotherapy. *Psychiatria Danubina, 17*, 97–100. PMID: 16395851

McElroy, S., Keck, P. E.Jr, & Pope, H. G.Jr. (1994). Compulsive buying: A report of 20 cases. *The Journal of Clinical Psychiatry, 55*, 242–248. PMID: 8071278

Mitchell, J. E., Burgard, M., Faber, R., Crosby, R. D., & deZwaan, M. (2006). Cognitive behavioral therapy for compulsive buying disorder. *Behaviour Research and Therapy, 44*(12), 1859–1865. DOI: 10.1016/j.brat.2005.12.009 PMID: 16460670

Monahan, P., Black, D. W., & Gabel, J. (1996). Reliability and validity of a scale to measure change in persons with compulsive buying. *Psychiatry Research, 64*(1), 59–67. DOI: 10.1016/0165-1781(96)02908-3 PMID: 8888365

Mueller, A., Mitchell, J. E., Mertens, C., Mueller, U., Silbermann, A., Burgard, M., & deZwaan, M. (2007). Comparison of treatment seeking compulsive buyers in Germany and the United States. *Behaviour Research and Therapy, 45*(7), 1629–1638. DOI: 10.1016/j.brat.2006.08.005 PMID: 17049486

Mueller, A., Mueller, U., Silbermann, A., Reinecker, H., Bleich, S., Mitchell, J. E., & deZwaan, M. (2008). A randomized, controlled trial of group cognitive-behavioral therapy for compulsive buying disorder: Posttreatment and 6-month follow-up results. *The Journal of Clinical Psychiatry, 69*(7), 1131–1138. DOI: 10.4088/JCP.v69n0713 PMID: 18557665

Müller, A., Claes, L., Birlin, A., Georgiadou, E., Laskowski, N. M., Steins-Loeber, S., Brand, M., Brand, M., & de Zwaan, M. (2020). Associations of buying-shopping disorder symptoms with identity confusion, materialism, and socially undesirable personality features in a community sample. *European Addiction Research, 27*(2), 142–150. DOI: 10.1159/000511078 PMID: 33120395

Müller, A., & de Zwaan, M. (2010). Pathological buying. A review of the current knowledge regarding this condition of behavioral excess. *Bundesgesundheitsblatt, Gesundheitsforschung, Gesundheitsschutz, 53*(4), 289–294. PMID: 20182679

Müller, A., Laskowski, N. M., Trotzke, P., Ali, K., Fassnacht, D. B., de Zwaan, M., Brand, M., Häder, M., & Kyrios, M. (2021). Proposed diagnostic criteria for compulsive buying-shopping disorder: A Delphi expert consensus study. *Journal of Behavioral Addictions, 10*(2), 208–222. DOI: 10.1556/2006.2021.00013 PMID: 33852420

Müller, A., Laskowski, N. M., Wegmann, E., Steins-Loeber, S., & Brand, M. (2021). Problematic Online Buying-Shopping: Is it Time to Consider the Concept of an Online Subtype of Compulsive Buying-Shopping Disorder or a Specific Internet-Use Disorder? *Current Addiction Reports*, *8*(4), 494–499. DOI: 10.1007/s40429-021-00395-3

Müller, A., Mitchell, J. E., & de Zwaan, M. (2015). Compulsive buying. *Journal of Behavioral Addictions*, *4*(3), 132–137. PMID: 26551898

Narayanan, A. H., Rajasekar, V. D., Danasekaran, R., Surya, B., Manoj, P., Kumar, S., Syed, R. N., & Ramesh, H. (2025). Compulsive buying disorder among medicine, dentistry, and nursing undergraduate students from Chengalpattu District, Tamil Nadu, India: A cross-sectional study. *Journal of Clinical and Diagnostic Research : JCDR*. Advance online publication. DOI: 10.7860/JCDR/2025/76372.20551

Ordabayeva, N., Lisjak, M., & Jones, A. C. (2022). How social perceptions influence consumption for self, for others, and within the broader system. *Current Opinion in Psychology*, *43*, 30–35. DOI: 10.1016/j.copsyc.2021.06.009 PMID: 34274563

Qureshi, F. H., Sokić, K., & Khawaja, S. (2024). Impulsive buying tendencies and personality: Cognitive and affective aspects. https://doi.org/DOI: 10.20944/preprints202409.2097.v1

Raab, G., Elger, C. E., Neuner, M., & Weber, B. (2011). A neurological study of compulsive buying behaviour. *Journal of Consumer Policy*, *34*(4), 401–413. DOI: 10.1007/s10603-011-9168-3

Rachubińska, K., Cybulska, A. M., Szylińska, A., Kupcewicz, E., Ćwiek, D., Walaszek, I., & Grochans, E. (2024). Psychosocial functioning of individuals at risk of developing compulsive buying disorder. *Journal of Clinical Medicine*, *13*(5), 1339. DOI: 10.3390/jcm13051339 PMID: 38592171

Rachubińska, K., Cybulska, A. M., Szylińska, A., Kupcewicz, E., Ćwiek, D., Walaszek, I., & Grochans, E. (2024). Psychosocial Functioning of Individuals at Risk of Developing Compulsive Buying Disorder. *Journal of Clinical Medicine*, *13*(5), 1339. DOI: 10.3390/jcm13051339 PMID: 38592171

Rana, M., & Malik, P. (2023). Determinants of compulsive buying behavior: Psychosomatic- social analysis of maladaptive spending. *Journal of Positive School Psychology*, *7*, 204–224.

Ridgway, N. M., Kukar-Kinney, M., & Monroe, K. B. (2008). An expanded conceptualization and a new measure of compulsive buying. *The Journal of Consumer Research*, *35*(4), 622–639. DOI: 10.1086/591108

Roberts, J. A., Manolis, C., & Tanner, J. F.Jr. (2003). Family structure, materialism, and compulsive buying: A reinquiry and extension. *Journal of Technological Advancements*, *31*(3), 300–311. DOI: 10.1177/0092070303031003007

Sathya, J., Babu, M., Gayathri, J., Indhumathi, G., Samad, Z. A., & Anandhi, E. (2023). Compulsive buying behavior and online shopping addiction of women. *Information Science Letters*, *12*(5), 1641–1650. DOI: 10.18576/isl/120512

Sharif, S. P., & Yeoh, K. K. (2018). Excessive Social Networking Sites Use and Online Compulsive Buying in Young Adults: The Mediating Role of Money Attitude. *Young Consumers*, *19*(3), 310–327. DOI: 10.1108/YC-10-2017-00743

Shehzadi, K., Ahmad-ur-Rehman, M., Cheema, A. M., & Ahkam, A. (2016). Impact of personality traits on compulsive buying behavior: Mediating role of impulsive buying. *Journal of Service Science and Management*, *9*(5), 416–432. DOI: 10.4236/jssm.2016.95046

Singh, R., & Nayak, J. K. (2016). Effect of family environment on adolescent compulsive buying: Mediating role of self-esteem. *Asia Pacific Journal of Marketing and Logistics*, *28*(3), 396–419. DOI: 10.1108/APJML-05-2015-0082

Strizhak, A., & Mancheva, I. K. (2022). The impact of sociocultural factors on demonstrative consumption: A theoretical analysis. *Vestnik Tomskogo Gosudarstvennogo Universiteta.Ekonomika (Nis)*, *58*(58), 5–23. DOI: 10.17223/19988648/58/1

Tarka, P., & Harnish, R. J. (2023). Toward better understanding the materialism-hedonism and the Big Five personality-compulsive buying relationships: A new consumer cultural perspective. *Journal of Global Marketing*, *36*(3), 165–192. DOI: 10.1080/08911762.2023.2188509

Tavares, H., Sabbatini, D., Lobo, S., & Fuentes, D. (2008). Compras compulsivas: uma revisão e um relato de caso Compulsive buying disorder: a review and a Case Vignette. *Revista Brasileira de Psiquiatria : Orgão Oficial da Associação Brasileira de Psiquiatria, Asociación Psiqui´trica de la América Latina*, •••, 30.

Trotzke, P., Starcke, K., Pedersen, A., & Brand, M. (2021). Dorsal and ventral striatum activity in individuals with buying-shopping disorder during cue-exposure: A functional magnetic resonance imaging study. *Addiction Biology*, *26*(6), e13073. DOI: 10.1111/adb.13073 PMID: 34156751

Ünübol, B., Ünsalver, B. Ö., Ünübol, H., & Hızlı Sayar, G. (2022). The prevalence and psychological relation of problem shopping: Data from a large-scale sample from Turkey. *BMC Psychology*, *10*(1), 1. Advance online publication. DOI: 10.1186/s40359-021-00711-6 PMID: 34980253

Valence, G., d'Astous, A., & Fortier, L. (1988). Compulsive buying: Concept and measurement. *Journal of Consumer Policy*, *11*(4), 419–433. DOI: 10.1007/BF00411854

Vasiliu, O. (2022). Therapeutic management of buying/shopping disorder: A systematic literature review and evidence-based recommendations. *Frontiers in Psychiatry*, *13*, 1047280. DOI: 10.3389/fpsyt.2022.1047280 PMID: 36405896

Vasiliu, O., & Vasile, D. (2017). Compulsive buying disorder: A review of current data. *02*.https://www.iaras.org/iaras/home/caijems/compulsive-buying-disorder-a-review-of-current-data

Weinstein, A., Maraz, A., Griffiths, M. D., Lejoyeux, M., & Demetrovics, Z. (2016). Compulsive buying—features and characteristics of addiction. In *Neuropathology of drug addictions and substance misuse* (pp. 993–1007). Academic Press. DOI: 10.1016/B978-0-12-800634-4.00098-6

Workman, L., & Paper, D. (2010). Compulsive Buying: A Theoretical Framework. *Journal of Business Inquiry*, •••, 9.

Chapter 7
Exercise Addiction

Tiffany Lee
https://orcid.org/0000-0001-8177-8225
Western Michigan University, USA

Lyndsay R. Nuyen
https://orcid.org/0009-0005-7056-1019
Western Michigan University, USA

Blaire Zielke
Western Michigan University, USA

ABSTRACT

This chapter provides an overview of the history and evolution of exercise addiction (EA), including current prevalence rates. Neurobiological and physiological features of EA are discussed as well as the characteristics of individuals who fit the proposed criteria of EA. The authors introduce screening and assessment instruments and the available psychotherapeutic and pharmacological approaches for treating this addictive behavior. The next section explores the overlap between EA and conditions such as eating disorders, body dysmorphic disorder, shopping addiction, substance use, and other psychiatric issues. The chapter also highlights cultural considerations and concludes with advocacy goals, and proposals for further research.

INTRODUCTION

The history and evolution of how researchers and professionals have defined Exercise Addiction (EA) has been documented for decades. Over the past 50 years, there has been a remarkable increase in attention to the identification of, and treatment for, excessive exercise as a behavioral disorder. There was little mention of EA

DOI: 10.4018/979-8-3373-0518-9.ch007

in the mental health field until the 1970s (Adams, 2013) when the term "exercise dependence" began to be noted in the literature. During that time, it was mostly viewed as a positive, beneficial phenomenon. In 1987, however, diagnostic criteria were proposed, and advocacy was emerging for the recognition of exercise as a potentially compulsive, harmful behavior (Veale, 1987).

Since 2010, the number of peer-reviewed publications on this topic has sky-rocketed and continues to highlight the diversity of ideology and interpretations of exercise as a distinct addictive behavior (Weinstein & Szabo, 2023). For instance, questions continue to arise regarding how to classify whether a person is exhibiting an addiction to exercise with normal, healthy levels of eating behaviors (i.e., primary dependence), or is showing manifestations of behaviors associated with unhealthy, eating disturbances such as anorexia nervosa (i.e., secondary dependence). In addition to inquiries related to eating behaviors, professionals screening for EA may also be required to separate excessive exercise from other pathologies, including Body Dysmorphic Disorder (Lim, 2021).

Nomenclature And Classification

Physical exercise is defined as "planned, structured, repetitive, and purposive activity" (Marques et al., 2019, p. 319) that can be harmful when excessive. Excessive exercise has been classified in a variety of ways. Despite the recent attention of its existence, there are contrasting opinions surrounding exercise as a distinct category which warrants its inclusion in future editions of the American Psychiatric Association's (APA) *Diagnostic and Statistical Manual of Mental Disorders (DSM)*. If exercise is a behavior to be considered in the *DSM,* there must be agreement on: (1) whether it is a dependence or an addiction, (2) if it falls into the obsessive-compulsive category, and (3) if it is a primary or secondary problem.

Engagement in sports, exercise, and other physical activities can result in symptoms that mirror the criteria employed to screen and assess for substance use disorders. Inquiries remain unanswered about whether to define exercise as a dependence and/or addiction and what criteria should be used in determining such behavior. Some scholars report that "excessive exercise is most usually described as a dependence on exercise rather than as an addiction" (Adams, 2013, p. 829), while others have used these two terms interchangeably. For instance, Marques et al. (2019) describes exercise as a dependency and included words such as "compulsive" and "consequences" in its definition—which are terms used in association with the four Cs of addiction (i.e., compulsion, consequences, control and craving). They go further to indicate that dependency on exercise can cause a person to exhibit signs similar to addiction such as mood disturbance, dedicating too much time to the behavior, and tolerance. Other aspects have been identified that also reflect addiction symptomology including withdrawals, continuing physical activity despite illness or injury, and negative affect and anxiety when abstaining from exercise (Colledge et al., 2019). Many authors have used the terminology "exercise addiction" specifically in the title of the works (e.g., Colledge et al., 2019; Landolfi, 2013; Weinstein & Szabo, 2023) and claim it as such. The variation in the terminology used in the field will become quite evident later in this chapter when the components of screening and assessment instruments are presented, as they are based on different conceptual frameworks.

One important framework to highlight when reviewing classifications of excessive exercise is the differentiation between a "primary" or "secondary" dependence. Primary dependence is when an individual (a) has a dependency on exercise, based on endorsed criteria, and (b) there is no presence of a co-occurring disorder such as an eating disorder or Body Dysmorphic Disorder. Thus, there are normal eating patterns, and the reward is directly associated with fulfilling the activity (Adams, 2013). Secondary dependence to exercise, on the other hand, is when another co-occurring disorder exists that drives the physical activity. In essence, exercise is instrumental in meeting the other objective (e.g., losing weight, gaining muscle mass). Recently, two scholars in the field recommended the phrase "instrumental exercise" to refer to secondary dependence (Szabo & Demetrovics, 2022) as the term helps to differentiate it from addiction and lessen the confusion which surrounds how to define this type of behavior.

In summary, exercise that is deemed harmful, compulsive, and excessive is not a behavioral disorder outlined in the most recent edition of the *DSM* and there is not a universally accepted definition. For the purposes of this chapter, Exercise Addiction is considered a pattern of behavior in which the individual loses control over their exercise habits and acts compulsively, exhibits primary dependence, and experiences negative consequences. Moreover, to remain consistent with the terminology cited more frequently in the current literature and to reflect the title of this publication, the current authors will use the term Exercise Addiction (EA) in lieu of exercise dependence.

Prevalence

With the increased number of publications over the last two decades on EA, researchers have been able to conduct more systematic reviews and meta-analyses to ascertain prevalence rates. Moreover, these results have shown differences among various demographic characteristics (e.g., gender, age, college students/non-athletes, country) and types of exercise (e.g., cross-fit, marathon running, cycling, power disciplines). This section will highlight findings found in the last 10 years.

While the rates of EA have widely varied, systematic reviews have indicated that 0.3-6.4% of the U.S. general population may have an EA and up to 9% of athletes (Di Lodovico et al., 2019; Marques et al., 2019). One meta-analysis of 13 studies on EA, with over 3600 participants, showed a 6.2% prevalence rate; the highest was among general exercisers (8.1%) compared to amateur competitive athletes (5.0%; Trott et al., 2020). Another U.S. study of 1,285 triathletes (53.7% female) estimated 20% of the sample had an EA (Youngman & Simpson, 2014). Gym/health club users show an even higher rate of EA. For example, one investigation found the prevalence of EA among those who use health clubs was 30.7% (Trott et al., 2020). It was noted that their sample consisted of 85% female participants.

With regard to gender, EA seems to be more prevalent in males. In fact, one recent systematic review of 27 studies, found that only two studies reported that the prevalence for EA was higher in women than men (Dumitru et al., 2018). It should also be noted that comparisons between genders suggest that males are more likely to have a primary EA than females (Adams, 2013; Nogueira et al., 2019).

When distinguishing between primary dependence versus secondary dependence (i.e., instrumental exercise) among the general population, the prevalence for primary EA is estimated to be 1.4%, while instrumental exercise is approximately 5.0% (Marques et al., 2019). Within the health club setting, primary dependence is significantly higher. For instance, one meta-analysis found 11.4% of health club users had a primary EA, or an EA in the absence of an eating disorder (Trott et al., 2020). When researchers studied instrumental exercise as a behavior linked to an eating disorder, participants with an indicated eating disorder were over 3.5 times more likely to also have an addiction to exercise compared to their counterparts that do not have an indicated eating disorder (Trott et al., 2021).

Studies conducted outside of the United States have produced findings worth noting; some countries have similar prevalence rates. Corazza and colleagues (2019), for example, surveyed over 1,600 participants who have memberships at fitness centers in four different countries. Of these countries, the presence of EA was highest in the Netherlands (20.9%), followed by the United Kingdom (16.1%), Hungary (9.3%) and Italy (7.9%). Exercise Addiction was detected in 11.7% of the overall sample, with a higher prevalence demonstrated in males (15%) versus females (10%). These data reflect some of the results cited above from the U.S. related to gender and fitness center EA rates (e.g., Nogueira et al., 2019; Trott et al., 2020). Researchers outside the U.S. have also determined prevalence rates among different populations and their activities. Table 1 highlights some of these results. For consistency, the current authors only included data that were collected from two specific instruments (i.e., Exercise Addiction Inventory and Exercise Dependence Scale).

Table 1. Prevalence of EA by Activity and Country

Country	Number	Prevalence
Italy	317 Runners [a]	15.4%
Spain	1014 Indoor cyclists	13.3%
Germany	1008 Fitness club users	10.2%
Australia	345 Ironman athletes [b]	9.0%
Germany	72 Marathon runners [c]	6.9%
Brazil	251 University students	6.4%
Spain	330 Cyclists [d]	6.1%
Denmark	603 Cross-fit athletes	5.0%

Note. As cited by Magee et al. (2016), Marques et al. (2019), and Weinstein & Szabo (2023).
[a] 39% ultra-trail, 32% road marathon, 29% mountain marathon
[b] 187 Australia country of birth; 71% male
[c] 19% female
[d] 9% female

The validity of the prevalence rates cited above may be impacted by several factors. These factors include how EA is being defined (e.g., primary versus secondary) and what criteria and instruments are employed to determine if a person has an EA. Researchers caution there could be an overestimation of the number of individuals that have an addiction to exercise due to these research limitations (Weinstein & Szabo, 2023).

Neurobiological And Physiological Features

The neurobiological and physiological features of EA are important to consider before exploring symptomology, which is described in the next section of this chapter, as they provide a foundational understanding of the biological processes driving the behavior. While there is a shortage of investigations related to these aspects (Weinstein & Szabo, 2023), there are theories regarding excessive exercise and associated impacts on the brain (e.g., endogenous opioid systems and β-endorphins, prefrontal cortex and impulsivity, ventral striatum and depressive symptoms). One of the earlier theories posits that the endogenous opioid systems are the reason for EA and connect exercise with elevations of β-endorphins in the bloodstream (i.e., achieving a "runners' high"). Studies on rats have been conducted to investigate this theory; however, researchers assert that sufficient evidence has not been demonstrated (Adams, 2013).

Of the etiological frameworks documented, the modification to the mesolimbic dopamine system (MDS) due to exercise is one worth noting. The MDS is referred to as the "pleasure center" of the brain and rewards behaviors related to survival through dopamine. When activated by behaviors such as exercise (or sex, gambling, overeating, taking psychoactive substances, etc.), these non-essential behaviors can become deemed essential (Lewis et al., 2021). Prolonged increases in dopamine cause the brain to self-modify and reduce the availability of post-synaptic dopamine receptors. Thus, abrupt decreases in frequency can result in strong cravings to engage in the behavior again. Additionally, when there are modifications to the MDS due to exercise, the person can be unable to experience pleasure in the absence of that behavior. This can result in anhedonia. Human and rat studies on certain behaviors such as video games and exercise have supported this theory, demonstrating connections to cravings, tolerance, anhedonia, and withdrawal (Adams, 2013) similar to those with chemical addictions.

Lastly, brain imaging studies demonstrate a possible correlation between an individual having an addiction and the amount of gray matter volume (GMV) in their brain, specifically in the orbitofrontal cortex (OFC). The OFC is found to play a crucial role in inhibition, information processing, and decision making related to reward. Furthermore, deficits in the OFC are related to the impairment of goal-directed behavior and impulsivity (Zhang et al., 2023). Neuroimaging studies have shown that a reduction in GMV may be connected to addictive behaviors, such as internet use (Lee et al., 2018) and gambling (Yip et al., 2018). A reduced GMV in the right OFC has also been found in those with EAs. For example, Zhang and colleagues (2023) conducted a study with 130 individuals who had EA symptomology. The images and scatterplot in Figure 1 illustrate their results which found the correlation between EA (x-axis) and a smaller amount of GMV in the right OFC (y-axis).

Figure 1. The Gray Matter Volume (GMV) Associated with Exercise Addiction

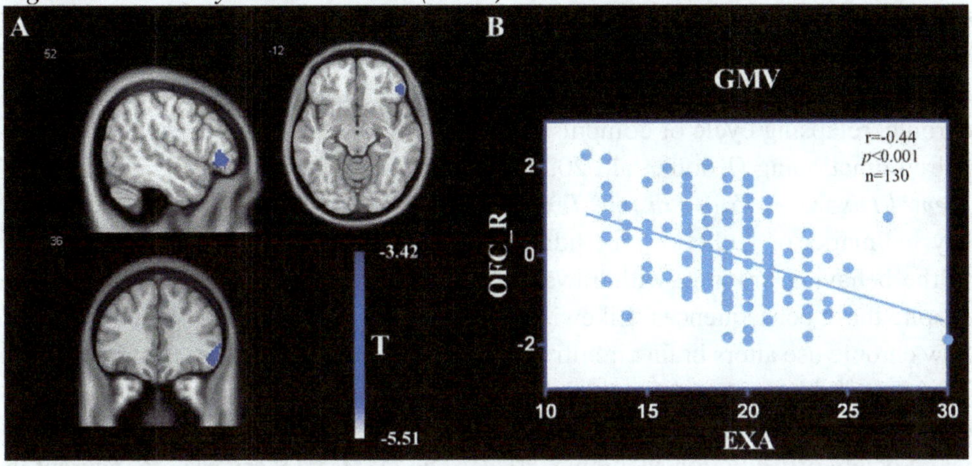

Note. (A) Brain image showed that the GMV in the right OFC was negatively correlated with exercise addiction (EXA); (B) Scatter plots depict the correlation between EXA and GMV in the right OFC. From Zhang et al. (2023). The role of the orbitofrontal cortex in exercise addiction and exercise motivation: A brain imaging study based on multimodal magnetic resonance imaging. Journal of Affective Disorders, 325, p. 244.

Interestingly, research has also shown less GMV of the OFC is found more often in men than in women and EA tends to be more prevalent among men. Thus, the presence of EA may be more often indicated in men due to the smaller GMV of the OFC (Zhang et al., 2023).

SCREENING AND ASSESSMENT

Key Features of Exercise Addiction

Exercise Addiction includes certain discernable characteristics that make it recognizable as a standalone disorder, despite there being no universally accepted definition. This section explores the features specific to EA as well as how to differentiate EA from commonly co-occurring conditions through the lens of screening and assessment. But first, with behavioral addictions receiving more and more attention in research and practice settings, it is important to begin by addressing the misconception that EA (or any behavior classified as "addictive") is a "positive addiction." In fact, the term "negative addiction" was introduced as an antonym to represent the devastating effects of all addictions, including behavioral addictions (Szabo & Rendi, 2008). This section will discuss criteria that are common across addictions, with a focus on symptoms specific to EA. These include the function of exercise in the individual's life, personality traits, risk factors, and consequences associated with EA. Additionally, screening and assessment questions and tools for evaluating EA will be presented.

Classifying compulsive exercise as an addiction underscores the similarities between behavioral addictions and substance use disorders (SUDs), namely the chronic, relapsing cycle of compulsive behavior that leads to dependence and impaired functioning (Koob et al., 2023). The *Diagnostic and Statistical Manual of Mental Disorders-Fifth Edition, Text Revision* (*DSM-5-TR;* APA, 2022) identifies key hallmarks of addiction, including tolerance, loss of control, time dedicated to the behavior, craving, withdrawal, negative consequences, and continued use despite these consequences. Likewise, the disease model of addiction emphasizes how chronic use alters brain circuitry involved in reward, motivation, and memory, driving individuals to seek increasing amounts of a substance to achieve the desired effect (i.e., tolerance) and cessation of use results in withdrawal symptoms (American Society of Addiction Medicine, 2024). The *DSM-5-TR* criteria are inherent in the etiology of addiction and are applicable when assessing for an EA, which are further explicated below.

The Components Model outlines six key features associated with addiction and was developed to highlight commonalities across various addictions, including behavioral addictions (Griffiths, 2005). The model posits all addictions involve: (1) *salience*, where the activity becomes central to the individual's life, characterized by preoccupation, cognitive distortions, cravings, and deteriorating social behavior; (2) *mood modification*, referring to the positive emotional, physical, or psychological effects after engagement in the activity; (3) *tolerance*, or the increasing amounts of the activity required to achieve desired effects; (4) *withdrawal*, or the unpleasant physical or emotional symptoms that occur when the activity ceases or is drastically reduced; (5) *conflict*, typically interpersonal, social, occupational, or intrapsychic; and (6) *relapse*, or the tendency to revert to earlier patterns of the behavior, with a rapid restoration to the addiction's intensity, even after extended abstinence.

Veale (1995) first proposed and later refined criteria specific to EA, advocating for its inclusion in the *DSM*. The criteria included: (1) preoccupation with exercise that becomes stereotyped and routine; (2) significant withdrawal symptoms in the absence of exercise, such as mood swings, irritability, and insomnia; (3) preoccupation with exercise causes clinically significant distress or impairment in physical, social, occupational, or other areas of functioning; and (4) preoccupation that is not better accounted for by another mental disorder (e.g., using exercise as a means of controlling weight, as seen in eating disorders). These criteria are congruent with SUDs, particularly regarding withdrawal and impairment of functioning, which provide a clear differentiation between commitment and dependence.

When assessing individuals for EA, application of the proposed criteria provides a comprehensive understanding of specific behaviors and their impact on those affected. Although EA is not defined by the number of hours spent exercising, it is notable that the Centers for Disease Control and Prevention (2023) recommends 150 minutes of moderate to vigorous exercise per week for healthy adults ages 18-64, or 30 minutes daily over five days. In contrast, those experiencing EA typically devote considerably more time to physical activity than the suggested recommendations (Landolfi, 2013). Moreover, they often continue exercising despite having met their stated goal, such as weight loss or performance targets; this pattern can be likened to alcohol use disorder, where drinking persists long after the desired effect has been achieved (Freimuth et al., 2011). This behavior can be attributed to the insatiable craving for exercise, or to the increasing amount of physical activity required over time to satisfy the individual's needs, known as tolerance (Hausenblas & Downs, 2002a).

The criteria discussed can be assessed by examining individual thought patterns and cognitive processes. For example, they may describe feeling out of control over their behavior while simultaneously believing they cannot live without physical activity (i.e., preoccupation). This may manifest as an inability to accept limits or setting unrealistic goals (Egorov & Szabo, 2013). Szabo's (1995) cognitive appraisal hypothesis suggests an association arises between exercise and stress reduction, leading to gradually increased amounts of exercise. This progression highlights both the tolerance aspect of EA and the role of brain circuitry involved in learning, which reinforces addictive behavior. One such distorted, learned belief that gets reinforced is: '*exercise is the only way to feel good or achieve happiness*.'

Beliefs that maintain EA are often related to attempts to avoid withdrawal. For example, those affected by EA are more likely to exercise despite bad weather, discomfort, or injury compared to exercisers that are not addicted (Hausenblas & Downs, 2002a). When exercise is reduced or halted, many experience withdrawal symptoms such as restlessness, tics, fatigue, insomnia, irritability, severe feelings of deprivation, anxiety, depression, muscle tension and soreness, decreased appetite, and irregular bowel movements (Lichtenstein et al., 2021). Many people with EA are aware of the centrality of exercise in their lives and report a loss of pleasure, intrinsic reward, and coping ability when it is removed, consistent with the self-medication hypothesis of addiction. Key features of EA also include: (a) an inability to control exercise volume; and (b) persistent, compulsive exercise despite negative consequences, such as health concerns, strained relations, financial instability, personal inconvenience, work interference, and a lack of time for other activities (Landolfi, 2013).

Differentiating Exercise Addiction

Since the initial proposal of criteria for EA, research has expanded to include aspects such as functionality, risk factors, and criteria to differentiate EA from disorders with similar presentations. New research indicates the need to rule out other potential causes when diagnosing EA (Pálfi et al., 2021). Like SUDs, studies suggest EA may function to modulate mood, enhance self-worth, fulfill identity, or satisfy a void.

Mood modification is an essential feature of EA and helps distinguish EA from healthy committed exercise. Specifically, individuals with EA use exercise to avoid negative emotions and daily difficulties of life, whereas healthy committed exercisers experience the inherent joy of physical activity (Berczik et al., 2014a). Individuals who are predisposed to developing EA often strongly identify as exercisers, have low self-esteem, or lack positive reinforcement from other social means, and use exercise as their primary measure of personal success (Despres, 1997). It is postulated these individuals seek to fill a "thought vacuum" or "vacuum of affection," using exercise as a coping mechanism for emotional distress while basing their self-worth and identity on the results of their physical activity (Weinstein & Weinstein, 2013).

While healthy levels of exercise can effectively help manage depression, individuals with EA who are unable to exercise may find symptoms of pre-existing mental health conditions resurfacing and worsening. This is often a result when exercise is used for coping, and compulsive behaviors have developed (Andreassen et al., 2013). Moreover, individuals who compulsively exercise as a means of managing mental health symptoms are at risk of worsened pre-existing symptoms if: (1) exercise-related activities have become a major way the individual identifies themselves and/or (2) the exerciser describes feelings of loss of control over their exercise. For example, an individual who strongly identifies as a "semiprofessional athlete," may experience increased internal pressure to exercise, which in turn, feeds the identification as a serious athlete and leads to compulsivity, tolerance, and loss of control. Together, the cessation of exercise when it is experienced as integral to identity or out of one's immediate control, can exacerbate the severity of pre-existing conditions. In these cases, it is important to distinguish between co-occurring mood disorders (e.g., depression), and withdrawal symptoms resulting from a disruption in exercise.

Risk Factors

Extensive research has determined risk profiles of those who develop EA (Szabo & Kovacsik, 2019). Although profiles pose no diagnostic value, familiarity with traits that predispose individuals to EA is valuable in screening, assessing, educating, and preventing dysfunctional exercise. Major behavioral risks in those who go on to exhibit EA include excessive training, staleness, distorted perception of exercise volume, training when injured, and missed social engagements.

When ritualized, obsessive repetition of exercise becomes compulsive, and may create feelings of staleness, described as burnout or chronic fatigue (Szabo, 2010). Staleness often results from both tolerance and perfectionism, driven by rigid expectations of oneself (Egorov & Szabo, 2013). Distorted perceptions of the necessary amount of training one requires makes a person vulnerable to overuse injuries; and those who exercise despite injury are found to be at risk for developing EA (Pálfi et al., 2021). The high priority given to exercise often leads to missed social engagements. These traits help differentiate EA from committed exercisers, who engage in physical activity for extrinsic rewards and do not experience severe withdrawal symptoms, thereby avoiding many negative consequences associated with EA (Landolfi, 2013).

Psychological profiles often underlie the behavioral risk factors for EA. It is hypothesized that individuals who are perfectionistic and highly driven are more prone to EA due to their intolerance of flaws and ongoing dissatisfaction with performance (Stoliaroff, 2003). High levels of neuroticism, which predisposes individuals to negative emotions and instability, are also common in EA. Narcissism is another risk factor, as individuals may prioritize excessive exercise over other obligations (Miller & Mesagno, 2014). Likewise, low agreeableness alongside high extraversion is typical in EA profiles, contributing to a need to "burn off" energy and resistance to reducing exercise intensity (Lichtenstein et al., 2014). Most notably, obsessive compulsive traits are prevalent in EA, often seen as an obsessive "need to work out" paired with severe distress if disrupted (Freimuth et al., 2011).

Individuals with a formal diagnosis of obsessive-compulsive disorder (OCD) are at greater risk for developing EA, since these individuals may lose sight of their original 'purpose' for exercising and become fixated on the 'act' of working out (Szabo & Griffiths, 2020). While OCD and addictive behaviors share similar presentations, one distinguishing feature is that addiction has the capacity to simultaneously increase positive feelings while decreasing negative affect. The overlapping symptomology has led to debates about the co-occurrence of OCD and EA, with emphasis on distinguishing primary and secondary disorders. Cunningham and others (2016), for instance, differentiated between excessive exercise driven by compulsion and that driven by addiction, with the latter identified as primary EA.

Individuals with eating disorders, or who exhibit significant concerns about weight or body image, are at increased risk for developing EA. This has led to differentiation between primary and secondary EA. As stated earlier, primary EA involves exercise as a goal in and of itself, while secondary EA occurs when exercise is driven by an underlying goal, like body transformation (Cunningham et al., 2016).

These findings support a relationship between EA and eating disorders, while noting a higher degree of EA does not lead to greater disordered eating. In fact, swimmers scored high on EA and low on eating disorders, while dancers scored high on both. Controlling for competitiveness, pressure to exercise, and level of EA, dancers were found to have the highest risk for developing EA among athletes; the key difference between groups being social pressure to be thin, which more accurately reflects secondary EA (McDonald, 1994; Pierce et al., 1993).

A key distinction between primary and secondary EA lies in the motivation behind exercise. Individuals with primary EA focus on performance more than body image and thus typically consume calories sufficient to support performance (Freimuth et al., 2011). In contrast, secondary EA involves a need for control over the body, often driven by eating disorders, including excessive exercise to lose weight (Hausenblas & Downs, 2002a). As such, a clear differential for primary EA is the absence of an eating disorder (Veale, 1987). Research has also proposed criteria for secondary EA (Allegre et al., 2009).

Shared symptomology and risk factors underlie multiple disorders. The overlapping presentations of EA, OCD, and disordered eating may be indicative of a personality profile that emerges from genetics, environment, and internal/external stimuli (Lichtenstein et al., 2017). Comorbid EA and eating disorders are found in 39%-48% of individuals who engage in compulsive exercise and also score high on addiction scales (Freimuth et al., 2011).

Conducting a Clinical Interview

Without formally established *DSM* criteria, diagnosis relies on clinical judgment, informed by a thorough interview that explores the client's current and historical relationship with exercise. This includes examining their exercise patterns, motivation, and impact on daily life. Refer to the proposed criteria and stay mindful of typical presentations and risk factors to guide effective assessment questions. See Table 2, informed by Hausenblaus et al. (2017), for a list of recommended questions for clinicians to use when they suspect an individual may have an EA.

Table 2.

Recommended EA Screening Questions for Clinicians
Explore the frequency, intensity, and duration of exercise, listening for signs of tolerance and assessing motivation: • *How often and how long do you exercise?* • *How do you measure success?*
Distinguish similarly presenting conditions: • *What motivates you to exercise?* • *What role does exercise have in your life?* • *How do you decide what type of exercise to do?*
A critical focus is on the client's ability to regulate exercise. These questions can reveal patterns of overcommitment, loss of control, and staleness: • *How do you decide when to stop?* • *Have you ever tried cutting back, and if so, what happened?* • *Do you ever get bored of your exercise, or feel tired of it?*
Assess for withdrawal symptoms when exercise is disrupted: • *How do you feel physically or emotionally when you can't exercise?* • *Do you take recovery days and what do those look like?*
Explore injury and response to injury: • *Do you exercise when you are sick or injured?* • *How do you modify your routine for these times?*
Assess the impact of exercise on daily functioning. These questions can help identify broader effects of exercise on major life domains: • *How do you feel during and after a workout?* • *What are your thoughts when you can't work out?* • *How do you spend your free time?* • *Has anyone ever expressed concern about your exercise habits?*

The goal of the assessment is to engage the client in a dialogue that provides a comprehensive understanding of their exercise behaviors and the context in which they occur. This allows the clinician to evaluate the impact of exercise on the client's daily functioning and make necessary referrals. A client may be experiencing EA if the person experiences significant distress around exercise; consistently increases their volume; exercises despite pain; fails to fulfill obligations; is reluctant to (or has difficulty in) taking time off; and experiences withdrawal without exercise (Colledge et al., 2020).

Screening Tools

Validated instruments are available to determine the risk and severity of EA, though these tools are limited to screening for, rather than diagnosing, EA. Two widely used tools are the Exercise Addiction Inventory (EAI) and the Exercise Dependence Scale (EDS). The EAI is congruent with proposed EA criteria and measures risk of EA. It has demonstrated internal consistency, convergent validity, and test-retest reliability (Khoshro et al., 2024). The EDS is rooted in theoretical foundations associated with SUDs from the *DSM-IV.* The instrument addresses the psychological and physiological aspects of EA and uses seven subscales to differentiate between individuals who are (a) at risk for developing EA, (b) nondependent but symptomatic, and (c) nondependent and asymptomatic. When at least three subscales are denoted 'at risk,' an EA profile is met (Granziol et al., 2023; Hausenblas & Downs, 2002b).

A multitude of validated questionnaires are also available to assess different aspects of EA. For instance, the Exercise Beliefs Questionnaire (EBQ) evaluates exercise withdrawal, function of exercise, and underlying psychological profiles of exercises by examining maladaptive beliefs associated with not exercising, personal appearance, social desirability, and emotion vulnerability (Sicilia et al., 2021). Another frequently cited instrument is the Running Addiction Scale (RAS), a self-report addiction scale of behaviors congruent to EA but specific to running. Items include questions about frequency of runs, running despite injury, prioritizing running over other activities, financial cost of running, running in poor weather, and experience of urges to run daily (Maceri et al., 2019). The Exercise Dependence Questionnaire (EDQ) assesses the multifaceted impact of EA by screening interference in daily life, withdrawal, function of exercise (e.g., weight control; social; health), insight, positive reinforcement, and stereotyped behavior (Berczik et al., 2014b) exercise, and consequences of addiction (Weinstein & Weinstein, 2013). It is positively correlated with the Exercise Dependence Scale. Though these tools are useful, it is recommended they be combined with a comprehensive clinical interview to avoid false positives and negatives. An example of a false positive would be when an elite athlete scores high without having an EA and a false negative would be when an individual with significant EA problems scores low. Technologies alone cannot capture the psychological nuances of EA, and a full assessment of how exercise controls a person's life is essential (Lichtenstein & Hinze, 2020), especially if a treatment recommendation is offered.

CLINICAL INTERVENTION

Recommendations for clinical intervention should consider relevant key variables, including the individual's stage of change, motivation for treatment, the progression of the addiction, and any co-occurring disorders (Freimuth et al., 2011). If EA is a coping strategy for an underlying psychological condition, treatment should target the root cause. If EA is the primary diagnosis, assessing the individual's stage of change is critical for appropriate intervention selection.

According to the Transtheoretical Model, behavior change occurs in five stages, beginning with precontemplation, where individuals are not yet considering change, and ending with maintenance, defined as at least six months of sustained change (Prochaska & DiClemente, 1983). Individuals with EA may remain in precontemplation for years, often viewing excessive exercise as a form of dedication or integral to their identity. They may see it as a problem to be solved later or feel resigned to it, rarely seeking treatment on their own volition, though they may present for medical or health concerns.

In contemplation, the second stage of change, individuals experience ambivalence and begin weighing reasons to stay the same with reasons to change. While behaviors may not yet change, they acknowledge that change may be necessary. Motivational Interviewing (MI), an evidence-based intervention, is recommended for individuals in this stage and its use is empirically supported for behavioral addictions (Garcia-Caballero et al., 2018). The next stage, preparation, occurs when individuals commit to modify behavior, begin exploring options for how to do so, and start taking steps. Interventions such as psychoeducation, addressing exercise-related myths, exploring attitudes, and considering who to involve in treatment (e.g., therapists, dieticians, fitness professionals) are recommended during this stage (Draeger et al., 2005).

For individuals in the action stage of change, cognitive behavioral and mindfulness-based approaches are recommended for treating EA, though evidence supporting their effectiveness is limited (Weinstein & Szabo, 2023). Cognitive behavioral interventions focus on eliciting and modifying automatic thoughts, maladaptive beliefs, and problematic behaviors related to exercise. For example, beliefs arising from low frustration tolerance (e.g., "I must exercise; I cannot miss a workout") generate guilt and anxiety when routines are disrupted (Outar et al., 2018). Cognitive restructuring, which reframes these beliefs into healthier alternatives, can reduce compulsive behaviors and promote balanced exercise habits. Other strategies include (a) exposure-response prevention to disrupt compulsive behavior; (b) self-management; (c) contingency management; (d) building support systems; (e) identifying healthy coping alternatives; and (f) cognitive processing (Adams et al., 2003). An important consideration for behavioral addictions like EA is that abstinence may not be the goal. Instead, focusing on moderation, pattern recognition, and reducing rigidity by introducing rest days, cross training, or transitioning to new forms of exercise may be more acceptable (Berczik et al., 2014a).

One specific cognitive behavioral approach, Rational Emotive Behavior Therapy (REBT), has been found to reduce low-frustration tolerance, maladaptive beliefs, and EA scores while increasing self-acceptance (Outar et al., 2018). However, research on REBT for EA is limited, with only two studies found demonstrating its effectiveness. Furthermore, despite findings suggesting that women with EA exhibit higher symptoms of anxiety, depression, and irrational beliefs compared to men, women were largely underrepresented in the studies (Turner et al., 2019).

Medication

Research on pharmacological intervention for EA is also limited. One case study explored the use of Quetiapine, an antipsychotic typically prescribed for bipolar I disorder, in treating comorbid EA and compulsive buying. After 12 weeks of treatment, behavioral symptoms improved significantly, and by 24 weeks, were completely resolved. EAI scores dropped from 28 at admission to 12 following treatment. Quetiapine is believed to act on the D1 and D2 dopamine receptor, adrenergic receptors, and serotonin receptors (5-HT1A, 5-HT2), effectively reducing obsessions and compulsive behavior by regulating mood (Maan et al., 2023).

Selective Serotonin Reuptake Inhibitors (SSRIs), which affect the serotoninergic system, may also have potential for treating EA. Off-label use of SSRIs, which refers to their application for conditions not explicitly approved by regulatory agencies, has shown promise in improving compulsive behaviors, particularly in pathological gambling, compulsive shopping, sex addiction, and video game cravings.

Another promising drug is Naltrexone, an opioid antagonist used in the treatment of opioid and alcohol dependence. Neurochemical and genetic evidence suggest dysregulated glutamate may contribute to compulsive behavior. As a glutamatergic modulator, Naltrexone effectively reduces reward-seeking behavior and thus may have implications for the treatment of behavioral addictions such as EA (Corazza & Dores, 2023).

CONSIDERATIONS

In further exploring Exercise Addiction (EA), it is imperative to consider its intersection with other mental health and behavioral conditions and the cultural and social pressures that normalize and exacerbate EA. Understanding those factors lends to the importance of advocacy and the crucial need to change public messaging, cultural expectations, and social influence to reduce the appeal of visual ideals that are upheld by EA. Additionally, future research is essential to deepen understanding, refine diagnostics, and promote interdisciplinary approaches to treatment. This section will consist of four subsections: (1) co-occurring conditions, (2) cultural and societal norms, (3) advocacy, and (4) future research.

Co-Occurring Conditions

Exercise Addiction frequently overlaps with other mental health and behavioral disorders, creating multifaceted clinical presentations that require integrated treatment approaches. In fact, research has found that *nearly one-third of individuals with EA meet criteria for another behavioral addiction* (Lichtenstein et al., 2017). The most prevalent co-occurring disorders include eating disorders, body and muscle dysmorphia, pathological buying, substance use, and psychiatric conditions. As noted previously, it is imperative to identify whether the dependence is a "primary" or "secondary" to determine a proper treatment protocol.

Eating Disorders

Exercise Addiction is most often linked to eating disorders, namely anorexia nervosa and bulimia nervosa in which excessive exercise is used as a compensatory behavior (Meyer et al., 2011; Trott et al., 2021). A study examining the prevalence of compulsive exercise in individuals with an eating disorder found that 45.5% of patients were identified as compulsive exercisers. The occurrence was highest in restricting-type anorexia nervosa (80%); moderate in binge/purging anorexia nervosa (43.3%) and purging-type bulimia nervosa (39.3%); and lowest in eating disorders, not otherwise specified (31.9%; Dalle Grave et al., 2008). Additionally, bulimia has been found to be significantly more frequent among individuals with exercise dependence (70%) than those without (47%; Lejoyeux et al., 2008). Moreover, those affected also experienced a higher number of weekly bulimic episodes (2.5 versus 1.3 respectively) (Lejoyeux et al., 2008). The connection between EA and eating disorders is acutely alarming in groups like athletes, as performance-related pressures can exacerbate restrictive eating habits and compulsive exercise behaviors. Research further indicates that *EA is over three and a half times more likely to co-occur with an eating disorder* than in individuals without a diagnosed eating disorder (Trott et al., 2021).

Body and Muscle Dysmorphia

In a culture that often focuses on appearance and associates a fit body with success and achievement, the pressure to conform to these ideals creates a societal environment that encourages the development of Exercise Addiction. According to research, EA often co-occurs with Body Dysmorphic Disorder (BDD) and its specifier, Muscle Dysmorphia (MD). The *DSM-5-TR* defines BDD as a preoccupation with a perceived physical flaw that is either minimal or unnoticeable to others; compulsions due to the preoccupation with perceived physical flaws; and the preoccupation causes clinically significant distress or impairment in functioning (APA, 2022). Muscle Dysmorphia, a subtype of BDD, is characterized by persistent, distressing and intrusive thoughts about not being muscular enough, along with a pervasive fear of losing muscle mass (APA, 2022). Research supports the notable link between MD and EA. In comparing those with and without MD, Babusa et al. (2015) found that individuals with MD had the highest levels of EA and participated in longer, more frequent exercise sessions. Similarly, another study observed that as MD symptoms increased, so did the risk of EA (Olave et al., 2019). This, in turn, worsened muscle dissatisfaction and amplified behaviors associated with MD. Notably, Hale and colleagues (2013) emphasized that female bodybuilders are particularly at risk for exercise dependence and muscle dysmorphia symptoms, more so than female recreational weightlifters.

Pathological Buying

Among the other mental health and behavioral disorders that EA overlaps, pathological buying (PB) is also frequently noted. Pathological buying, commonly referred to as shopping addiction, involves compulsive and excessive purchasing behaviors that result in significant distress or impairment in daily functioning (Black, 2007). This is an often-overlooked co-occurring condition that warrants attention due to its shared underlying mechanisms with EA.

Research suggests that EA and shopping addiction potentially share similar neurobiological, psychological, and sociocultural factors (Freimuth et al., 2011; Lejoyeux et al., 2008; Müller et al., 2015; Villella et al., 2011). Exercise Addiction often co-occurs with PB due to shared traits like impulsivity, compulsivity, and reward system dysregulation. Both conditions serve as maladaptive coping mechanisms for emotional distress that provide temporary relief but also reinforce dependence. Sociocultural influences, such as consumerism and fitness ideals, further link these behaviors by glorifying material success and physical perfection (Corazza et al., 2019; Lejoyeux et al., 2008). Recognizing this overlap is vital for comprehensive screening and integrated treatment approaches, including cognitive-behavioral therapy and mindfulness interventions (Andreassen et al., 2013; Weinstein & Szabo, 2023).

Substance Use

While substance use disorders (SUDs) and Exercise Addiction share characteristics such as reward system dysregulation and compulsive behaviors, research has not consistently demonstrated a strong overlap between the two conditions. As stated earlier in the chapter, the "runner's high," linked to endorphins and cannabinoids, highlights the shared neurobiological mechanisms that may contribute to addictive tendencies (Weinstein & Weinstein, 2013). Additionally, genetic studies suggest that the same genes influencing drug preferences also govern preferences for naturally rewarding behaviors like exercise, which further connects the two (Weinstein & Weinstein, 2013). These potential overlaps emphasize the importance of considering shared mechanisms when screening individuals for EA and the potential comorbidities that may exist, such as SUDs.

When researchers investigated substance use specifically, no significant differences were found in alcohol, nicotine, or illicit drug use among individuals classified as asymptomatic, symptomatic, or at risk for EA (Szabo et al., 2018). Similarly, other researchers found that individuals with exercise dependence smoked nicotine less than those without exercise dependence and alcohol consumption was equivalent between the two groups (Lejoyeux et al., 2008). However, Sussman and colleagues (2011) speculated that 15% of those addicted to exercise are also addicted to nicotine, alcohol, or illicit drugs, which suggests that while the overlap may not be widespread, there is a subset of individuals with co-occurring addictions.

Risky substance use can also be found alongside EA, particularly in individuals attempting to enhance their performance but feel they cannot do so without using performance-enhancing drugs (PEDs). Competition participants are more likely to use substances such as anabolic steroids, cocaine, and protein drinks, while non-athletes have also been found to use both addictive and performance-enhancing substances (Lim, 2021). PEDs, including anabolic-androgenic steroids (AAS) and caffeine, have been associated with EA (Lim, 2021). PED use is particularly linked to EA in individuals striving for hyper-muscular physiques or peak performance goals. A strong association between EA and steroid use in gym settings has been identified, where users exhibited an obsessive focus on achieving idealized body types (Corazza et al., 2019). Similarly, another study found that AAS misuse reinforced compulsive exercise behaviors, driven by the perceived benefits of increased muscle mass and strength (Kanayama et al., 2009). These findings highlight the need for further research to better understand the nuanced relationship between exercise dependence and substance use behaviors.

Psychiatric Conditions

Psychiatric conditions, particularly anxiety and depression, are common co-morbidities of EA, creating a bidirectional relationship that worsens symptoms and complicates recovery. People with EA often use exercise to manage stress or improve mood, as suggested by the self-medication hypothesis (Lichtenstein et al.,

2014). However, over-reliance on exercise can worsen psychiatric symptoms when routines are disrupted and create a cycle of dependency and emotional instability.

Research supports this connection. For instance, in a study of 123 participants, 23.6% were classified as at risk for EA. After controlling for weekly exercise hours, individuals at risk for EA scored higher on measures of depression, attention deficit hyperactivity disorder, and childhood trauma compared to those not at risk, showing greater psychological and emotional challenges in this group (Colledge et al., 2022).

Comparably, Meyer and colleagues (2021) examined 156 individuals who exercised more than 10 hours per week despite illness or injury and discovered that 75% of participants met the criteria for at least one psychiatric disorder, with depressive disorders (56.3%), personality disorders (46.9%), and obsessive-compulsive disorders (31.3%) being the most prevalent. Notably, the study found a positive correlation between the severity of EA and the number of co-occurring psychiatric disorders, illustrating the intertwined nature of EA and mental health. Additionally, Weinstein and fellow research collaborators (2015) identified a strong association between compulsive exercise behaviors and symptoms of anxiety and depression among individuals exercising for both professional and recreational purposes.

In conclusion, addressing any identified psychiatric conditions with those individuals who have an addiction to exercise is vitally important in an effort to break the cycle of emotional instability and dependency.

Cultural and Societal Norms

Fitspiration and Societal Standards

Cultural and societal norms surrounding fitness and body image significantly contribute to the development and persistence of Exercise Addiction. The "fitspiration" movement on social media epitomizes this influence, as it showcases content that glorifies extreme fitness routines and unattainable body ideals. Although intended to inspire healthier lifestyles, fitspiration often leads to negative psychological outcomes such as body dissatisfaction, anxiety, and compulsive exercise behaviors. In fact, a 2021 study emphasized that younger individuals, who are more likely to engage with these platforms, are particularly vulnerable to these pressures (Cataldo et al., 2021). Exposure to fitspiration content has been shown to increase body dissatisfaction, negative mood, and appearance-based social comparison in women, which may reinforce compulsive exercise behaviors and contribute to the development or maintenance of exercise addiction (Tiggemann & Zaccardo, 2015). These effects are often accompanied by a stronger drive for thinness, muscularity, and excessive exercise, suggesting that fitspiration can serve as a digital trigger that exacerbates underlying vulnerabilities related to body image and compulsivity

(Holland & Tiggemann, 2017). Similarly, a recent publication by Minutillo and colleagues (2024) asserted that the highly edited and curated nature of social media content exacerbates these behaviors by setting unrealistic standards that encourage people to make compulsive attempts to achieve them.

The influence of social media on EA extends beyond the posting of pictorial ideals. Social media platforms often act as echo chambers that validate and normalize compulsive exercise behaviors, generally unintentionally. Through social media features such as "likes," comments, and follower counts, the users are rewarded for showcasing extreme fitness dedication, which further reinforces unhealthy patterns. This phenomenon mirrors trends in pop culture, where extreme dedication to fitness is often glamorized by celebrity figures, influencers, and fitness challenges that go viral. One prominent fitness challenge example is the "75 Hard Challenge," a popular online program requiring two workouts per day, drinking a gallon of water, a strict diet, no rest days, taking daily progress pictures, and daily progress tracking for 75 consecutive days. While promoted as a mental toughness regimen, health professionals have raised concerns about its potential to trigger or worsen exercise addiction, particularly among individuals with a history of disordered eating, perfectionism, or body image issues. Dr. Kiki Ramsey, a psychologist, warns that "the strict, all-or-nothing approach may not be beneficial for those who have a history of disordered eating or feel overwhelmed by rigid routines," while licensed clinical social worker Caitlin Weese explains that the challenge's inflexibility may increase anxiety, fear of failure, and compulsive behaviors (Nazish, 2024). Both emphasize that, if taken too far, the challenge can lead to burnout, distorted self-image, and compulsive exercise patterns that resemble or reinforce symptoms of EA.

Research has highlighted that problematic social media use is a significant predictor of EA and is mediated by heightened body image concerns and compulsive tendencies (Akbari et al., 2024). This bidirectional relationship not only may worsen EA but also can perpetuate associated mental health challenges, such as anxiety and depression. The cycle of validation and comparison that these platforms create makes social media a significant factor in the cultural landscape of EA and needs to be considered in prevention and intervention efforts.

Fitness apps (e.g., MyFitnessPal: Calorie Counter, Strava, Peloton: Fitness & Workouts, and Lose It! – Calorie Counter) and wearable trackers (e.g. Apple Watch, Fitbit, Garmin, Oura ring) may have a significant impact on compulsive exercise behaviors. While these technologies are designed to track and promote health and fitness, they also risk reinforcing unhealthy exercise habits. Arora and Razavian (2021) discussed the gamification in health and fitness tracking, including "points and rewards for health activity as well as social elements like competitions and challenges with other people" (p. 1). A study by Blackstone and Herrmann (2020) found that fitness tracking wearables may exacerbate harmful compulsions, including exercise dependence, and the researchers suggest that wearables should be cautiously recommended by health education specialists. This poses as a significant consideration due to the amount of use and consumption of these products. Given that the global fitness tracker market generated approximately $46.3 billion USD in 2023 (Pangarkar, 2025), their influence on exercise behaviors is both widespread and significant.

Beyond social media and fitness trackers, broader cultural and societal standards also play a significant role in the normalization of EA. Western ideals emphasize hyper-muscularity and leanness, and frame these physical traits as markers of success, discipline, and self-worth (De Luca et al., 2017). These ideals often mask the pathological nature of EA by presenting excessive exercise as a virtuous or desirable behavior. Consequently, individuals exhibiting EA are frequently praised for their commitment and dedication, complicating the recognition and treatment of this condition. As societal norms continue to glorify extreme fitness behaviors, there is an urgent need to challenge these harmful ideals and promote a balanced approach to fitness and body image. By addressing the cultural drivers of EA, we can better understand and mitigate the factors that contribute to its development and persistence.

Gender

Gender differences significantly influence the prevalence and expression of Exercise Addiction. A review of 27 studies concluded that men are generally more likely than women to exhibit EA, although this tendency may vary depending on study methods and criteria (Dumitru et al., 2018). Men often experience primary EA or present with higher risk of EA, focused on athletic performance and muscularity, and driven by societal norms emphasizing strength and masculinity (Bueno-Antequera et al., 2020; Cunningham et al., 2016; Dumitru et al., 2018; Manfredi, 2022). In contrast, women are more likely to experience secondary EA, often linked to body dissatisfaction and eating disorders, where exercise serves as a compensatory mechanism for weight control (Cunningham et al., 2016; Manfredi, 2022; Szabo et al., 2022). While men tend to exhibit higher EA scores overall, it is important to consider that women report greater emotional distress, including depression and anxiety, alongside EA behaviors (Bueno-Antequera et al., 2020; Modolo et al., 2011; Weinstein & Szabo, 2023). Recent research by Szabo et al. (2022) also found that when a minimum weekly training volume of three hours is used as a recruitment criterion, no significant gender differences in EA are observed. These findings suggest that the perceived gender gap in EA may be influenced by study designs and recruitment strategies.

The complex interplay between cultural pressures, psychological factors, and study methodologies underscores the need for gender-sensitive prevention and treatment approaches. Further research is essential to better understand these patterns and develop tailored interventions for diverse populations.

Access

The COVID-19 pandemic significantly disrupted exercise routines and highlighted the influence of accessibility and cultural norms on EA. Exercise Addiction scores were found to have decreased during lockdown due to limited gym access, while leisure-time exercise increased and eating disorder symptoms worsened (Trott et al., 2021). Some individuals experienced heightened anxiety and panic from the inability to exercise outside, whereas others reassessed their habits and discovered the benefits of moderation and loosening their attachment to compulsive exercise (Lim, 2021).

During COVID lockdown, 4.1% of physically active Italians exhibited EA, driven by factors such as higher appearance anxiety, lower self-compassion, and increased perceived benefits of exercise (Ceci et al., 2022). Individuals with EA reported stronger motivations for physical wellness, psychological well-being, and confidence in relationships, while 84.2% noted significant changes in fitness routines. A review of global behavioral addiction rates during the pandemic found the prevalence of EA to be 7%, influenced by factors like accessibility, age, and internet use (Alimoradi et al., 2022). Behavioral addictions like food, gaming, and social media addiction were more prevalent during lockdowns, further emphasizing the role of pandemic-induced lifestyle disruptions as well as the necessity for holistic approaches addressing psychological, cultural, and contextual factors to support individuals at risk of EA.

Advocacy

Advocacy for recognizing Exercise Addiction as a distinct and serious behavioral health condition is critical to addressing gaps in awareness, screening, and treatment. Despite growing evidence, EA remains under-recognized in both clinical and fitness settings and is often dismissed as a sign of dedication or discipline. To combat this, healthcare professionals and fitness experts must receive targeted training to identify and address EA. This includes distinguishing between healthy exercise habits and compulsive behaviors, as well as understanding the nuanced interplay between EA and co-occurring disorders such as eating disorders, body and muscle dysmorphia, and anxiety (Lichtenstein et al., 2017).

Public health campaigns are essential to shift societal attitudes that glorify excessive exercise. Platforms like social media often reinforce harmful behaviors by rewarding extreme fitness dedication, which normalizes EA under the guise of discipline and health (Akbari et al., 2024). Advocacy efforts should emphasize the importance of balance and moderation, targeting fitness organizations, gyms, and digital platforms to reframe exercise as a holistic component of well-being rather than an obsessive pursuit of perfection. Strategic collaborations with organizations that support mental health, eating disorder awareness, and body positivity could amplify these messages and promote a cultural shift that values health over visual ideals.

For these efforts to be effective, advocacy must also engage public health agencies, media outlets, and influencers to reshape how exercise is portrayed across various communication channels. Public service announcements, educational campaigns, and policy initiatives should be developed to counteract the glorification of overtraining and to promote sustainable, balanced activity. Advocacy groups can partner with content creators and journalists to develop narratives that humanize rest, recovery, and joyful movement—encouraging individuals to prioritize their unique health needs over societal pressures.

A strong example of evidence-based messaging is the *Move Your Way®* campaign, developed by the Office of Disease Prevention and Health Promotion. It provides accessible, research-backed guidelines from the Physical Activity Guidelines for Americans, emphasizing that all forms of movement count whether it's dancing, walking the dog, or doing yard work. This approach shifts the focus away from aesthetics and performance and instead reinforces that consistent, moderate activity improves overall health. By shifting the focus away from aesthetics and performance, and instead promoting consistent, moderate activity, the campaign models how inclusive, evidence-informed messaging can support a more realistic and compassionate understanding of fitness.

In addition to advocacy and education, policymakers and public health stakeholders should also focus on standardizing EA assessment protocols and integrating EA into diagnostic frameworks like the *DSM*. Integrating EA into formal diagnostic systems could enhance its visibility in clinical practice and support the development of more precise treatment pathways. Enhanced clinical guidelines could encourage early detection and interdisciplinary treatment approaches, combining psychological, nutritional, and medical support.

Future Research

Future research must delve deeper into the complexities of Exercise Addiction to enhance prevention, screening, and treatment efforts. One priority is establishing universally accepted diagnostic criteria for EA to address inconsistencies in its definition and measurement. These criteria should clearly differentiate between primary EA, where exercise is the primary pathology, and secondary EA, driven by underlying conditions such as eating disorders or body dysmorphia. Without this distinction, clinical assessments and research outcomes remain fragmented, limiting the applicability of findings. Moreover, creating a standardized diagnostic tool that integrates psychological, behavioral, and neurobiological markers could improve early identification and treatment (Trott et al., 2021).

Another critical area of inquiry is the neurobiological underpinnings of EA. Research into the mesolimbic dopamine system and its role in reinforcing addictive behaviors is essential, as these mechanisms parallel those observed in substance use disorders (Adams, 2013; Zhang et al., 2023). For instance, understanding how exercise affects dopamine receptor availability and β-endorphin release could inform pharmacological interventions. As reported earlier in the chapter, current evidence suggests that medications such as SSRIs and Naltrexone may have potential for treating EA, particularly in cases of severe compulsive behaviors. However, rigorous clinical trials are needed to confirm their efficacy and safety for individuals with EA (Corazza & Dores, 2023).

The impact of digital fitness culture also warrants further exploration. With the proliferation of fitness apps, wearable trackers, and social media, these technologies play a significant role in shaping exercise behaviors. Research should examine how these tools contribute to the development and maintenance of EA through mechanisms such as performance tracking, social comparison through gamification, and validation (Akbari et al., 2024; Cataldo et al., 2021). Longitudinal studies could assess how the use of these technologies affects individuals at different stages of EA which would provide valuable insights into targeted interventions to mitigate their potential harms.

Additionally, there is a pressing need to investigate the intersection of EA with co-occurring conditions such as eating disorders, substance use, and mental health. Studies should explore how these conditions reinforce one another and affect treatment outcomes. For example, individuals with diagnoses of EA and an eating disorder may require integrated treatment models that address both simultaneously (Lichtenstein et al., 2017; Trott et al., 2021). Similarly, research should examine the role of performance-enhancing drugs (PEDs) and other substances in EA, particularly in athletic populations where competitive pressures may exacerbate compulsive exercise behaviors (Corazza et al., 2019).

Gender differences in EA also remain an underexplored area. While men are more likely to exhibit primary EA, women often present with secondary EA tied to eating disorders and body dissatisfaction (Dumitru et al., 2018; Manfredi, 2022). Future studies should investigate the psychological, social, and cultural factors that influence these gendered patterns to develop tailored prevention and intervention strategies. For instance, research should explore how societal norms surrounding masculinity and femininity contribute to the distinct manifestations of EA in men and women.

Finally, interdisciplinary research is needed to address the broader societal and cultural factors that perpetuate EA. Collaborations across psychology, neuroscience, sociology, and public health should illuminate the systemic drivers of EA, from fitness industry norms to media portrayals of idealized body types. By fostering a holistic understanding of EA and its multifaceted causes, future research can inform more effective prevention, diagnosis, and treatment efforts.

Chapter Questions

1. What are your thoughts on how excessive exercise is categorized (e.g., obsessive-compulsive, dependence, addiction)?
2. What distinguishes primary dependence from secondary dependence in EA, and why is this distinction important?
3. Identify at least five different co-occurring conditions that are frequently found among those with EA.
4. How do cultural and societal norms, such as the "fitspiration" movement, contribute to the development and perpetuation of EA?
5. How prepared and confident would you be to provide clinical services to someone with EA? What instruments might you use in practice?

Case Study

Matt is a 35-year-old, single, white, heterosexual male (he/his) who has never been married and has no children. He lives alone in an apartment and is employed as a fitness trainer at a local gym. He is attending his first therapy session at the recommendation of his sister due to feeling alone and having thoughts of suicide recently, which he has never experienced before. He denies any plans or intent but "just wondered who would care if he was not here anymore." Matt reports no history of "serious" mental health concerns but "probably should have gone to see someone years ago." He also mentioned that he started having major sleep difficulties within the last year.

Matt stated that lately he has felt "without purpose" and is "dissatisfied with where his life is at his age." He wants to be in a relationship and have a family. His sister has three children, and they have a very close relationship. Matt reports little difficulty with starting relationships but has "issues with keeping" a partner. He stated that since his early 20s, his focus has been on his health, and it has caused the dissolution of several past relationships. His last relationship was with Liz and it lasted eight months, which is the longest Matt has had in the past 10 years. He stated that she initiated the breakup, and it ended three months ago.

When asked for more details about the issues in their relationship, he stated that Liz did not support his "workout routine and lifestyle." Matt starts every morning at 4am and either runs outside or goes to the gym. He works as a trainer during the day and if he has a client after work, he will work out again with them. He said Liz was unhappy with how frequently he would work out each day, especially if it was in the evening because it interfered with them spending time together. They would get into arguments when Liz would laugh at or joke about his diet or supplement routine, or because she was annoyed that he would talk about the details of his food intake and workouts. Matt also stated he has specific products that he "needs in order to continue to be in peak performance." Liz asked him to stop using them as she believed they affected intimacy. Matt denied that they caused any of these issues but did report that he has always had difficulty with physical intimacy. He felt uncomfortable talking more about it, but he knows the cause. He stated that "it is something he has tried to give up but can't seem to stop doing" even when he is in a relationship, and it has been the reason for breakups in the past.

Matt reports plantar fasciitis and severe knee pain recently but has still exercised every day for the past three months except for a family funeral which required him to travel. When asked what it was like for him, Matt stated that he "thought about running all day and was very angry at having to drive to Indiana with his sister." Matt tracks his runs every day on his phone on various apps and "broke his running streak." Matt stated that his anxiety "skyrocketed," and he was unable to sleep at all because he did not post any content on his social media during this time, causing him to feel like he "let his followers down." He has a 50-mile ultramarathon race in a week, his second ultra in five months and the fourth event since he and Liz broke up. The training has taken his mind off Liz, and he thinks that competing in this longer distance race will help him "get back to himself." This year has been the "most active he has been in his life," and he continues to set personal records. He plans on more events next year and he wants to "get even faster and stronger." He denied having any friends outside of the gym or fitness community. About once every two weeks, he will go visit his sister and her children.

Matt stated that he is 6 ft 1 and 163 pounds. He presented mostly with a flat affect, was noted to be fidgety, and picked at his fingernails frequently. When asked about goals for therapy, he stated he wants to "be happy" and "should probably talk about some issues from childhood." He does not want to change his exercise routine drastically but thinks he should consider spending more time with a partner in the future. He wants to "work on his temper" as this has impacted a few interactions with clients at the gym.

Questions

1. Would you classify Matt's behavior as an exercise addiction? Why or why not?
   a. What symptoms did you note?
   b. Is his behavior possibly instrumental exercise or a primary dependency?
2. What would you screen or assess for with this case? Which screening or assessment instrument(s) would you use?
3. What stage of change is Matt in about his exercise at this time?
4. Are there any potential co-occurring issues (e.g., related to mental health, substance use, other addictive behaviors)?
5. What information would you want to gather and consider if you were Matt's therapist?
6. What are your recommendations for Matt?

REFERENCES

Abel, N. (2019). Do It, don't feel it, and be invincible: A prolog of exercise addiction in endurance sports. *Frontiers in Psychology*, *10*, 1–9. DOI: 10.3389/fpsyg.2019.02692 PMID: 31920780

Adams, J. (2013). Exercise dependence. *Principles of Addiction*, *1*, 827–835. DOI: 10.1016/B978-0-12-398336-7.00083-8

Adams, J. M., Miller, T. W., & Kraus, R. F. (2003). Exercise dependence: Diagnostic and therapeutic issues for patients in psychotherapy. *Journal of Contemporary Psychotherapy*, *33*(2), 93–107. DOI: 10.1023/A:1022883104269

Akbari, M., Seydavi, M., Zamani, E., & Griffiths, M. D. (2024). The risk of exercise addiction mediates the relationship between social media use and mental health indices among young Iranians. *Addiction Research and Theory*, *32*(1), 27–37. DOI: 10.1080/16066359.2022.2149742

Alimoradi, Z., Lotfi, A., Lin, C.-Y., Griffiths, M. D., & Pakpour, A. H. (2022). Estimation of behavioral addiction prevalence during COVID-19 pandemic: A systematic review and meta-analysis. *Current Addiction Reports*, *9*(4), 486–517. DOI: 10.1007/s40429-022-00435-6 PMID: 36118286

Allegre, B., Souville, M., Therme, P., & Griffiths, M. (2009). Definitions and measures of exercise dependence. *Addiction Research and Theory*, *14*(6), 631–646. DOI: 10.1080/16066350600903302

American Psychiatric Association. (2022). *Diagnostic and statistical manual of mental disorders* (5th ed., text rev.)., DOI: 10.1176/appi.books.9780890425787

American Society of Addiction Medicine. (2024). *American Society of Addiction Medicine*. https://www.asam.org/

Andreassen, C. S., Griffiths, M. D., Gjertsen, S. R., Krossbakken, E., Kvam, S., & Pallesen, S. (2013). The relationships between behavioral addictions and the five-factor model of personality. *Journal of Behavioral Addictions*, *2*(2), 90–99. DOI: 10.1556/JBA.2.2013.003 PMID: 26165928

Arora, C., & Razavian, M. (2021). Ethics of gamification in health and fitness-tracking. *International Journal of Environmental Research and Public Health*, *18*(21), 11052. DOI: 10.3390/ijerph182111052 PMID: 34769570

Babusa, B., Czeglédi, E., Túry, F., Mayville, S. B., & Urbán, R. (2015). Differentiating the levels of risk for muscle dysmorphia among Hungarian male weightlifters: A factor mixture modeling approach. *Body Image*, *12*, 14–21. DOI: 10.1016/j.bodyim.2014.09.001 PMID: 25280243

Berczik, K., Griffiths, M. D., Szabo, A., Kurimay, T., Kokonyei, G., Urban, R., & Demetrovics, Z. (2014a). Exercise addiction—The emergence of a new disorder. *Australasian Epidemiologist*, *21*(2), 36–40.

Berczik, K., Griffiths, M. D., Szabó, A., Kurimay, T., Urban, R., & Demetrovics, Z. (2014b). Exercise addiction. *Behavioral Addictions*, 317–342. DOI: 10.1016/B978-0-12-407724-9.00013-6

Black, D. W. (2007). A review of compulsive buying disorder. *World Psychiatry; Official Journal of the World Psychiatric Association (WPA)*, *6*(1), 14–18. PMID: 17342214

Blackstone, S. R. & Herrmann, L. K. (2020). Fitness wearables and exercise dependence in college women: Considerations for university health education specialists. *American Journal of Health Education, 51*(4), 225–233. https://doi.org/.2020.1767004DOI: 10.1080/19325037

Bueno-Antequera, J., Mayolas-Pi, C., Reverter-Masià, J., López-Laval, I., Oviedo-Caro, M. Á., Munguía-Izquierdo, D., Ruidíaz-Peña, M., & Legaz-Arrese, A. (2020). Exercise addiction and its relationship with health outcomes in indoor cycling practitioners in fitness centers. *International Journal of Environmental Research and Public Health*, *17*(11), 4159. DOI: 10.3390/ijerph17114159 PMID: 32545197

Cataldo, I., De Luca, I., Giorgetti, V., Cicconcelli, D., Bersani, F. S., Imperatori, C., Abdi, S., Negri, A., Esposito, G., & Corazza, O. (2021). Fitspiration on social media: Body-image and other psychopathological risks among young adults. A narrative review. *Emerging Trends in Drugs, Addictions, and Health*, *1*, 100010. DOI: 10.1016/j.etdah.2021.100010

Ceci, F., Di Carlo, F., Burkauskas, J., Salone, A., De Luca, I., Cicconcelli, D., Giorgetti, V., La Fratta, I., Todaro, A., Simonato, P., Martinotti, G., di Giannantonio, M., & Corazza, O. (2022). Physical activity and exercise addiction during the COVID-19 pandemic in Italy. *International Journal of Mental Health and Addiction*, *21*(6), 3678–3698. DOI: 10.1007/s11469-022-00815-z PMID: 35469185

Centers for Disease Control and Prevention. (2023). *Physical activity basics.* U.S. Department of Health and Human Services. https://www.cdc.gov/physical-activity-basics/guidelines/adults.html

Colledge, F., Buchner, U., Schmidt, A., & Walter, M. (2019). Does exercise addiction exist? A brief review of current measurement tools and future directions. *Mental Health and Addiction Research*, *4*(2), 1–4. DOI: 10.15761/MHAR.1000181

Colledge, F., Buchner, U., Schmidt, A., Wiesbeck, G., Lang, U., Pühse, U., Gerber, M., & Walter, M. (2022). Individuals at risk of exercise addiction have higher scores for depression, adhd, and childhood trauma. *Frontiers in Sports and Active Living*, *3*, 761844–761844. DOI: 10.3389/fspor.2021.761844 PMID: 35156014

Colledge, F., Cody, R., Buchner, U. G., Schmidt, A., Pühse, U., Gerber, M., Wiesbeck, G., Lang, U. E., & Walter, M. (2020). Excessive exercise—A meta-review. *Frontiers in Psychiatry*, *11*, 521572. Advance online publication. DOI: 10.3389/fpsyt.2020.521572 PMID: 33329076

Corazza, D., & Dores, A. R. (2023). *The body in the mind: Exercise addiction, body image and the use of enhancement drugs*. Cambridge University Press., DOI: 10.1017/9781911623731

Corazza, O., Simonato, P., Demetrovics, Z., Mooney, R., van de Ven, K., Roman-Urrestarazu, A., Rácmolnár, L., De Luca, I., Cinosi, E., Santacroce, R., Marini, M., Wellsted, D., Sullivan, K., Bersani, G., Martinotti, G., & Annunziato, R. A. (2019). The emergence of exercise addiction, body dysmorphic disorder, and other image-related psychopathological correlates in fitness settings: A cross-sectional study. *PLoS One*, *14*(4), e0213060–e0213060. DOI: 10.1371/journal.pone.0213060 PMID: 30943200

Cunningham, H. E., Pearman, S.III, & Brewerton, T. D. (2016). Conceptualizing primary and secondary pathological exercise using available measures of excessive exercise. *International Journal of Eating Disorders*, *49*(8), 778–792. DOI: 10.1002/eat.22551 PMID: 27203379

Dalle Grave, R., Calugi, S., & Marchesini, G. (2008). Compulsive exercise to control shape or weight in eating disorders: Prevalence, associated features, and treatment outcome. *Comprehensive Psychiatry*, *49*(4), 346–352. DOI: 10.1016/j.comppsych.2007.12.007 PMID: 18555054

De Luca, I., Simonato, P., Mooney, R., Bersani, G., Corazza, O., Corazza, O., & Unit, N. P. S. (2017). Can exercise be an addiction? The evolution of 'fitspiration' in society. *Research and Advances in Psychiatry*, *4*, 27–34.

Despres, R. (1997). Burn, baby, burn: At what point does the quest for ultimate fitness turn into an unhealthy obsession? For women athletes, as it turns out, it's hard to tell. *Women's Sports and Fitness*, *19*, 38–44.

Di Lodovico, L., Poulnais, S., & Gorwood, P. (2019). Which sports are more at risk of physical exercise addiction: A systematic review. *Addictive Behaviors*, *93*, 257–262. DOI: 10.1016/j.addbeh.2018.12.030 PMID: 30595420

Draeger, J., Yates, A., & Crowell, D. (2005). The obligatory exerciser. *The Physician and Sportsmedicine*, *33*(6), 13–23. DOI: 10.3810/psm.2005.06.101 PMID: 20086364

Dumitru, D. C., Dumitru, T., & Maher, A. J. (2018). A systematic review of exercise addiction: Examining gender differences. *Journal of Physical Education and Sport*, *18*(3), 1738–1747. DOI: 10.7752/jpes.2018.03253

Egorov, A. Y., & Szabo, A. (2013). The exercise paradox: An interactional model for a clearer conceptualization of exercise addiction. *Journal of Behavioral Addictions*, *2*(4), 199–208. DOI: 10.1556/JBA.2.2013.4.2 PMID: 25215201

Freimuth, M., Moniz, S., & Kim, S. R. (2011). Clarifying exercise addiction: Differential diagnosis, co-occurring disorders, and phases of addiction. *International Journal of Environmental Research and Public Health*, *8*(10), 4069–4081. DOI: 10.3390/ijerph8104069 PMID: 22073029

Garcia-Caballero, A., Torrens-Lluch, M., Ramirez-Gendrau, I., Garrido, G., Valles, V., & Aragay, N. (2018). The efficacy of motivational interviewing and cognitive-behavioral therapy for pathological gambling. *Addictions*, *30*(3).

Granziol, U., Griffiths, M. D., Zou, L., Yang, P., Herschel, H. K., Junker, A., Akimoto, T., Stoll, O., Alpay, M., Aydın, Z., Zandonai, T., Di Lodovico, L., Lichtenstein, M. B., Trott, M., Portman, R. M., Schipfer, M., Cook, B., Cerea, S., Egorov, A. Y., & Szabo, A. (2023). The Expanded Exercise Addiction Inventory (EAI-3): Towards reliable and international screening of exercise-related dysfunction. *International Journal of Mental Health and Addiction*, *22*(6), 3559–3585. DOI: 10.1007/s11469-023-01066-2 PMID: 37363769

Griffiths, M. (2005). A 'components' model of addiction within a biopsychosocial framework. *Journal of Substance Use*, *10*(4), 191–197. DOI: 10.1080/14659890500114359

Hale, B. D., Diehl, D., Weaver, K., & Briggs, M. (2013). Exercise dependence and muscle dysmorphia in novice and experienced female bodybuilders. *Journal of Behavioral Addictions*, *2*(4), 244–248. DOI: 10.1556/JBA.2.2013.4.8 PMID: 25215207

Hausenblas, H. A., & Downs, D. S. (2002a). Exercise dependence: A systematic review. *Psychology of Sport and Exercise*, *3*(2), 89–123. DOI: 10.1016/S1469-0292(00)00015-7

Hausenblas, H. A., & Downs, D. S. (2002b). How much is too much? The development and validation of the exercise dependence scale. *Psychology & Health, 17*(4), 387–404. DOI: 10.1080/0887044022000004894

Hausenblas, H. A., Schreiber, K., & Smoliga, J. M. (2017). Addiction to exercise. *BMJ (Clinical Research Ed.)*, j1745. Advance online publication. DOI: 10.1136/bmj.j1745 PMID: 28446435

Holland, G., & Tiggemann, M. (2017). "Strong beats skinny every time": Disordered eating and compulsive exercise in women who post fitspiration on Instagram. *International Journal of Eating Disorders, 50*(1), 76–79. DOI: 10.1002/eat.22559 PMID: 27302867

Kanayama, G., Brower, K. J., Wood, R. I., Hudson, J. I., & Pope, H. G.Jr. (2009). Anabolic-androgenic steroid dependence: An emerging disorder. *Addiction (Abingdon, England), 104*(12), 1966–1978. DOI: 10.1111/j.1360-0443.2009.02734.x PMID: 19922565

Khoshro, S., Farhangi, M. A., & Jahangiry, L. (2024). Psychometric properties of the exercise addiction inventory (EAI) questionnaire among physically active young adults. *BMC Research Notes, 17*(1), 76. DOI: 10.1186/s13104-024-06722-x PMID: 38486222

Koob, G.F., Kandel, D.B., Baler, R.D., & Volkow, N.D. (2023). Neurobiology of addiction. *Tasman's Psychiatry,* 1-51. https://doi.org/DOI: 10.1007/978-3-030-42825-9_29-1

Landolfi, E. (2013). Exercise addiction. *Sports Medicine (Auckland, N.Z.), 43*(2), 111–119. DOI: 10.1007/s40279-012-0013-x PMID: 23329605

Lee, D., Namkoong, K., Lee, J., & Jung, Y. C. (2018). Abnormal gray matter volume and impulsivity in young adults with Internet gaming disorder. *Addiction Biology, 23*(5), 1160–1167. DOI: 10.1111/adb.12552 PMID: 28884950

Lejoyeux, M., Avril, M., Richoux, C., Embouazza, H., & Nivoli, F. (2008). Prevalence of exercise dependence and other behavioral addictions among clients of a Parisian fitness room. *Comprehensive Psychiatry, 49*(4), 353–358. https://doi.org/ . 2007.12.005DOI: 10.1016/j.comppsych

Lewis, R. G., Florio, E., Punzo, D., & Borrelli, E. (2021). The brain's reward system in health and disease. *Advances in Experimental Medicine and Biology, 1344*, 57–69. DOI: 10.1007/978-3-030-81147-1_4 PMID: 34773226

Lichtenstein, M. B., Christiansen, E., Elklit, A., Bilenberg, N., & Støving, R. K. (2014). Exercise addiction: A study of eating disorder symptoms, quality of life, personality traits and attachment styles. *Psychiatry Research, 215*(2), 410–416. DOI: 10.1016/j.psychres.2013.11.010 PMID: 24342179

Lichtenstein, M. B. & Hinze, C. J. (2020). Exercise addiction. *Adolescent Addiction*, 265–288. DOI: 10.1016/B978-0-12-818626-8.00010-4

Lichtenstein, M. B., Hinze, C. J., Emborg, B., Thomsen, F., & Hemmingsen, S. D. (2017). Compulsive exercise: Links, risks and challenges faced. *Psychology Research and Behavior Management, 10*, 85–95. DOI: 10.2147/PRBM.S113093 PMID: 28435339

Lichtenstein, M. B., Melin, A. K., Szabo, A., & Holm, L. (2021). The prevalence of exercise addiction symptoms in a sample of national level elite athletes. *Frontiers in Sports and Active Living*, *3*, 635418. Advance online publication. DOI: 10.3389/fspor.2021.635418 PMID: 34179773

Lim, M. A. (2021). Exercise addiction and COVID-19-associated restrictions. *Journal of Mental Health (Abingdon, England), 30*(2), 135–137. DOI: 10.1080/09638237.2020.1803234 PMID: 32755432

Maan, J. S., Ershadi, M., Khan, I., & Saadabadi, A. (2023). Quetiapine. In *StatPearls*. StatPearls Publishing., https://www.ncbi.nlm.nih.gov/books/NBK459145

Maceri, R. M., Cherup, N. P., Buckworth, J., & Hanson, N. J. (2019). Exercise addiction in long distance runners. *International Journal of Mental Health and Addiction*, *19*(1), 62–71. DOI: 10.1007/s11469-019-00122-0

Magee, C. A., Buchman, I., & Barrie, L. (2016). Profiles of exercise dependence symptoms in ironman participants. *Psychology of Sport and Exercise*, *24*, 48–55. DOI: 10.1016/j.psychsport.2016.01.005

Manfredi, P. (2022). Benefits, risks and gender differences in sport, and exercise dependence: Key role of alexithymia. *International Journal of Environmental Research and Public Health*, *19*(9), 5288. DOI: 10.3390/ijerph19095288 PMID: 35564683

Marques, A., Peralta, M., Sarmento, H., Loureiro, V., Gouveia, É. R., & de Matos, M. G. (2019). Prevalence of risk for exercise dependence: A systematic review. *Sports Medicine (Auckland, N.Z.), 49*(2), 319–330. DOI: 10.1007/s40279-018-1011-4 PMID: 30374944

Meyer, C., Taranis, L., Goodwin, H., & Haycraft, E. (2011). Compulsive exercise and eating disorders. *European Eating Disorders Review*, *19*(3), 174–189. DOI: 10.1002/erv.1122 PMID: 21584911

Meyer, M., Sattler, I., Schilling, H., Lang, U. E., Schmidt, A., Colledge, F., & Walter, M. (2021). Mental disorders in individuals with exercise addiction—A cross-sectional study. *Frontiers in Psychiatry*, *12*, 751550–751550. DOI: 10.3389/fpsyt.2021.751550 PMID: 34955915

Miller, K. J., & Mesagno, C. (2014). Personality traits and exercise dependence: Exploring the role of narcissism and perfectionism. *International Journal of Sport and Exercise Psychology*, *12*(4), 368–381. DOI: 10.1080/1612197X.2014.932821

Minutillo, A., Di Trana, A., Aquilina, V., Ciancio, G. M., Berretta, P., & La Maida, N. (2024). Recent insights in the correlation between social media use, personality traits and exercise addiction: A literature review. *Frontiers in Psychiatry*, *15*, 1392317–1392317. DOI: 10.3389/fpsyt.2024.1392317 PMID: 38800058

Modolo, V. B., Antunes, H. K. M., de Gimenez, P. R. B., De Mello Santiago, M. L., Tufik, S., & de Mello, M. T. (2011). Negative addiction to exercise: Are there differences between genders? *Clinics (São Paulo, Brazil)*, *66*(2), 255–260. https://doi.org/DOI: 10.1590/S1807-59322011000200013

Müller, A., Loeber, S., Söchtig, J., Te Wildt, B. T., & De Zwaan, M. (2015). Risk for exercise dependence, eating disorder pathology, alcohol use disorder and addictive behaviors among clients of fitness centers. *Journal of Behavioral Addictions*, *4*(4), 273–280. DOI: 10.1556/2006.4.2015.044 PMID: 26690622

Nazish, N. (2024, December 30). *Is the TikTok-viral 75 Hard Challenge right for you? Experts explain.* Verywell Mind. https://www.verywellmind.com/75-hard-challenge-8750715

Olave, L., Momeñe, J., Rodríguez Pérez, J. G., Estévez, A., & Iruarrizaga, I. (2019). ¿Existen diferencias en los esquemas cognitivos y en la autoestima entre las personas con adicción al ejercicio físico o con dismorfia muscular? [Are there differences in cognitive patterns and self-esteem among people with exercise addiction or muscle dysmorphia?]. *Revista Española de Drogodependencias*, *44*(2), 43–61. https://www.aesed.com/upload/files/v44n2_art2-dismorfia.pdf

Outar, L., Turner, M. J., Wood, A. G., & Lowry, R. (2018). "I need to go to the gym": Exploring the use of rational emotive behaviour therapy upon exercise addiction, irrational and rational beliefs. *Performance Enhancement & Health*, *6*(2), 82–93. DOI: 10.1016/j.peh.2018.05.001

Pálfi, V., Kovacsik, R., & Szabo, A. (2021). Symptoms of exercise addiction in aerobic and anaerobic exercises: Beyond the components model of addiction. *Psychology of Sport and Exercise*, *57*, 101952. DOI: 10.1016/j.psychsport.2021.101952 PMID: 34938830

Pangarkar, T. (2025, January 13). *Fitness tracker statistics 2025 by health activities.* Market.us News. https://www.news.market.us/fitness-tracker-statistics/

Pierce, E. F., Daleng, M. L., & McGowan, R. W. (1993). Scores on exercise dependence among dancers. *Perceptual and Motor Skills*, *76*(2), 531–535. DOI: 10.2466/pms.1993.76.2.531 PMID: 8483663

Prochaska, J. O., & DiClemente, C. C. (1983). Stages and processes of self-change of smoking: Toward an integrative model of change. *Journal of Consulting and Clinical Psychology*, *51*(3), 390–395. DOI: 10.1037/0022-006X.51.3.390 PMID: 6863699

Sicilia, Á., Paterna, A., Alcaraz-Ibáñez, M., & Griffiths, M. D. (2021). Theoretical conceptualisations of problematic exercise in Psychometric Assessment Instruments: A systematic review. *Journal of Behavioral Addictions*, *10*(1), 4–20. DOI: 10.1556/2006.2021.00019 PMID: 33822749

Stoliaroff, S. (2003). Know the signs of unhealthy exercise addiction. *Running Fit News*, *18*(6), 4–5.

Sussman, S., Lisha, N., & Griffiths, M. (2011). Prevalence of the addictions: A problem of the majority or the minority? *Evaluation & the Health Professions*, *34*(1), 3–56. DOI: 10.1177/0163278710380124 PMID: 20876085

Szabo, A. (1995). The impact of exercise deprivation on well-being of habitual exercises. *Australian Journal of Science and Medicine in Sport*, *27*, 68–75. PMID: 8599747

Szabo, A. (2010). *Addiction to exercise: A symptom or a disorder?* Nova Science Publishers, Incorporated.

Szabo, A., de la Vega, R., Kovácsik, R., Jiménez Almendros, L., Ruíz-Barquín, R., Demetrovics, Z., Boros, S., & Köteles, F. (2022). Dimensions of passion and their relationship to the risk of exercise addiction: Cultural and gender differences. *Addictive Behaviors Reports*, *16*, 100451–100451. DOI: 10.1016/j.abrep.2022.100451 PMID: 36092546

Szabo, A., & Demetrovics, Z. (2022). *Passion and addiction in sports and exercise.* Routledge. DOI: 10.4324/9781003173595

Szabo, A., & Griffiths, M. D. (2020). Exercise addiction: Prevalence, diagnosis, and treatment. In *Handbook of sport psychology* (pp. 153–165). Elsevier., DOI: 10.1016/B978-0-12-818626-8.00010-4

Szabo, A., Griffiths, M. D., Aarhus Høglid, R., & Demetrovics, Z. (2018). Drug, nicotine, and alcohol use among exercisers: Does substance addiction co-occur with exercise addiction? *Addictive Behaviors Reports, 7*, 26–31. https://doi.org/. 2017.12.001DOI: 10.1016/j.abrep

Szabo, A., & Kovacsik, R. (2019). When passion appears, exercise addiction disappears. *Swiss Journal of Psychology*, *78*(3–4), 137–142. DOI: 10.1024/1421-0185/a000228

Szabo, A., & Rendi, M. (2008). Exercise addiction. In Lane, A. (Ed.), *Sport and exercise psychology: Topics in applied psychology* (pp. 186–203). Hodder Education., https://perpus.univpancasila.ac.id/repository/EBUPT180160.pdf#page=186

Tiggemann, M., & Zaccardo, M. (2015). "Exercise to be fit, not skinny": The effect of fitspiration imagery on women's body image. *Body Image*, *15*, 61–67. DOI: 10.1016/j.bodyim.2015.06.003 PMID: 26176993

Trott, M., Jackson, S. E., Firth, J., Jacob, L., Grabovac, I., Mistry, A., Stubbs, B., & Smith, L. (2020). A comparative meta-analysis of the prevalence of exercise addiction in adults with and without indicated eating disorders. *Eating and Weight Disorders*, *26*(1), 37–46. DOI: 10.1007/s40519-019-00842-1 PMID: 31894540

Trott, M., Johnstone, J., Pardhan, S., Barnett, Y., & Smith, L. (2021). Changes in body dysmorphic disorder, eating disorder, and exercise addiction symptomology during the COVID-19 pandemic: A longitudinal study of 319 health club users. *Psychiatry Research*, *298*, 113831–113831. DOI: 10.1016/j.psychres.2021.113831 PMID: 33652248

Turner, M. J., Carrington, S., & Miller, A. (2019). Psychological distress across sport participation groups: The mediating effects of secondary irrational beliefs on the relationship between primary irrational beliefs and symptoms of anxiety, anger, and depression. *Journal of Clinical Sport Psychology*, *13*(1), 17–40. DOI: 10.1123/jcsp.2017-0014

Veale, D. M. (1987). Exercise dependence. *British Journal of Addiction*, *82*(7), 735–740. DOI: 10.1111/j.1360-0443.1987.tb01539.x PMID: 3311101

Veale, D. M. (1995). Does primary exercise dependence really exist? In Annett, J., Cripps, B., & Steinberg, H. (Eds.), *Exercise addiction: Motivation for participation in sport and exercise: Proceedings of British Psychology, Sport and Exercise Psychology Section* (pp. 71–75). British Psychological Society.

Villella, C., Martinotti, G., Di Nicola, M., Cassano, M., La Torre, G., Gliubizzi, M. D., Messeri, I., Petruccelli, F., Bria, P., Janiri, L., & Conte, G. (2011). Behavioural addictions in adolescents and young adults: Results from a prevalence study. *Journal of Gambling Studies*, *27*(2), 203–214. DOI: 10.1007/s10899-010-9206-0 PMID: 20559694

Weinstein, A. & Szabo, A. (2023). Exercise addiction: A narrative overview of research issues. *Dialogues in Clinical Neuroscience, 25*(1), 1–13. https://doi.org/. 2023.2164841DOI: 10.1080/19585969

Weinstein, A., & Weinstein, Y. (2013). Exercise addiction- diagnosis, bio-psychological mechanisms and treatment issues. *Current Pharmaceutical Design*, *20*(25), 4062–4069. DOI: 10.2174/13816128113199990614 PMID: 24001300

Weinstein, A., Weinstein, Y., & Maayan, G. (2015). A study on the relationship between compulsive exercise, depression and anxiety. *Journal of Behavioral Addictions*, *4*(4), 315–318. DOI: 10.1556/2006.4.2015.034 PMID: 26690627

Yip, S. W., Worhunsky, P. D., Xu, J., Morie, K. P., Constable, R. T., Malison, R. T., Carroll, K. M., & Potenza, M. N. (2018). Gray-matter relationships to diagnostic and transdiagnostic features of drug and behavioral addictions. *Addiction Biology*, *23*(1), 394–402. DOI: 10.1111/adb.12492 PMID: 28150390

Youngman, J., & Simpson, D. (2014). Risk for exercise addiction: A comparison of triathletes training for sprint-, olympic-, half-ironman-, and ironman-distance triathlons. *Journal of Clinical Sport Psychology*, *8*(1), 19–37. DOI: 10.1123/jcsp.2014-0010

Zhang, F., Xie, H., Wang, S., Li, F., Gong, Q., & Jia, Z. (2023). The role of the orbitofrontal cortex in exercise addiction and exercise motivation: A brain imaging study based on multimodal magnetic resonance imaging. *Journal of Affective Disorders*, *325*, 240–247. DOI: 10.1016/j.jad.2023.01.030 PMID: 36638963

Conclusion

The examination of behavioral addiction articulated in this volume underscores a paradigm shift within the scientific and clinical communities regarding the recognition, classification, and treatment of these complex disorders. Historically, the concept of addiction was predominantly associated with substance misuse, often leading to skepticism about behaviors such as gambling, gaming, or pornography viewing being labeled as true addictions. However, burgeoning neuroscience research robustly affirms that addiction is fundamentally a brain-based disease, characterized by neuroplastic changes and dysregulation within the brain's reward circuitry (American Society of Addiction Medicine [ASAM], 2019; National Institute on Drug Abuse [NIDA], 2020; Widyanto & McMurran, 2004). This evidence challenges older stigmatized notions and broadens the scope to include behaviors that, although without chemical substances, can produce similar neurobiological and psychological hallmarks of addiction.

The neurobiological framework emphasizes that addictive behaviors—whether related to internet use, gambling, shopping, or pornography—activate the mesolimbic dopamine pathway, a core neural substrate involved in processing reward, motivation, and reinforcement. As ASAM articulates, addiction is a treatable, chronic medical condition where individuals engage in behaviors that become compulsive, often persisting despite significant adverse consequences (ASAM, 2019). This understanding not only informs diagnosis and treatment but also fosters compassion and reduces moral judgment, acknowledging that these behaviors stem from brain dysregulation rather than simply moral failings.

Groundbreaking contributions by scholars like Stanton Peele broaden the conceptualization of addiction to include maladaptive coping strategies that are not necessarily substance related. Peele's perspective emphasizes that addiction is fundamentally related to the reliance on certain experiences or activities—such as compulsive gaming, overeating, or social media use—to manage emotional distress or fulfill unmet psychological needs (Peele & Brodsky, 1975). This aligns with current research demonstrating that behavioral addictions often serve as attempts to regulate affect, manage boredom, or escape pain, thereby integrating emotional and cognitive dimensions into understanding these disorders (Shaffer & Shaffer, 2023; Sussman & Tsi, 2020).

A growing body of evidence supports the argument that behavioral addictions share core features with substance use disorders, including salience, euphoria, tolerance, withdrawal, conflict, and relapse (Alimoradi et al., 2022; Fournier et al., 2023; Shaffer & Shaffer, 2023). These features are critical for diagnosis and intervention planning. For example, the prevalence of such disorders is significant—albeit variable—yet recent meta-analyses of a global population sample indicate that approximately 11.1% of populations experience some form of behavioral addiction, with higher rates observed among adolescents and young adults (Alimoradi et al., 2022). Furthermore, national surveys within the United States reveal widespread engagement with potentially addictive behaviors, raising the urgency for mental health professionals to be equipped with a nuanced understanding of these conditions.

Treatment Considerations

Several authors articulate research-based interventions in the different chapters. In addition, the editors would like to caution behavioral and other health care professionals working within clinical, educational, and community settings that they must remain vigilant against the risks of over-pathologizing behaviors due to personal biases or moral judgments. The history of stigma within marginalized communities, such as the kink community, exemplifies how moralistic perspectives can interfere with objective assessment and ethical treatment (Wright, 2008). As outlined by Kardefelt-Winther et al. (2017), behaviors should only be classified as addictions when they produce significant functional impairment or distress, and when other underlying psychiatric conditions do not better account for the presentation. This cautions against simplistic or moralistic diagnoses, fostering a scientific, respectful, and culturally sensitive approach.

Directions for Future Research

The chapters on internet use, exercise, gambling, social media, shopping, and pornography illustrate a standard research focus on behavioral addiction and its impact on individuals' mental health and society. There is a consensus that behavioral addictions continue to have devastating effects, negatively affecting human relationships and overall well-being. These chapters explore the scope, symptomatology, prevalence, assessment, and treatment options for various behavioral addictions. While the authors identify emerging trends within this field, it remains crucial to advocate for ongoing and repeated research efforts to enhance our understanding of screening, assessment, and intervention strategies.

Recent studies increasingly examine how specific addictions influence individuals, families, and communities. We recommend longitudinal research that allows for the observation of particular variables over extended periods within targeted populations. Such studies should encompass diverse demographics, including age, gender, and ethnicity, to assess how these behaviors affect individuals and society over time. For example, the concept of Exercise Addiction, as described by Lee, Nuyen, and Zielke (in this volume), provides a valuable basis for future longitudinal studies. Comparative research could explore differences between athletes and non-athletes or between types of exercise, such as marathon running versus CrossFit, to understand their influence on physical and mental development from emerging adulthood into late adulthood.

These longitudinal studies would also facilitate the development of more effective assessment tools. Similarly, research into the complexities of social media use could focus on diverse populations worldwide, especially considering cultural and socioeconomic differences. Given the challenges of studying such diverse groups, it is essential to compare populations with access to affordable internet with those without such resources. Variables such as cognitive, social, and physical development should also be considered to explore how internet and social media use affect overall growth, social interaction, and mental health.

For instance, the chapter on internet use and unregulated social media, particularly regarding video game addiction and its impact on adolescent mental health (included in this volume), highlights significant implications. This area opens the door to numerous longitudinal and experimental studies aimed at informing educators, counselors, parents, policymakers, and other stakeholders about concerns surrounding social interaction among minors, particularly those related to online anonymity and gaming, which require further investigation. Questions arise about striking a balance between supervising teens' autonomy and promoting outdoor physical activities. If these issues are valid for families, there is a clear need to assess potential risks, develop effective coping strategies, establish support groups for affected youth and their families, and enhance treatments.

There is a pressing need for providers to learn how to incorporate emerging technologies and innovative treatment approaches. Many individuals now use mobile applications to identify and manage mental health issues. However, challenges such as privacy concerns and limited integration of empirically validated techniques persist. Finding practical and functional apps suitable for individuals struggling with behavioral addictions remains a critical task for health professionals (Magee et al., 2018).

Policy and Advocacy Considerations

Significant work remains to raise awareness about the existence and harmful effects of behavioral addictions. Those affected are often stigmatized and face discrimination in various social contexts. Community engagement and advocacy can help combat these biases. Additionally, educators should proactively incorporate prevention strategies and destigmatization efforts into curricula.

Health professionals—behavioral health specialists, addiction counselors, educators, and other stakeholders—must stay informed about the evolving landscape of behavioral addiction research. Further investigation is necessary to deepen the understanding of non-substance addictive behaviors and improve assessment and treatment protocols.

The editors and contributors hope this volume not only educates and informs but also motivates further training and advocacy efforts. Understanding the needs of clients experiencing behavioral addictions is essential for developing compassionate and effective interventions and policies. One client, asked by Dr. Johnson what it would mean to feel no longer addicted to pornography, responded: "Freedom! I would be free." May the insights provided in this work help individuals in distress find relief and liberation from their out-of-control behaviors.

Rommel Johnson
Reuben Mwangi

REFERENCES

Alimoradi, Z., Lotfi, A., Lin, C.-Y., Griffiths, M. D., & Pakpour, A. H. (2022). Estimation of Behavioral Addiction Prevalence During COVID-19 Pandemic: A Systematic Review and Meta-analysis. *Current Addiction Reports*, *9*(4), 486–517. Advance online publication. DOI: 10.1007/s40429-022-00435-6 PMID: 36118286

American Society of Addiction Medicine. (2019, September 15). Definition of Addiction. https://www.asam.org/docs/default-source/quality-science/asam's-2019-definition-of-addiction-(1).pdf?sfvrsn=b8b64fc2_2

Fournier, L., Schimmenti, A., Musetti, A., Boursier, V., Flayelle, M., Cataldo, I., Starcevic, V., & Billieux, J. (2023). Deconstructing the components model of addiction: An illustration through "addictive" use of social media. *Addictive Behaviors*, *143*, 107694. DOI: 10.1016/j.addbeh.2023.107694 PMID: 36940658

Kardefelt-Winther, D., Heeren, A., Schimmenti, A., van Rooij, A., Maurage, P., Carras, M., Edman, J., Blaszczynski, A., Khazaal, Y., & Billieux, J. (2017). How can we conceptualize behavioural addiction without pathologizing common behaviours? *Addiction (Abingdon, England)*, *112*(10), 1709–1715. DOI: 10.1111/add.13763 PMID: 28198052

Magee, J. C., Adut, S., Brazil, K. & Warnick, S. (2018). Mobile App Tools for Identifying and Managing Mental Health Disorders in Primary Care. Curr Treat Options Psychiatry. 16;5(3):345–362. DOI: 10.1007/s40501-018-0154-0

National Institute on Drug Abuse. (2020). *Drug Misuse and Addiction*. National Institute on Drug Abuse; National Institutes of Health. https://nida.nih.gov/publications/drugs-brains-behavior-science-addiction/drug-misuse-addiction

Peele, S., & Brodsky, A. (1975). *Love and Addiction*. Taplinger.

Shaffer, H. J., & Shaffer, P. M. (2023). Behavioral Addiction. In Friedman, H. S. (Ed.), *Encyclopedia of Mental Health* (3rd ed., Vol. 1, pp. 180–187). Academic Press., DOI: 10.1016/B978-0-323-91497-0.00001-1

Sussman, S., & Tsai, J. Y. (2020). Sexual addiction. *Adolescent Addiction*, 241–263. https://doi.org/DOI: 10.1016/B978-0-12-818626-8.00009-8

Widyanto, L., & McMurran, M. (2004). The psychometric properties of the internet addiction test. *Cyberpsychology & Behavior*, *7*(4), 443–450. DOI: 10.1089/cpb.2004.7.443 PMID: 15331031

Wright, S. (2008). Second national survey of violence & discrimination against sexual minorities. *National coalition for sexual freedom*, 19. https://secureservercdn.net/198.71.233.68/9xj.1d5.myftpupload.com/wp-content/uploads/2019/12/Violence-Discrimination-Against-Sexual-Minorities-Survey.pdf

Compilation of References

Aarseth, E., Bean, A. M., Boonen, H., Colder Carras, M., Coulson, M., Das, D., Deleuze, J., Dunkels, E., Edman, J., Ferguson, C. J., Haagsma, M. C., Helmersson Bergmark, K., Hussain, Z., Jansz, J., Kardefelt-Winther, D., Kutner, L., Markey, P., Nielsen, R. K. L., Prause, N., & Van Rooij, A. J. (2017). Scholars' open debate paper on the World Health Organization ICD-11 Gaming Disorder proposal. *Journal of Behavioral Addictions*, *6*(3), 267–270. DOI: 10.1556/2006.5.2016.088 PMID: 28033714

Abel, N. (2019). Do It, don't feel it, and be invincible: A prolog of exercise addiction in endurance sports. *Frontiers in Psychology*, *10*, 1–9. DOI: 10.3389/fpsyg.2019.02692 PMID: 31920780

Aboujaoude, E. (2014). Compulsive buying disorder: A review and update. *Current Pharmaceutical Design*, *20*(25), 4021–4025. DOI: 10.2174/13816128113199990618 PMID: 24001296

Abreu, R. L., & Kenny, M. C. (2018). Cyberbullying and LGBTQ youth: A systematic literature review and recommendations for prevention and intervention. *Journal of Child & Adolescent Trauma*, *11*(1), 81–97. DOI: 10.1007/s40653-017-0175-7 PMID: 32318140

Abu Khait, A., Mrayyan, M. T., Al-Rjoub, S., Rababa, M., & Al-Rawashdeh, S. (2023). Cyberchondria, anxiety sensitivity, hypochondria, and internet addiction: Implications for mental health professionals. *Current Psychology (New Brunswick, N.J.)*, *42*(31), 27141–27152. DOI: 10.1007/s12144-022-03815-3 PMID: 36254213

Adams, J. (2013). Exercise dependence. *Principles of Addiction*, *1*, 827–835. DOI: 10.1016/B978-0-12-398336-7.00083-8

Adams, J. M., Miller, T. W., & Kraus, R. F. (2003). Exercise dependence: Diagnostic and therapeutic issues for patients in psychotherapy. *Journal of Contemporary Psychotherapy*, *33*(2), 93–107. DOI: 10.1023/A:1022883104269

Adu-Akoh, P. J. (2022). Problem Gambling Correlates and Their Effects on Study Habits of Students" Sport Bettors in the University of Cape Coast (Doctoral dissertation, University of Cape Coast).

Ajewumi, O. E., Magbagbeola, V., Kalu, O. C., Ike, R. A., Folajimi, O., & Diyaolu, C. O. (2024). The impact of social media on mental health and well-being. *World Journal of Advanced Research and Reviews*, *24*(1), 107–121. DOI: 10.30574/wjarr.2024.24.1.3027

Akbari, M., Seydavi, M., Zamani, E., & Griffiths, M. D. (2024). The risk of exercise addiction mediates the relationship between social media use and mental health indices among young Iranians. *Addiction Research and Theory*, *32*(1), 27–37. DOI: 10.1080/16066359.2022.2149742

Alavi, S. S., Ghanizadeh, M., Mohammadi, M. R., Jannatifard, F., Esmaeeli Alamooti, S., & Farahani, M. (2021). The effects of cognitive-behavioral group therapy on reducing the symptoms of internet addiction disorder and promoting the quality of life and mental health. *Trends in Psychiatry and Psychotherapy*, *43*(1). Advance online publication. DOI: 10.47626/2237-6089-2020-0010 PMID: 33681908

Alavi, S. S., Maracy, M. R., Jannatifard, F., & Eslami, M. (2011). The effect of psychiatric symptoms on the internet addiction disorder in Isfahan's University students. *Journal of Research in Medical Sciences : the Official Journal of Isfahan University of Medical Sciences*, *16*(6), 793. PMID: 22091309

Albrecht, U., Kirschner, N. E., & Grüsser, S. M. (2007). Diagnostic instruments for behavioural addiction: an overview. GMS Psycho-Social Medicine, 4.

Alimoradi, Z., Lotfi, A., Lin, C.-Y., Griffiths, M. D., & Pakpour, A. H. (2022). Estimation of behavioral addiction prevalence during COVID-19 pandemic: A systematic review and meta-analysis. *Current Addiction Reports*, *9*(4), 486–517. DOI: 10.1007/s40429-022-00435-6 PMID: 36118286

Allegre, B., Souville, M., Therme, P., & Griffiths, M. (2009). Definitions and measures of exercise dependence. *Addiction Research and Theory*, *14*(6), 631–646. DOI: 10.1080/16066350600903302

Amemiya, S., Takao, H., & Abe, O. (2024). Resting-State fMRI: Emerging Concepts for Future Clinical Application. *Journal of Magnetic Resonance Imaging*, *59*(4), 1135–1148. DOI: 10.1002/jmri.28894 PMID: 37424140

American Psychiatric Association (APA). (2013). *Diagnostic and Statistical Manual of Mental Disorders* (5th ed.). American Psychiatric Publishing.

American Psychiatric Association. (2013). *Diagnostic and statistical manual of mental disorders* (5th ed.). American Psychiatric Publishing.

American Psychiatric Association. (2023, January). Internet gaming. *James Sherer, M.D.*https://www.psychiatry.org/patients-families/internet-gaming

American Psychological Association. (2015). *APA Dictionary of Psychology* (2nd ed.). American Psychological Association.

American Society of Addiction Medicine. (2024). *American Society of Addiction Medicine*. https://www.asam.org/

Amichai-Hamburger, Y., & Vinitzky, G. (2010). Social network use and personality. *Computers in Human Behavior, 26*(6), 1289–1295. DOI: 10.1016/j.chb.2010.03.018

Amin, H. S., Nagshabandi, K., & Alhammad, S. (2022). Compulsive buying disorder (CBD) among medical students in colleges of medicine, dentistry and pharmacy at King Saud University in Riyadh. *Journal of Family Medicine and Primary Care, 11*(11), 6876–6884. DOI: 10.4103/jfmpc.jfmpc_769_22 PMID: 36993053

Anderson, R. (2017). Understanding video game mechanics as a tool in creating a sustainable relationship with digital media. In J. Christenson & A. Merritts (Eds.), *Family therapy with adolescents in residential treatment* (pp. 49□70). Springer, Cham. https://doi.org/DOI: 10.1007/978-3-319-51747-6_4

Andic, S., & Durak Batigun, A. (2019). *Development of Internet Addiction Scale Based on DSM-5 Diagnostic Criteria: An Evaluation in Terms of Internet Gaming Disorder*. Turkish Journal of Psychiatry., DOI: 10.5080/u23194

Andreassen, C. S. (2015). Online social network site addiction: A comprehensive review. *Current Addiction Reports, 2*(2), 175–184. DOI: 10.1007/s40429-015-0056-9

Andreassen, C. S., Griffiths, M. D., Gjertsen, S. R., Krossbakken, E., Kvam, S., & Pallesen, S. (2013). The relationships between behavioral addictions and the five-factor model of personality. *Journal of Behavioral Addictions, 2*(2), 90–99. DOI: 10.1556/JBA.2.2013.003 PMID: 26165928

Andreassen, C. S., Griffiths, M. D., Pallesen, S., Bilder, R. M., Torsheim, T., & Aboujaoude, E. (2015). The Bergen Shopping Addiction Scale: Reliability and validity of a brief screening test. *Frontiers in Psychology, 6*, 1374. DOI: 10.3389/fpsyg.2015.01374 PMID: 26441749

Andreassen, C. S., Torsheim, T., Brunborg, G. S., & Pallesen, S. (2012). Development of a Facebook Addiction Scale. *Psychological Reports, 110*(2), 501–517. DOI: 10.2466/02.09.18.PR0.110.2.501-517 PMID: 22662404

Antoniac, L.-D., Hu ul, T.-D., Karner-Hu uleac, A., & Hu ul, A. (2024). Addressing Internet Addiction Among Adolescents: A Literature Review and a Proposal of Guidelines for Psychotherapists and Mental Health Workers. *The American Journal of Family Therapy, 1*(16). Advance online publication. DOI: 10.1080/01926187.2024.2434850

Arora, C., & Razavian, M. (2021). Ethics of gamification in health and fitness-tracking. *International Journal of Environmental Research and Public Health, 18*(21), 11052. DOI: 10.3390/ijerph182111052 PMID: 34769570

Arrigoni, C. L. E. (2019). Are loot boxes gambling? A crate start for a new gambling framework.

Arzani-Birgani, A., Zarei, J., Favaregh, L., & Ghanaatiyan, E. (2021). Internet addiction, mental health, and sleep quality in students of medical sciences, Iran: A cross-sectional study. *Journal of Education and Health Promotion, 10*(1), 409. DOI: 10.4103/jehp.jehp_1506_20 PMID: 35071615

Astuti, S. A. T., & Winarti, Y. (2022). A scoping review: the impact of pornography addiction on adolescents. *Proceeding of Muhammadiyah International Public Health and Medicine Conference (MIPHMC), 2*(1), 366-381. DOI: 10.61811/miphmp.v1i2.265

Attwood, F. (2004). Pornography and objectification. *Feminist Media Studies, 4*(1), 7–19. DOI: 10.1080/14680770410001674617

Aziz, M., Chemnad, K., Al-Harahsheh, S., Abdelmoneium, A. O., Bagdady, A., Hassan, D. A., & Ali, R. (2024). The influence of adolescents essential and non-essential use of technology and Internet addiction on their physical and mental fatigues. *Scientific Reports, 14*(1), 1745. DOI: 10.1038/s41598-024-51655-x PMID: 38242916

Babusa, B., Czeglédi, E., Túry, F., Mayville, S. B., & Urbán, R. (2015). Differentiating the levels of risk for muscle dysmorphia among Hungarian male weightlifters: A factor mixture modeling approach. *Body Image, 12*, 14–21. DOI: 10.1016/j.bodyim.2014.09.001 PMID: 25280243

Bae, M. (2023). Coping strategies initiated by COVID-19-related stress, individuals' motives for social media use, and perceived stress reduction. *Internet Research, 33*(1), 124–151. DOI: 10.1108/INTR-05-2021-0269

Baer, R. A., & Huss, D. B. (2008). Mindfulness-and acceptance-based therapy. Twenty-first century psychotherapies: Contemporary approaches to theory and practice, 123-166.

Baik, J. H. (2020). Stress and the dopaminergic reward system. *Experimental & Molecular Medicine*, *52*(12), 1879–1890. DOI: 10.1038/s12276-020-00532-4 PMID: 33257725

Baloğlu, M., Şahin, R., & Arpaci, I. (2020). A review of recent research in problematic internet use: Gender and cultural differences. *Current Opinion in Psychology*, *36*, 124–129. DOI: 10.1016/j.copsyc.2020.05.008 PMID: 32629412

Bancroft, J., Janssen, E., Strong, D., Carnes, L., Vukadinovic, Z., & Long, J. S. (2003). The relation between mood and sexuality in heterosexual men. *Archives of Sexual Behavior*, *32*(3), 217–230. DOI: 10.1023/A:1023409516739 PMID: 12807294

Bannon, S., McGlynn, T., McKenzie, K., & Quayle, E. (2015). The Internet and young people with Additional Support Needs (ASN): Risk and safety. *Computers in Human Behavior*, *53*, 495–503. DOI: 10.1016/j.chb.2014.12.057

Bautovich, A. (2017). Pharmacological Management of Problem Gambling. In C. McIntosh & K. O'Neill, Evidence-Based Treatments for Problem Gambling (p. 85-93). Springer International Publishing. DOI: 10.1007/978-3-319-62485-3_9

Belk, R. W. (1988). Possessions and the extended self. *The Journal of Consumer Research*, *15*(2), 139–168. DOI: 10.1086/209154

Belujon, P., & Grace, A. A. (2017). Dopamine system dysregulation in major depressive disorders. *The International Journal of Neuropsychopharmacology*, *20*(12), 1036–1046. DOI: 10.1093/ijnp/pyx056 PMID: 29106542

Benson, A. L. (Ed.). (2000). *I shop, therefore I am: Compulsive buying and the search for self.* Jason Aronson.

Berczik, K., Griffiths, M. D., Szabó, A., Kurimay, T., Urban, R., & Demetrovics, Z. (2014b). Exercise addiction. *Behavioral Addictions*, 317–342. DOI: 10.1016/B978-0-12-407724-9.00013-6

Berczik, K., Griffiths, M. D., Szabo, A., Kurimay, T., Kokonyei, G., Urban, R., & Demetrovics, Z. (2014a). Exercise addiction—The emergence of a new disorder. *Australasian Epidemiologist*, *21*(2), 36–40.

Berryman, C., Ferguson, C. J., & Negy, C. (2018). Social media use and mental health among young adults. *The Psychiatric Quarterly*, *89*(2), 307–314. DOI: 10.1007/s11126-017-9535-6 PMID: 29090428

Beyari, H. (2023). The relationship between social media and the increase in mental health problems. *International Journal of Environmental Research and Public Health*, *20*(3), 2383. DOI: 10.3390/ijerph20032383 PMID: 36767749

Bickel, W. K., Mellis, A. M., Snider, S. E., Athamneh, L. N., Stein, J. S., & Pope, D. A. (2018). 21st century neurobehavioral theories of decision making in addiction: Review and evaluation. *Pharmacology, Biochemistry, and Behavior*, *164*, 4–21. DOI: 10.1016/j.pbb.2017.09.009 PMID: 28942119

Bickham, D. S., Vandewater, E. A., Huston, A. C., Lee, J. H., Caplovitz, A. G., & Wright, J. C. (2003). Predictors of children's electronic media use: An examination of three ethnic groups. *Media Psychology*, *5*(2), 107–137. DOI: 10.1207/S1532785XMEP0502_1

Billieux, J., Schimmenti, A., Khazaal, Y., Maurage, P., & Heeren, A. (2015). Are we overpathologizing everyday life? A tenable blueprint for behavioral addiction research. *Journal of Behavioral Addictions*, *4*(3), 119–123. DOI: 10.1556/2006.4.2015.009 PMID: 26014667

Błachnio, A., Przepiórka, A., Gorbaniuk, O., Benvenuti, M., Ciobanu, A. M., Senol-Durak, E., Durak, M., Giannakos, M. N., Mazzoni, E., Pappas, I. O., Popa, C., Seidman, G., Wu, A. M. S., Yu, S., & Ben-Ezra, M. (2019). Cultural Correlates of Internet Addiction. *Cyberpsychology, Behavior, and Social Networking*, *22*(4), 258–263. DOI: 10.1089/cyber.2018.0667 PMID: 30958038

Blac, K. D. W. (2007). A review of compulsive buying disorder. *World Psychiatry; Official Journal of the World Psychiatric Association (WPA)*, *6*(1), 14–18. PMID: 17342214

Black, D. W. (2001). Compulsive buying disorder: Definition, assessment, epidemiology and clinical management. *CNS Drugs*, *15*(1), 17–27. DOI: 10.2165/00023210-200115010-00003 PMID: 11465011

Black, D. W. (2007). Compulsive buying disorder: A review of the evidence. *CNS Spectrums*, *12*(2), 124–132. DOI: 10.1017/S1092852900020630 PMID: 17277712

Black, D. W., Shaw, M., McCormick, B., Bayless, J. D., & Allen, J. (2012). Neuropsychological performance, impulsivity, ADHD symptoms, and novelty seeking in compulsive buying disorder. *Psychiatry Research*, *200*(2-3), 581–587. DOI: 10.1016/j.psychres.2012.06.003 PMID: 22766012

Blackstone, S. R. & Herrmann, L. K. (2020). Fitness wearables and exercise dependence in college women: Considerations for university health education specialists. *American Journal of Health Education, 51*(4), 225–233. https://doi.org/. 2020.1767004DOI: 10.1080/19325037

Blackwell, D., Leaman, C., Tramposch, R., Osborne, C., & Liss, M. (2017). Extraversion, neuroticism, attachment style and fear of missing out as predictors of social media use and addiction. *Personality and Individual Differences*, *116*, 69–72. DOI: 10.1016/j.paid.2017.04.039

Bleuler, E. (1930). *Textbook of psychiatry*. Macmillan.

Bliss, C. (2024, January 22). Beyond the screens: Discover engaging activities with screen time management tips. *Color Bliss*. https://colorbliss.com/blog/beyond-the-screens-discover-engaging-activities-with-screen-time-management-tips

Block, J. J. (2008). Issues for dsm-v: Internet addiction. *The American Journal of Psychiatry*, *165*(3), 306–307. DOI: 10.1176/appi.ajp.2007.07101556 PMID: 18316427

Borges, G., Orozco, R., Benjet, C., Martínez, K., Contreras, E. V., Pérez, A., Cedrés, A., Uribe, P., Couder, M., Gutiérrez-García, R., Chávez, G., Albor, Y., Méndez, E., Medina-Mora, M. E., Mortier, P., & Ayuso-Mateos, J. (2021). (Internet) Gaming disorder in DSM-5 and ICD-11: A case of the glass half empty or half full. *Canadian Journal of Psychiatry*, *66*(5), 477–484. DOI: 10.1177/0706743720948431 PMID: 32806957

Bowen, S., Chawla, N., Grow, J., & Marlatt, G. A. (2021). Mindfulness-based relapse prevention for addictive behaviors. Guilford Publications. https://books.google.com/books?hl=fr&lr=&id=nOj3DwAAQBAJ&oi=fnd&pg=PP1

Brahma, A., & Brahma, M. C. (2023). An overview of internet pornography addiction. *Eastern Journal of Psychiatry*, *20*(1), 3–6. DOI: 10.5005/EJP-20-1-3

Brand, M., Antons, S., Bőthe, B., Demetrovics, Z., Fineberg, N. A., Jimenez-Murcia, S., King, D. L., Mestre-Bach, G., Moretta, T., Müller, A., Wegmann, E., & Potenza, M. N. (2025). Current Advances in Behavioral Addictions : From Fundamental Research to Clinical Practice. *The American Journal of Psychiatry*, *182*(2), 155–163. DOI: 10.1176/appi.ajp.20240092 PMID: 39659159

Breault, A. A. (2020). *L'hyperphagie boulimique et la dépendance alimentaire: comparaison des profils* (Doctoral dissertation, Université Laval).

Brewer, J. A., & Potenza, M. N. (2008). The neurobiology and genetics of impulse control disorders : Relationships to drug addictions. *Biochemical Pharmacology*, *75*(1), 63–75. DOI: 10.1016/j.bcp.2007.06.043 PMID: 17719013

Bridges, A. J., Wosnitzer, R., Scharrer, E., Sun, C., & Liberman, R. (2010). Aggression and sexual behavior in best-selling pornography videos: A content analysis update. *Violence Against Women*, *16*(10), 1065–1085. DOI: 10.1177/1077801210382866 PMID: 20980228

Brooke, S. (2021, November 16). What to make of the new regulations in China's gaming industry. *China Briefing*. https://www.china-briefing.com/news/what-to-make-of-the-new-regulations-in-china-online-gaming-industry/

Bueno-Antequera, J., Mayolas-Pi, C., Reverter-Masià, J., López-Laval, I., Oviedo-Caro, M. Á., Munguía-Izquierdo, D., Ruidíaz-Peña, M., & Legaz-Arrese, A. (2020). Exercise addiction and its relationship with health outcomes in indoor cycling practitioners in fitness centers. *International Journal of Environmental Research and Public Health, 17*(11), 4159. DOI: 10.3390/ijerph17114159 PMID: 32545197

Buijs, P., Boot, E., Shugar, A., Fung, W. L. A., & Bassett, A. S. (2017). Internet safety issues for adolescents and adults with intellectual disabilities. *Journal of Applied Research in Intellectual Disabilities, 30*(2), 416–418. DOI: 10.1111/jar.12250 PMID: 26914835

Burtăverde, V., Jonason, P. K., Giosan, C., & Ene, C. (2021). Why do people watch porn? An evolutionary perspective on the reasons for pornography consumption. *Evolutionary Psychology, 19*(2). Doi.org .DOI: 10.1177/14747049211028798

Bussone, S., Trentini, C., Tambelli, R., & Carola, V. (2020). Early-life interpersonal and affective risk factors for pathological gaming. *Frontiers in Psychiatry, 11*, 423. DOI: 10.3389/fpsyt.2020.00423 PMID: 32499728

Camardese, G., Leone, B., Walstra, C., Janiri, L., & Guglielmo, R. (2015). Pharmacological Treatment of Internet Addiction. In Montag, C., & Reuter, M. (Eds.), *Internet Addiction* (pp. 151–165). Springer International Publishing., DOI: 10.1007/978-3-319-07242-5_10

Camilleri, C., Perry, J. T., & Sammut, S. (2021). Compulsive Internet Pornography Use and Mental Health: A Cross-Sectional Study in a Sample of University Students in the United States. *Frontiers in Psychology, 11*, 613244. Doi.org/10./fpsyg.2020.613244. DOI: 10.3389/fpsyg.2020.613244 PMID: 33510691

Campana, B., Brasiel, P. G., de Aguiar, A. S., & Dutra, S. C. P. L. (2019). Obesity and food addiction: Similarities to drug addiction. *Obesity Medicine, 16*, 100136. DOI: 10.1016/j.obmed.2019.100136

Caplan, S. E. (2006). Relations among loneliness, social anxiety, and problematic Internet use. *Cyberpsychology & Behavior, 10*(2), 234–242. DOI: 10.1089/cpb.2006.9963 PMID: 17474841

Carson, N., Lê Cook, B., Chen, C. N., & Alegria, M. (2012). Racial/ethnic differences in video game and Internet use among US adolescents with mental health and educational difficulties. *Journal of Children and Media*, *6*(4), 450–468. DOI: 10.1080/17482798.2012.724592 PMID: 29167696

Carvalheira, A., Træen, B., & Stulhofer, A. (2015). Masturbation and pornography use among coupled heterosexual men with decreased sexual desire: How many roles of masturbation? *Journal of Sex & Marital Therapy*, *41*(6), 626–635. DOI: 10.1080/0092623X.2014.958790 PMID: 25189834

Cash, H. D., Rae, C. H., Steel, A., & Winkler, A. (2012). Internet addiction: A brief summary of research and practice. *Current Psychiatry Reviews*, *8*(4), 292–298. DOI: 10.2174/157340012803520513 PMID: 23125561

Cataldo, I., De Luca, I., Giorgetti, V., Cicconcelli, D., Bersani, F. S., Imperatori, C., Abdi, S., Negri, A., Esposito, G., & Corazza, O. (2021). Fitspiration on social media: Body-image and other psychopathological risks among young adults. A narrative review. *Emerging Trends in Drugs, Addictions, and Health*, *1*, 100010. DOI: 10.1016/j.etdah.2021.100010

Cauce, A. M., & Domenech-Rodriguez, M. (2002). Latino families: Myths and realities. *Latino children and families in the United States: Current research and future directions*, 3-25.

Ceceli, A. O., King, S. G., McClain, N., Alia-Klein, N., & Goldstein, R. Z. (2023). The neural signature of impaired inhibitory control in individuals with heroin use disorder. *The Journal of Neuroscience : The Official Journal of the Society for Neuroscience*, *43*(1), 173–182. DOI: 10.1523/JNEUROSCI.1237-22.2022 PMID: 36396402

Ceci, F., Di Carlo, F., Burkauskas, J., Salone, A., De Luca, I., Cicconcelli, D., Giorgetti, V., La Fratta, I., Todaro, A., Simonato, P., Martinotti, G., di Giannantonio, M., & Corazza, O. (2022). Physical activity and exercise addiction during the COVID-19 pandemic in Italy. *International Journal of Mental Health and Addiction*, *21*(6), 3678–3698. DOI: 10.1007/s11469-022-00815-z PMID: 35469185

Centers for Disease Control and Prevention. (2023). *Physical activity basics.* U.S. Department of Health and Human Services. https://www.cdc.gov/physical-activity-basics/guidelines/adults.html

Chadha, Y., Patil, R., Toshniwal, S., & Sinha, N. (2024). Internet Addiction Management: A Comprehensive Review of Clinical Interventions and Modalities. *Cureus*, *16*(3). Advance online publication. DOI: 10.7759/cureus.55466 PMID: 38571828

Chakravarthy, S., Balasubramani, P. P., Mandali, A., Jahanshahi, M., & Moustafa, A. A. (2018). The many facets of dopamine: Toward an integrative theory of the role of dopamine in managing the body's energy resources. *Physiology & Behavior*, *195*, 128–141. DOI: 10.1016/j.physbeh.2018.06.032 PMID: 30031088

Chanda, C., & Surepalli, S. (2019). Dopaminergic dysfunction in neuropsychiatric disorders. Pathophysiology, current therapeutics, and future perspectives. *Neuropsychiatria i Neuropsychologia/Neuropsychiatry and Neuropsychology, 14*(1), 39-47.

Chang, M. L., & Lee, I. O. (2024). Functional connectivity changes in the brain of adolescents with internet addiction: A systematic literature review of imaging studies. *PLOS Mental Health, 1*(1), e0000022. Advance online publication. DOI: 10.1371/journal.pmen.0000022

Chang, Y. H., Chang, K. C., Hou, W. L., Lin, C. Y., & Griffiths, M. D. (2021). Internet gaming as a coping method among schizophrenic patients facing psychological distress. *Journal of Behavioral Addictions*, *9*(4), 1022–1031. DOI: 10.1556/2006.2020.00081 PMID: 33128519

Chen, M., Sun, Y., Lu, L., & Shi, J. (2017). Similarities and differences in neurobiology. Substance and Non-substance Addiction, 45-58.

Chen, E., Wood, D., & Ysseldyk, R. (2022). Online social networking and mental health among older adults: A scoping review. *Canadian Journal on Aging*, *41*(1), 26–39. DOI: 10.1017/S0714980821000040 PMID: 33736725

Chen, J., Li, X., Zhang, Q., Zhou, Y., Wang, R., Tian, C., & Xiang, H. (2021). Impulsivity and response inhibition related brain networks in adolescents with internet gaming disorder: A preliminary study utilizing resting-state fMRI. *Frontiers in Psychiatry*, *11*, 618319. DOI: 10.3389/fpsyt.2020.618319 PMID: 33519558

Chen, L., & Nath, R. (2016). Understanding the underlying factors of Internet addiction across cultures: A comparison study. *Electronic Commerce Research and Applications*, *17*, 38–48. DOI: 10.1016/j.elerap.2016.02.003

Chen, W., Gao, Y., Ren, R., Bi, Y., & Liao, Y. (2025). Socioeconomic status and internet addiction: Double-mediated moderation. *BMC Public Health*, *25*(1), 48. Advance online publication. DOI: 10.1186/s12889-024-21153-w PMID: 39762803

Chen, Z., Ge, J., Gan, Q., Fu, Y., & Chen, Z. (2025). Protocol for a Randomized Controlled Trial to Enhance Executive Function via Brief Mindfulness Training in Individuals with Internet Gaming Disorder. *PLoS One*, *20*(4), e0320305. DOI: 10.1371/journal.pone.0320305 PMID: 40168432

China Legal Experts. (2024, July 9). China gaming laws. *China Legal Experts.* https://www.chinalegalexperts.com/news/china-gaming-laws

Choudhury, M., & Ali, A. (2020). Social media addiction among youth: A gender comparison. *International Journal of Indian Psychology*, *8*(3), 740–748.

Christenson, G. A., Faber, R. J., De Zwaan, M., Raymond, N. C., Specker, S. M., Ekern, M. D., & Eckert, E. D. (1994). Compulsive buying: Descriptive characteristics and psychiatric comorbidity. *The Journal of Clinical Psychiatry*, *55*(1), 5–11. PMID: 8294395

Chu, G. C., Chan, L. Y., Do, C. W., Tse, A. C., Cheung, T., Szeto, G. P., So, B. C. L., Lee, R. L. T., & Lee, P. H. (2023). Association between time spent on smartphones and digital eye strain: A 1-year prospective observational study among Hong Kong children and adolescents. *Environmental Science and Pollution Research International*, *30*(20), 58428–58435. DOI: 10.1007/s11356-023-26258-0 PMID: 36991204

Chung, S., Lee, J., & Lee, H. K. (2019). Personal Factors, Internet Characteristics, and Environmental Factors Contributing to Adolescent Internet Addiction: A Public Health Perspective. *International Journal of Environmental Research and Public Health*, *16*(23), 4635. DOI: 10.3390/ijerph16234635 PMID: 31766527

Cillero, I. H., & Jago, R. (2010). Systematic review of correlates of screen-viewing among young children. *Preventive Medicine*, *51*(1), 3–10. DOI: 10.1016/j.ypmed.2010.04.012 PMID: 20417227

Cinelli, M., De Francisci Morales, G., Galeazzi, A., Quattrociocchi, W., & Starnini, M. (2021). The echo chamber effect on social media. *Proceedings of the National Academy of Sciences of the United States of America*, *118*(9), e2023301118. DOI: 10.1073/pnas.2023301118 PMID: 33622786

Clark, L., Smith, T., & Johnson, R. (2022). Ethical game design: Industry promises and consumer realities. *Journal of Behavioral Addictions*, *11*(3), 456467.

Cleveland Clinic. (2022, May 27). Video game addiction. *Cleveland Clinic.* https://my.clevelandclinic.org/health/diseases/23124-video-game-addiction

Colder Carras, M., Aljuboori, D., Shi, J., Date, M., Karkoub, F., Ortiz, K. G., Abreha, F. M., & Thrul, J. (2024). Prevention and Health Promotion Interventions for Young People in the Context of Digital Well-Being: Rapid Systematic Review. *Journal of Medical Internet Research*, *26*, e59968. Advance online publication. DOI: 10.2196/59968 PMID: 39693138

Colledge, F., Buchner, U., Schmidt, A., & Walter, M. (2019). Does exercise addiction exist? A brief review of current measurement tools and future directions. *Mental Health and Addiction Research*, *4*(2), 1–4. DOI: 10.15761/MHAR.1000181

Colledge, F., Buchner, U., Schmidt, A., Wiesbeck, G., Lang, U., Pühse, U., Gerber, M., & Walter, M. (2022). Individuals at risk of exercise addiction have higher scores for depression, adhd, and childhood trauma. *Frontiers in Sports and Active Living*, *3*, 761844–761844. DOI: 10.3389/fspor.2021.761844 PMID: 35156014

Colledge, F., Cody, R., Buchner, U. G., Schmidt, A., Pühse, U., Gerber, M., Wiesbeck, G., Lang, U. E., & Walter, M. (2020). Excessive exercise—A meta-review. *Frontiers in Psychiatry*, *11*, 521572. Advance online publication. DOI: 10.3389/fpsyt.2020.521572 PMID: 33329076

Colledge, F., Sattler, I., Schilling, H., Gerber, M., Pühse, U., & Walter, M. (2020). Mental disorders in individuals at risk for exercise addiction–A systematic review. *Addictive Behaviors Reports*, *12*, 100314. DOI: 10.1016/j.abrep.2020.100314 PMID: 33364322

Collins, A. L., & Saunders, B. T. (2020). Heterogeneity in striatal dopamine circuits: Form and function in dynamic reward seeking. *Journal of Neuroscience Research*, *98*(6), 1046–1069. DOI: 10.1002/jnr.24587 PMID: 32056298

Colwell, J., & Kato, M. (2003). Investigation of the relationship between social isolation, self-esteem, aggression and computer game play in Japanese adolescents. *Asian Journal of Social Psychology*, *6*(2), 149–158. DOI: 10.1111/1467-839X.t01-1-00017

Cooper, A., Putnam, D., Planchon, L., & Boies, S. (1999). Online sexual compulsivity: Getting tangled in the net. *Sexual Addiction & Compulsivity*, *6*(2), 79–104. DOI: 10.1080/10720169908400182

Cooper, S., Robison, A. J., & Mazei-Robison, M. S. (2017). Reward circuitry in addiction. *Neurotherapeutics; the Journal of the American Society for Experimental NeuroTherapeutics*, *14*(3), 687–697. DOI: 10.1007/s13311-017-0525-z PMID: 28324454

Corazza, D., & Dores, A. R. (2023). *The body in the mind: Exercise addiction, body image and the use of enhancement drugs*. Cambridge University Press., DOI: 10.1017/9781911623731

Corazza, O., Simonato, P., Demetrovics, Z., Mooney, R., van de Ven, K., Roman-Urrestarazu, A., Rácmolnár, L., De Luca, I., Cinosi, E., Santacroce, R., Marini, M., Wellsted, D., Sullivan, K., Bersani, G., Martinotti, G., & Annunziato, R. A. (2019). The emergence of exercise addiction, body dysmorphic disorder, and other image-related psychopathological correlates in fitness settings: A cross-sectional study. *PLoS One*, *14*(4), e0213060–e0213060. DOI: 10.1371/journal.pone.0213060 PMID: 30943200

Corey, G. (2017). *Theory and practice of counselling and psychotherapy*. Cengage Learning.

Corey, G. (2023). *Theory & practice of group counseling*. Cengage.

Coyne, S. M., Rogers, A. A., Zurcher, J. D., Stockdale, L., & Booth, M. (2020). Does time spent using social media impact mental health?: An eight year longitudinal study. *Computers in Human Behavior*, *104*, 106160. DOI: 10.1016/j.chb.2019.106160

Cunningham, H. E., Pearman, S.III, & Brewerton, T. D. (2016). Conceptualizing primary and secondary pathological exercise using available measures of excessive exercise. *International Journal of Eating Disorders*, *49*(8), 778–792. DOI: 10.1002/eat.22551 PMID: 27203379

Da Silva, F. L. (2023). EEG: origin and measurement. In *EEG-fMRI: physiological basis, technique, and applications* (pp. 23–48). Springer International Publishing.

Dalle Grave, R., Calugi, S., & Marchesini, G. (2008). Compulsive exercise to control shape or weight in eating disorders: Prevalence, associated features, and treatment outcome. *Comprehensive Psychiatry*, *49*(4), 346–352. DOI: 10.1016/j.comppsych.2007.12.007 PMID: 18555054

Dalley, J. W., & Ersche, K. D. (2019). Neural circuitry and mechanisms of waiting impulsivity: relevance to addiction. *Philosophical Transactions of the Royal Society B, 374*(1766), 20180145.

Daneback, K., Månsson, S. A., Ross, M. W., & Markham, C. M. (2012). The internet as a source of information about sexuality. *Sex Education*, *12*(5), 583–598. DOI: 10.1080/14681811.2011.627739

Daneback, K., Ross, M. W., & Månsson, S. A. (2006). Characteristics and behaviors of sexual compulsives who use the internet for sexual purposes. *Sexual Addiction & Compulsivity*, *13*(1), 53–67. DOI: 10.1080/10720160500529276

Danesh, M. R. A., Taklavi, S., & Kazemi, R. (2021). The Effectiveness of Acceptance and Commitment Therapy on Emotional Self-Control, Emotional Flexibility, and the Valued Living among Women with Compulsive Buying Disorder.

Daniyal, M., Javaid, S. F., Hassan, A., & Khan, M. A. (2022). The relationship between cellphone usage on the physical and mental wellbeing of university students: A cross-sectional study. *International Journal of Environmental Research and Public Health, 19*(15), 9352. DOI: 10.3390/ijerph19159352 PMID: 35954709

Darrat, A. A., Darrat, M., & Darrat, M. A. (2022). Does wanting more lead to losing control? Examining the psychological drivers of compulsive buying. *Young Consumers, 24*(1), 56–73. DOI: 10.1108/YC-01-2022-1453

Davis, R. A. (2001). A cognitive-behavioral model of pathological Internet use. *Computers in Human Behavior, 17*(2), 187–195. DOI: 10.1016/S0747-5632(00)00041-8

De Alarcón, R., de la Iglesia, J. I., Casado, N. M., & Montejo, A. L. (2019). Online Porn Addiction: What We Know and What We Don't-A Systematic Review. *Journal of Clinical Medicine, 8*(1), 91. Doi.org/10.3390/jcm8010091. DOI: 10.3390/jcm8010091 PMID: 30650522

De Luca, I., Simonato, P., Mooney, R., Bersani, G., Corazza, O., Corazza, O., & Unit, N. P. S. (2017). Can exercise be an addiction? The evolution of 'fitspiration' in society. *Research and Advances in Psychiatry, 4*, 27–34.

De Sousa, A., & Lodha, P. (2017). Neurobiology of pornography addiction – a clinical review. *Telangana Journal of Psychiatry, 3*(2), 66–67. DOI: 10.18231/2455-8559.2017.0016

Deloy, J. (2006). Patterns of relationship satisfaction and sexual behavior as a function of pornography use among college men. *Theses and Dissertations*. 2532. https://commons.und.edu/theses/2532

Despres, R. (1997). Burn, baby, burn: At what point does the quest for ultimate fitness turn into an unhealthy obsession? For women athletes, as it turns out, it's hard to tell. *Women's Sports and Fitness, 19*, 38–44.

Di Chiara, G., Bassareo, V., Fenu, S., De Luca, M. A., Spina, L., Cadoni, C., Acquas, E., Carboni, E., Valentini, V., & Lecca, D. (2004). Dopamine and drug addiction: The nucleus accumbens shell connection. *Neuropharmacology, 47*(1), 227–241. DOI: 10.1016/j.neuropharm.2004.06.032 PMID: 15464140

Di Lodovico, L., Poulnais, S., & Gorwood, P. (2019). Which sports are more at risk of physical exercise addiction: A systematic review. *Addictive Behaviors, 93*, 257–262. DOI: 10.1016/j.addbeh.2018.12.030 PMID: 30595420

Dieris-Hirche, J., Bottel, L., Pape, M., te Wildt, B. T., Wölfling, K., Henningsen, P., Timmesfeld, N., Neumann, A., Neusser, S., Beckers, R., & Herpertz, S. (2021). Effects of an online-based motivational intervention to reduce problematic internet use and promote treatment motivation in internet gaming disorder and internet use disorder (OMPRIS): Study protocol for a randomised controlled trial. *BMJ Open, 11*(8), e045840. DOI: 10.1136/bmjopen-2020-045840 PMID: 34344675

Dingemans, A., Danner, U., & Parks, M. (2017, November 22). Emotion Regulation in Binge Eating Disorder: A Review. *Nutrients*, *9*(11), 1274. DOI: 10.3390/nu9111274 PMID: 29165348

Ding, K., & Li, H. (2023). Digital addiction intervention for children and adolescents: A scoping review. *International Journal of Environmental Research and Public Health*, *20*(6), 4777. DOI: 10.3390/ijerph20064777 PMID: 36981687

Dom, G., & Moggi, F. (Eds.). (2015). *Co-occurring Addictive and Psychiatric Disorders : A Practice-Based Handbook from a European Perspective*. Springer Berlin Heidelberg., DOI: 10.1007/978-3-642-45375-5

Domoff, S. E., Harrison, K., Gearhardt, A. N., Gentile, D. A., Lumeng, J. C., & Miller, A. L. (2019). Development and validation of the Problematic Media Use Measure: A parent report measure of screen media "addiction" in children. *Psychology of Popular Media Culture*, *8*(1), 2–11. DOI: 10.1037/ppm0000163 PMID: 30873299

Donahue, C. B., Odlaug, B. L., & Grant, J. E. (2011). Compulsive buying treated with motivational interviewing and imaginal desensitization. *Annals of Clinical Psychiatry*, *23*, 226–227. PMID: 21808756

Dong, G., Zheng, H., Liu, X., Wang, Y., Du, X., & Potenza, M. N. (2018). Gender-related differences in cue-elicited cravings in Internet gaming disorder: The effects of deprivation. *Journal of Behavioral Addictions*, *7*(4), 953–964. DOI: 10.1556/2006.7.2018.118 PMID: 30556781

Dowling, N. A., Cowlishaw, S., Jackson, A. C., Merkouris, S. S., Francis, K. L., & Christensen, D. R. (2015). Prevalence of psychiatric co-morbidity in treatment-seeking problem gamblers : A systematic review and meta-analysis. *The Australian and New Zealand Journal of Psychiatry*, *49*(6), 519–539. DOI: 10.1177/0004867415575774 PMID: 25735959

Draeger, J., Yates, A., & Crowell, D. (2005). The obligatory exerciser. *The Physician and Sportsmedicine*, *33*(6), 13–23. DOI: 10.3810/psm.2005.06.101 PMID: 20086364

Dumitru, D. C., Dumitru, T., & Maher, A. J. (2018). A systematic review of exercise addiction: Examining gender differences. *Journal of Physical Education and Sport, 18*(3), 1738–1747. DOI: 10.7752/jpes.2018.03253

Dunlop, S., Freeman, B., & Perez, D. (2016). Exposure to internet-based tobacco advertising and branding: Results from population surveys of Australian youth 2010-2013. *Journal of Medical Internet Research, 18*(6), e104. DOI: 10.2196/jmir.5595 PMID: 27338761

Educational Advancement. (2022, May 21). The good and the bad effects of video games on children. *Educational Advancement*. https://educationaladvancement.org/blog-the-good-and-the-bad-effects-of-video-games-on-children/#:~:text=Discourage%20children%20to%20do%20well,detrimental%20to%20your%20child's%20development

Edwards, E. A. (1993). Edwards Compulsive Buying Scale. *Financial Counseling and Planning*.

Egorov, A. Y., & Szabo, A. (2013). The exercise paradox: An interactional model for a clearer conceptualization of exercise addiction. *Journal of Behavioral Addictions, 2*(4), 199–208. DOI: 10.1556/JBA.2.2013.4.2 PMID: 25215201

Ekhtiari, H., Sangchooli, A., Carmichael, O., Moeller, F. G., O'Donnell, P., Oquendo, M. A., & Brady, K. (2024). Neuroimaging biomarkers of addiction. *Nature Mental Health*, •••, 1–20. PMID: 39281741

El-Sherbini, H. H., & Abdou, R. A. (2020). Effect of Cognitive Behavioral Therapy on Internet Gaming Disorder and Quality of Life Among Preparatory School Students in Alexandria. *Assiut Scientific Nursing Journal, 8*(23), 22–38. DOI: 10.21608/asnj.2020.46217.1057

Esparza-Reig, J., Guillén-Riquelme, A., Martí-Vilar, M., & González-Sala, F. (2021). A reliability generalization meta-analysis of the south oaks gambling screen (SOGS). *Psicothema, 33*(3), 490–499. DOI: 10.7334/psicothema2020.449 PMID: 34297680

Evans, C., King, D. L., & Delfabbro, P. H. (2018). Effect of brief gaming abstinence on withdrawal in adolescent at-risk daily gamers: A randomized controlled study. *Computers in Human Behavior, 88*, 70–77. DOI: 10.1016/j.chb.2018.06.024

Faber, R. J., & O'guinn, T. C. (1992). A clinical screener for compulsive buying. *The Journal of Consumer Research, 19*(3), 459–469. DOI: 10.1086/209315

Feleke, N., Mihretu, A., Habtamu, K., Amare, B., & Teferra, S. (2024). Validation of the Amharic version of Internet Addiction Test-20: A cross-sectional study. *Frontiers in Psychiatry, 14*, 1243035. DOI: 10.3389/fpsyt.2023.1243035 PMID: 38264639

Ferracci, S., Manippa, V., D'Anselmo, A., Bovolon, L., Guagnano, M. T., Brancucci, A., Porcelli, P., & Conti, C. (2024). The role of impulsivity and binge eating in outpatients with overweight or obesity: An EEG temporal discounting study. *Journal of Eating Disorders, 12*(1), 130. DOI: 10.1186/s40337-024-01080-2 PMID: 39227881

Ferrer-Pérez, C., Montagud-Romero, S., & Blanco-Gandía, M. C. (2024). Neurobiological Theories of Addiction: A Comprehensive Review. *Psychoactives, 3*(1), 35–47. DOI: 10.3390/psychoactives3010003

Ferris, J., & Wynne, H. (2001). L'indice canadien du jeu excessif. Ottawa, Canada: Centre canadien de lutte contre l'alcoolisme et les toxicomanies.

Filomensky, T. Z., & Tavares, H. (2021). *Compulsive buying disorder*. Springer., DOI: 10.1007/978-3-030-36391-8_69

Fineberg, N. A., Menchón, J. M., Hall, N., Dell'Osso, B., Brand, M., Potenza, M. N., Chamberlain, S. R., Cirnigliaro, G., Lochner, C., Billieux, J., Demetrovics, Z., Rumpf, H. J., Müller, A., Castro-Calvo, J., Hollander, E., Burkauskas, J., Grünblatt, E., Walitza, S., Corazza, O., & Zohar, J. (2022). Advances in problematic usage of the internet research–A narrative review by experts from the European network for problematic usage of the internet. *Comprehensive Psychiatry, 118*, 152346. DOI: 10.1016/j.comppsych.2022.152346 PMID: 36029549

Firat, R. B. (2019). Opening the "Black Box": Functions of the frontal lobes and their implications for sociology. *Frontiers in Sociology, 4*, 3. DOI: 10.3389/fsoc.2019.00003 PMID: 33869331

First, M. B., Gaebel, W., Maj, M., Stein, D. J., Kogan, C. S., Saunders, J. B., Poznyak, V. B., Gureje, O., Lewis-Fernández, R., Maercker, A., Brewin, C. R., Cloitre, M., Claudino, A., Pike, K. M., Baird, G., Skuse, D., Krueger, R. B., Briken, P., Burke, J. D., & Reed, G. M. (2021). An organization-and category-level comparison of diagnostic requirements for mental disorders in ICD-11 and DSM-5. *World Psychiatry; Official Journal of the World Psychiatric Association (WPA), 20*(1), 34–51. DOI: 10.1002/wps.20825 PMID: 33432742

First, M. B., Reed, G. M., Hyman, S. E., & Saxena, S. (2015). The development of the ICD-11 clinical descriptions and diagnostic guidelines for mental and behavioural disorders. *World Psychiatry; Official Journal of the World Psychiatric Association (WPA), 14*(1), 82–90. DOI: 10.1002/wps.20189 PMID: 25655162

Flack, D. (2020, May). Engaging avoidant teens. https://www.counseling.org/publications/counseling-today-magazine/article archive/article/legacy/engaging-avoidant-teens

Fong, T. W., Reid, R. C., & Parhami, I. (2012). Behavioral Addictions Where to Draw the Lines? *The Psychiatric Clinics of North America*, *35*(2), 279–296. DOI: 10.1016/j.psc.2012.03.001 PMID: 22640756

Freimuth, M., Moniz, S., & Kim, S. R. (2011). Clarifying exercise addiction: Differential diagnosis, co-occurring disorders, and phases of addiction. *International Journal of Environmental Research and Public Health*, *8*(10), 4069–4081. DOI: 10.3390/ijerph8104069 PMID: 22073029

Frison, E., & Eggermont, S. (2016). Exploring the relationships between different types of Facebook use, perceived online social support, and adolescents' depressed mood. *Social Science Computer Review*, *34*(2), 153–171. DOI: 10.1177/0894439314567449

Galbraith, N., Rose, C., & Rose, P. (2022). The roles of motivational interviewing and self-efficacy on outcomes and cost-effectiveness of a community-based exercise intervention for inactive middle-older aged adults. *Health & Social Care in the Community*, *30*(4), e1048–e1060. DOI: 10.1111/hsc.13510 PMID: 34260782

Galea, S., Nandi, A., & Vlahov, D. (2004). The social epidemiology of substance use. *Epidemiologic Reviews*, *26*(1), 36–52. DOI: 10.1093/epirev/mxh007 PMID: 15234946

Gambling Commission. (2020). *Evaluating the impact of the Bet Regret campaign*. UK Gambling Commission.

Gambling Commission. (2021). *Credit card ban evaluation report*. UK Gambling Commission.

Gao, Y. X., Wang, J. Y., & Dong, G. H. (2022). The prevalence and possible risk factors of internet gaming disorder among adolescents and young adults: Systematic reviews and meta-analyses. *Journal of Psychiatric Research*, *154*, 35–43. DOI: 10.1016/j.jpsychires.2022.06.049 PMID: 35926424

Garcia-Caballero, A., Torrens-Lluch, M., Ramirez-Gendrau, I., Garrido, G., Valles, V., & Aragay, N. (2018). The efficacy of motivational interviewing and cognitive-behavioral therapy for pathological gambling. *Addictions*, *30*(3).

García-Castro, J., Cancela, A., & Cárdaba, M. A. (2023). Neural cue-reactivity in pathological gambling as evidence for behavioral addiction: A systematic review. *Current Psychology (New Brunswick, N.J.)*, *42*(32), 28026–28037. DOI: 10.1007/s12144-022-03915-0 PMID: 36373116

Gearhardt, A. N., White, M. A., & Potenza, M. N. (2011, September). Binge eating disorder and food addiction. *Current Drug Abuse Reviews*, *4*(3), 201–207. DOI: 10.2174/1874473711104030201 PMID: 21999695

Ge, M.-W., Hu, F.-H., Jia, Y.-J., Tang, W., Zhang, W.-Q., Zhao, D.-Y., Shen, W.-Q., & Chen, H.-L. (2023). The relationship between loneliness and internet or smartphone addiction among adolescents: A systematic review and meta-analysis. *Psychological Reports, 128*(3), 1429–1451. DOI: 10.1177/00332941231180119 PMID: 37261719

George, M., Maheshwari, S., Chandran, S., & Rao, T. S. S. (2019). Psychosocial aspects of pornography. *Journal of Psychosexual Health, 1*(1), 44–47. DOI: 10.1177/2631831818821535

German, D. C., & Manaye, K. F. (1993, May 15). Midbrain dopaminergic neurons (nuclei A8, A9, and A10): Three-dimensional reconstruction in the rat. *The Journal of Comparative Neurology, 331*(3), 297–309. DOI: 10.1002/cne.903310302 PMID: 8514911

Ghallab, Y. K., & Elassal, O. S. (2024). Biochemical and Neuropharmacology of Psychiatric Disorders. In *Nutrition and Psychiatric Disorders: An Evidence-Based Approach to Understanding the Diet-Brain Connection* (pp. 25–47). Springer Nature Singapore. DOI: 10.1007/978-981-97-2681-3_2

Giardina, A., Di Blasi, M., Schimmenti, A., King, D. L., Starcevic, V., & Billieux, J. (2021). Online gaming and prolonged self-isolation: Evidence from Italian gamers during the COVID-19 outbreak. *Clinical Neuropsychiatry, 18*(1), 65. PMID: 34909021

Giel, K. E., Bulik, C. M., Fernandez-Aranda, F., Hay, P., Keski-Rahkonen, A., Schag, K., Schmidt, U., & Zipfel, S. (2022). Binge eating disorder. *Nature Reviews. Disease Primers, 8*(1), 16. DOI: 10.1038/s41572-022-00344-y PMID: 35301358

Ginley, M. K., Zajac, K., Rash, C. J., & Petry, N. M. (2019). Pharmacological treatment of behavioral addictions. https://psycnet.apa.org/record/2019-20159-028

Gjoneska, B. B\Hothe, B., Potenza, M. N., Szabo, A., & Demetrovics, Z. (2024). Epidemiology of Behavioral Addictions. The Sage Handbook of Addiction Psychology, 47.

Goethe, O. (2019). Visual aesthetics in games and gamification. In *Gamification Mindset* (pp. 85–92). Springer., DOI: 10.1007/978-3-030-11078-9_8

Gola, M., Lewczuk, K., & Skorko, M. (2016). What matters: Quantity or quality of pornography use? Psychological and behavioral factors of treatment-seeking for problematic pornography use. *Journal of Sexual Medicine, 13*(5), 815–824. DOI: 10.1016/j.jsxm.2016.02.169 PMID: 27012817

Gómez-Gonzalvo, F., Devís-Devís, J., & Molina-Alventosa, P. (2020). Video game usage time in adolescents' academic performance. *Comunicar: Media Education Research Journal, 28*(65), 87–96. DOI: 10.3916/C65-2020-08

Gongora, M., Teixeira, S., Martins, L., Marinho, V., Velasques, B., Moraes, L., & Ribeiro, P. (2019). Neurobiological evidences, functional and emotional aspects associated with the amygdala: From "What is it?" to "What's to be done?". *Neuropsychiatry, 9*(3), 749–751.

González-Bueso, V., Santamaría, J. J., Fernández, D., Merino, L., Montero, E., & Ribas, J. (2018). Association between internet gaming disorder or pathological video-game use and comorbid psychopathology: A comprehensive review. *International Journal of Environmental Research and Public Health, 15*(4), 668. DOI: 10.3390/ijerph15040668 PMID: 29614059

González-Fuente, B., & de la Villa Moral Jiménez, M. (2024). Compra compulsiva online y offline y su relación con la ansiedad estado-rasgo y la impulsividad. *Behavioral Psychology–Psicologia Conductual,* 249–267. https://doi.org/DOI: 10.51668/bp.8324202s

Gordon-Larsen, P., McMurray, R. G., & Popkin, B. M. (2000). Determinants of adolescent physical activity and inactivity patterns. *Pediatrics, 105*(6), e83–e83. DOI: 10.1542/peds.105.6.e83 PMID: 10835096

Gottfried, J., & Sidoti, O. (2024, May 9). Adolescentss and video games today. *Pew Research Center.* https://www.pewresearch.org/internet/2024/05/09/adolescentss -and-video- gamestoday/#fnref-165467-1

Goulet-Kennedy, J., Labbe, S., & Fecteau, S. (2016). The involvement of the striatum in decision making. *Dialogues in Clinical Neuroscience, 18*(1), 55–63. DOI: 10.31887/DCNS.2016.18.1/sfecteau PMID: 27069380

Gouveia, A. (2024). On the concept, taxonomy, and transculturality of disordered grief. *Frontiers in Psychology, 14,* 1165421. DOI: 10.3389/fpsyg.2023.1165421 PMID: 38374931

Grant, J. E., & Chamberlain, S. R. (2016). Expanding the definition of addiction: DSM-5 vs. ICD-11. *CNS Spectrums, 21*(4), 300–303. DOI: 10.1017/S1092852916000183 PMID: 27151528

Grant, J. E., & Chamberlain, S. R. (2020). Gambling and substance use: Comorbidity and treatment implications. *Progress in Neuro-Psychopharmacology & Biological Psychiatry, 99,* 109852. DOI: 10.1016/j.pnpbp.2019.109852 PMID: 31881248

Grant, J. E., & Chamberlain, S. R. (2024). Compulsive buying disorder: Conceptualization based on addictive, impulsive, and obsessive-compulsive features and comorbidity. *Psychiatry Research Communications, 4*(4), 100199. DOI: 10.1016/j.psycom.2024.100199

Grant, J. E., Ioannidis, K., & Chamberlain, S. R. (2024). Defining treatment response in gambling disorder. *Journal of Psychiatric Research, 180*, 382–386. DOI: 10.1016/j.jpsychires.2024.11.006 PMID: 39522449

Grant, J. E., Odlaug, B. L., Chamberlain, S. R., Potenza, M. N., Schreiber, L. R., Donahue, C. B., & Kim, S. W. (2013). A randomized, placebo-controlled trial of N-acetylcysteine plus imaginal desensitization for nicotine-dependent pathological gamblers. *The Journal of Clinical Psychiatry, 74*(1), 16833. PMID: 24345329

Grant, J. E., Potenza, M. N., Weinstein, A., & Gorelick, D. A. (2010). Introduction to behavioral addictions. *The American Journal of Drug and Alcohol Abuse, 36*(5), 233–241. DOI: 10.3109/00952990.2010.491884 PMID: 20560821

Granziol, U., Griffiths, M. D., Zou, L., Yang, P., Herschel, H. K., Junker, A., Akimoto, T., Stoll, O., Alpay, M., Aydın, Z., Zandonai, T., Di Lodovico, L., Lichtenstein, M. B., Trott, M., Portman, R. M., Schipfer, M., Cook, B., Cerea, S., Egorov, A. Y., & Szabo, A. (2023). The Expanded Exercise Addiction Inventory (EAI-3): Towards reliable and international screening of exercise-related dysfunction. *International Journal of Mental Health and Addiction, 22*(6), 3559–3585. DOI: 10.1007/s11469-023-01066-2 PMID: 37363769

Greenwood, B. N. (2019). The role of dopamine in overcoming aversion with exercise. *Brain Research, 1713*, 102–108. DOI: 10.1016/j.brainres.2018.08.030 PMID: 30171838

Griffiths, M. D. (2018). The therapeutic and health benefits of playing video games.

Griffiths, M. (2005). A 'components' model of addiction within a biopsychosocial framework. *Journal of Substance Use, 10*(4), 191–197. DOI: 10.1080/14659890500114359

Griffiths, M. D., Kuss, D. J., Billieux, J., & Pontes, H. M. (2016). The evolution of internet addiction: A global Perspective. *Addictive Behaviors, 53*, 193–195. DOI: 10.1016/j.addbeh.2015.11.001 PMID: 26562678

Griffiths, M. D., & Meredith, A. (2009). Videogame addiction and its treatment. *Journal of Contemporary Psychotherapy, 39*(4), 247–253. DOI: 10.1007/s10879-009-9118-4

Grinspoon, P. (2020, December 22). *The health effects of too much gaming*. Harvard Health. https://www.health.harvard.edu/blog/the-health-effects-of-too-much-gaming-2020122221645

Grougiou, V., Moschis, G., & Kapoutsis, I. (2015). Compulsive buying: The role of earlier-in-life events and experiences. *Journal of Consumer Marketing*, *32*(4), 278–289. DOI: 10.1108/JCM-01-2015-1283

Grubbs, J. B., Exline, J. J., Pargament, K. I., Hook, J. N., & Carlisle, R. D. (2015). Transgression as addiction: Religiosity and moral disapproval as predictors of perceived addiction to pornography. *Archives of Sexual Behavior*, *44*(1), 125–136. DOI: 10.1007/s10508-013-0257-z PMID: 24519108

Grubbs, J. B., & Kraus, S. W. (2021). Pornography use and psychological science: A call for consideration. *Current Directions in Psychological Science*, *30*(1), 68–75. DOI: 10.1177/0963721420979594

Guedes, E., Nardi, A. E., Guimarães, F. M. C. L., Machado, S., & King, A. L. S. (2016). Social networking, a new online addiction: A review of Facebook and other addiction disorders. *MedicalExpress (São Paulo)*, *3*(1), M160101. DOI: 10.5935/MedicalExpress.2016.01.01

Guess, A. M., & Munger, K. (2023). Digital literacy and online political behavior. *Political Science Research and Methods*, *11*(1), 110–128. DOI: 10.1017/psrm.2022.17

Gustirini, R., & Putri, A. (2020). Peningkatan pengetahuan remaja tentang dampak negatif paparan pornografi di sma negeri 14 palembang. *Khidmah*, *2*(1), 96–101. DOI: 10.52523/khidmah.v2i1.308

Gwin, C. F., Roberts, J. A., & Martínez, C. R. (2004). Nature vs. Nurture: The Role of Family in Compulsive Buying. *Nature*.

Habibi, L. A. N., & Kurniawan, A. (2021). Loneliness relationship with cybersex behaviour in emerging adult. [BRPKM]. *Psychology and Mental Health Research Bulletin*, *1*(1), 722–733. DOI: 10.20473/brpkm.v1i1.26863

Hald, G. M., Seaman, C., & Linz, D. (2014). Sexuality and pornography. In D. L. Tolman, L. M. Diamond, J. A. Bauermeister, W. H. George, J. G. Pfaus, & L. M. Ward (Eds.), *APA handbook of sexuality and psychology, Vol. 2. Contextual approaches* (pp. 3–35). American Psychological Association. DOI: 10.1037/14194-001

Hald, M. G., & Malamuth, N. N. (2014). Experimental effects of exposure to pornography: The moderating effect of personality and mediating effect of sexual arousal. *Archives of Sexual Behavior*, *44*(1), 99–109. DOI: 10.1007/s10508-014-0291-5 PMID: 24729134

Hale, B. D., Diehl, D., Weaver, K., & Briggs, M. (2013). Exercise dependence and muscle dysmorphia in novice and experienced female bodybuilders. *Journal of Behavioral Addictions*, *2*(4), 244–248. DOI: 10.1556/JBA.2.2013.4.8 PMID: 25215207

Han, D. H., Bolo, N., Daniels, M. A., Arenella, L., Lyoo, I. K., & Renshaw, P. F. (2011). Brain activity and desire for Internet video game play. *Comprehensive Psychiatry, 52*(1), 88–95. DOI: 10.1016/j.comppsych.2010.04.004 PMID: 21220070

Han, H., Jeong, H., Jo, S. J., Son, H. J., & Yim, H. W. (2020). Relationship between the experience of online game genre and high risk of Internet gaming disorder in Korean adolescents. *Epidemiology and Health, 42*, e2020016. Advance online publication. DOI: 10.4178/epih.e2020016 PMID: 32272007

Han, J., Seo, Y., Hwang, H., Kim, S. M., & Han, D. H. (2020). Efficacy of cognitive behavioral therapy for internet gaming disorder. *Clinical Psychology & Psychotherapy, 27*(2), 203–213. DOI: 10.1002/cpp.2419 PMID: 31881100

Han, T. S., Cho, H., Sung, D., & Park, M. H. (2022). A systematic review of the impact of COVID-19 on the game addiction of children and adolescents. *Frontiers in Psychiatry, 13*, 976601. DOI: 10.3389/fpsyt.2022.976601 PMID: 36061296

Han, X., Wang, Y., Jiang, W., Bao, X., Sun, Y., Ding, W., Cao, M., Wu, X., Du, Y., & Zhou, Y. (2018). Resting-state activity of prefrontal-striatal circuits in internet gaming disorder: Changes with cognitive behavior therapy and predictors of treatment response. *Frontiers in Psychiatry, 9*, 341. DOI: 10.3389/fpsyt.2018.00341 PMID: 30123144

Harsej, Z., Mokhtari Lakeh, N., Sheikholeslami, F., & KazemnezhadLeili, E. (2021). Internet addiction and its relationship with family functioning in high school students. *Journal of Holistic Nursing and Midwifery, 31*(1), 44–52. DOI: 10.32598/jhnm.31.1.2025

Hausenblas, H. A., & Downs, D. S. (2002a). Exercise dependence: A systematic review. *Psychology of Sport and Exercise, 3*(2), 89–123. DOI: 10.1016/S1469-0292(00)00015-7

Hausenblas, H. A., & Downs, D. S. (2002b). How much is too much? The development and validation of the exercise dependence scale. *Psychology & Health, 17*(4), 387–404. DOI: 10.1080/0887044022000004894

Hausenblas, H. A., & Giacobbi, P. R.Jr. (2004). Relationship between exercise dependence symptoms and personality. *Personality and Individual Differences, 36*(6), 1265–1273. DOI: 10.1016/S0191-8869(03)00214-9

Hausenblas, H. A., Schreiber, K., & Smoliga, J. M. (2017). Addiction to exercise. *BMJ (Clinical Research Ed.)*, j1745. Advance online publication. DOI: 10.1136/bmj.j1745 PMID: 28446435

Hawi, N. S., Samaha, M., & Griffiths, M. D. (2018). Internet gaming disorder in Lebanon: Relationships with age, sleep habits, and academic achievement. *Journal of Behavioral Addictions, 7*(1), 70–78. DOI: 10.1556/2006.7.2018.16 PMID: 29486571

Heller, A. S., & Casey, B. J. (2016). The neurodynamics of emotion: Delineating typical and atypical emotional processes during adolescence. *Developmental Science, 19*(1), 3–18. DOI: 10.1111/desc.12373 PMID: 26548573

Heung, S., Jiang, L., Azenkot, S., & Vashistha, A. (2024, May). "Vulnerable, Victimized, and Objectified": Understanding Ableist Hate and Harassment Experienced by Disabled Content Creators on Social Media. In *Proceedings of the CHI Conference on Human Factors in Computing Systems* (pp. 1-19).

He, X., Chen, S., Yu, Q., Yang, P., & Yang, B. (2024). Correlations between problematic internet use and suicidal behavior among Chinese adolescents: A systematic review and meta-analysis. *Frontiers in Psychiatry, 15*, 1484809. DOI: 10.3389/fpsyt.2024.1484809 PMID: 39588549

Hill, J. P., & Lynch, M. E. (1983). The intensification of gender-related role expectations during early adolescence. In *Girls at Puberty: Biological and Psychosocial Perspectives* (pp. 201-228). Springer US. DOI: 10.1007/978-1-4899-0354-9_10

Hilton, D. L.Jr. (2013). Pornography addiction – a supranormal stimulus considered in the context of neuroplasticity. *Socioaffective Neuroscience & Psychology, 3*(1), 20767. DOI: 10.3402/snp.v3i0.20767 PMID: 24693354

Hiroi, N., & Agatsuma, S. (2005). Genetic susceptibility to substance dependence. *Molecular Psychiatry, 10*(4), 336–344. DOI: 10.1038/sj.mp.4001622 PMID: 15583701

Hollander, E. (Ed.). (1993). *Obsessive-compulsive related disorders*. American Psychiatric Press.

Holland, G., & Tiggemann, M. (2017). "Strong beats skinny every time": Disordered eating and compulsive exercise in women who post fitspiration on Instagram. *International Journal of Eating Disorders, 50*(1), 76–79. DOI: 10.1002/eat.22559 PMID: 27302867

Horigian, V. E., Anderson, A. R., & Szapocznik, J. (2016). Family-based treatments for adolescent substance use. *Child and Adolescent Psychiatric Clinics of North America, 25*(4), 603–628. DOI: 10.1016/j.chc.2016.06.001 PMID: 27613341

Hua, Y., Wang, W., Shi, J., Wang, H., Xu, K., Shi, G., Guo, L., & Lu, C. (2022). Childhood trauma and internet addiction among Chinese adolescents: The mediating role of coping styles. *Current Psychology (New Brunswick, N.J.), 42*(19), 16507–16517. DOI: 10.1007/s12144-022-02862-0

Hultman, R., Mague, S. D., Li, Q., Katz, B. M., Michel, N., Lin, L., Wang, J., David, L. K., Blount, C., Chandy, R., Carlson, D., Ulrich, K., Carin, L., Dunson, D., Kumar, S., Deisseroth, K., Moore, S. D., & Dzirasa, K. (2016). Dysregulation of prefrontal cortex-mediated slow-evolving limbic dynamics drives stress-induced emotional pathology. *Neuron*, *91*(2), 439–452. DOI: 10.1016/j.neuron.2016.05.038 PMID: 27346529

Hunicke, R., LeBlanc, M., & Zubek, R. (2004, July). MDA: A formal approach to game design and game research. In *Proceedings of the AAAI Workshop on Challenges in Game AI* (Vol. 4, No. 1, p. 1722).

Ioannidis, K., Huneke, N. T., Solly, J. E., Veronesi, G. F., Tzagarakis, C., Parlatini, V., Westwood, S. J., Del Giovane, C., Baldwin, D. S., & Grant, J. E. (2024). Placebo and nocebo effects in gambling disorder pharmacological trials : A meta-analysis. *Acta Neuropsychiatrica*, •••, 1–11. PMID: 39563187

Ivanova, V. (2020). Carpal tunnel syndrome symptoms in esports players. *Journal of Clinical Rehabilitation*, *34*(3), 115–123.

İzci, F., Sağlam, N. G. U., & Ergelen, M. (2022). Neurobiology and Genetics of Behavioral Addictions: A Brief Review. *Bağimlik Dergisi*, *23*(2), 233–241. DOI: 10.51982/bagimli.991533

Jain, N., Adams, E. A., Joyes, E. C., McLellan, G., Burrows, M., Paisi, M., McGowan, L. J., Iafrate, L., Landes, D., Watt, R., Sniehotta, F. F., Kaner, E., & Ramsay, S. E. (2024). Engagement and access to support for oral health, substance use, smoking and diet by people with severe and multiple disadvantage: A qualitative study. *PLoS One*, *19*(12), e0315254. Advance online publication. DOI: 10.1371/journal.pone.0315254 PMID: 39693306

Jameel, A., Khan, S., Alonazi, W. B., & Khan, A. A. (2024). Exploring the Impact of Social Media Sites on Compulsive Shopping Behavior: The Mediating Role of Materialism. *Psychology Research and Behavior Management*, *17*, 171–185. DOI: 10.2147/PRBM.S442193 PMID: 38250636

Jawad, L., Aboufatima, R., Aicha, O., Bezza, K., El Gabbas, Z., Mehdi, A. L., Fatimazahra, M., Aaziz, K., & Chait, A. (2019). Behavioral and histological characterization of the effects of cigarette smoke inhalation and withdrawal in rats. *Toxicological and Environmental Chemistry*, *101*(1-2), 129–147. DOI: 10.1080/02772248.2019.1628236

Jeong, E. J., & Kim, D. H. (2011). Social activities, self-efficacy, game attitudes, and game addiction. *Cyberpsychology, Behavior, and Social Networking*, *14*(4), 213–221. DOI: 10.1089/cyber.2009.0289 PMID: 21067285

Jiang, C., Li, C., Zhou, H., & Zhou, Z. (2020). Individuals with internet gaming disorder have similar neurocognitive impairments and social cognitive dysfunctions as methamphetamine-dependent patients. Adicciones, 1342(10.20882).

Johnson, K. (2023, February 13). Kids and video games: The good and the bad. *Akron Children's Hospital*. https://www.akronchildrens.org/inside/2023/02/13/kids-and-video-games-the-good-and-the-bad/#:~:text=Studies%20show%20playing%20video%20games,been%20linked%20with%20developing%20obesity

Johnson, D., Dupuis, G., Piche, J., Clayborne, Z., & Colman, I. (2018). Adult mental health outcomes of adolescent depression: A systematic review. *Depression and Anxiety*, *35*(8), 700–716. DOI: 10.1002/da.22777 PMID: 29878410

Johnson, M. E., Salvatore, M. F., Maiolo, S. A., & Bobrovskaya, L. (2018). Tyrosine hydroxylase as a sentinel for central and peripheral tissue responses in Parkinson's progression: Evidence from clinical studies and neurotoxin models. *Progress in Neurobiology*, *165*, 1–25. DOI: 10.1016/j.pneurobio.2018.01.002 PMID: 29331395

Jose, A. (2023). A study on the effects of compulsive buying behavior and shopping addiction on the self-esteem of college-going female students. *International Journal of Indian Psychology*, *11*(4), 585–592. DOI: 10.25215/1104.052

Kalon, E., Hong, J. Y., Tobin, C., & Schulte, T. (2016). Psychological and neurobiological correlates of food addiction. *International Review of Neurobiology*, *129*, 85–110. DOI: 10.1016/bs.irn.2016.06.003 PMID: 27503449

Kamate, R., Baliga, S., & Mallapur, M. D. (2019). Internet addiction among engineering students in Belagavi city: Cross sectional study. *International Journal of Community Medicine and Public Health*, *6*(4), 1488. DOI: 10.18203/2394-6040.ijcmph20191372

Kanayama, G., Brower, K. J., Wood, R. I., Hudson, J. I., & Pope, H. G.Jr. (2009). Anabolic-androgenic steroid dependence: An emerging disorder. *Addiction (Abingdon, England)*, *104*(12), 1966–1978. DOI: 10.1111/j.1360-0443.2009.02734.x PMID: 19922565

Kaptsis, D., King, D. L., Delfabbro, P. H., & Gradisar, M. (2016). Withdrawal symptoms in internet gaming disorder: A systematic review. *Clinical Psychology Review*, *43*, 58–66. DOI: 10.1016/j.cpr.2015.11.006 PMID: 26704173

Kar, S. K. (2016). Lost online, then lust online. *New Journal of Psychiatric Nursing*, *5*(3), 117–119. DOI: 10.21088/jpn.2277.9035.5316.4

Kbah, S. N. S., Tan, T. S., Sheikh, J., Al-Qazzaz, N. K., Salim, M. I. M., Hum, Y. C., & Qiu, F. (2025). Review on Fundamental of Electroencephalography and Detection Techniques in Substance and Behavioral Addiction. *Journal of Human Centered Technology*, *4*(1), 78–85. DOI: 10.11113/humentech.v4n1.98

Keilty, P. (2018). Desire by design: Pornography as technology industry. *Porn Studies*, *1–5*(3), 338–342. Advance online publication. DOI: 10.1080/23268743.2018.1483208

Khang, H., Kim, J. K., & Kim, Y. (2013). Self-traits and motivations as antecedents of digital media flow and addiction: The Internet, mobile phones, and video games. *Computers in Human Behavior*, *29*(6), 2416–2424. DOI: 10.1016/j.chb.2013.05.027

Khorrami, M. S., Esfidani, M. R., & Delavari, S. (2015). The effect of situational factors on impulse buying and compulsive buying: Clothing. International Journal of Management. *Accounting and Economics*, *2*(8), 823–837.

Khoshro, S., Farhangi, M. A., & Jahangiry, L. (2024). Psychometric properties of the exercise addiction inventory (EAI) questionnaire among physically active young adults. *BMC Research Notes*, *17*(1), 76. DOI: 10.1186/s13104-024-06722-x PMID: 38486222

Khubchandani, J., Sharma, S., & Price, J. H. (2021). COVID-19 Pandemic and the Burden of Internet Addiction in the United States. *Psychiatry International*, *2*(4), 402–409. DOI: 10.3390/psychiatryint2040031

Kim, S. M., Han, D. H., Lee, Y. S., & Renshaw, P. F. (2012). Combined cognitive behavioral therapy and bupropion for the treatment of problematic online game play in adolescents with major depressive disorder. *Computers in Human Behavior*, *28*(5), 1954–1959. DOI: 10.1016/j.chb.2012.05.015

Kim, S., & Chun, J. (2022). The impact of parental and peer attachment on gaming addiction among out-of-school adolescents in South Korea: The mediating role of social stigma. *International Journal of Environmental Research and Public Health*, *20*(1), 72. DOI: 10.3390/ijerph20010072 PMID: 36612398

King, C., Hayes, M., Maldonado, L., Monter, E., Aujla, R., Phlegar, E., Smith, C., Parker, L., Blome, K., Sandford, A., Douglas, E., & Guille, C. (2025). A perinatal psychiatry access program to address rural and medically underserved populations using telemedicine. *BMC Women's Health*, *25*(1), 30. Advance online publication. DOI: 10.1186/s12905-025-03561-1 PMID: 39838366

King, D. L., Chamberlain, S. R., Carragher, N., Billieux, J., Stein, D., Mueller, K., Potenza, M. N., Rumpf, H. J., Saunders, J., Starcevic, V., Demetrovics, Z., Brand, M., Lee, H. K., Spada, M., Lindenberg, K., Wu, A. M. S., Lemenager, T., Pallesen, S., Achab, S., & Delfabbro, P. H. (2020). Screening and assessment tools for gaming disorder: A comprehensive systematic review. *Clinical Psychology Review*, *77*, 101831. DOI: 10.1016/j.cpr.2020.101831 PMID: 32143109

King, D. L., Delfabbro, P. H., Doh, Y. Y., Wu, A. M., Kuss, D. J., Pallesen, S., Mentzoni, R., Carragher, N., & Sakuma, H. (2018). Policy and prevention approaches for disordered and hazardous gaming and Internet use: An international perspective. *Prevention Science*, *19*(2), 233–249. DOI: 10.1007/s11121-017-0813-1 PMID: 28677089

King, D. L., Haagsma, M. C., Delfabbro, P. H., Gradisar, M., & Griffiths, M. D. (2013). Toward a consensus definition of pathological video-gaming: A systematic review of psychometric assessment tools. *Clinical Psychology Review*, *33*(3), 331–342. DOI: 10.1016/j.cpr.2013.01.002 PMID: 23396015

King, D., & Delfabbro, P. (2019). Video game monetization: Psychological impacts. *Current Addiction Reports*, *6*(3), 323–330.

Ko, C. H., Kiraly, O., Demetrovics, Z., Chang, Y. M., & Yen, J. Y. (2020). Identifying individuals in need of help for their uncontrolled gaming: A narrative review of concerns and comments regarding gaming disorder diagnostic criteria. *Journal of Behavioral Addictions*, *9*(3), 572–588. DOI: 10.1556/2006.2020.00058 PMID: 33011711

Ko, C. H., Liu, G. C., Hsiao, S., Yen, J. Y., Yang, M. J., Lin, W. C., Yen, C.-F., & Chen, C. S. (2009). Brain activities associated with gaming urge of online gaming addiction. *Journal of Psychiatric Research*, *43*(7), 739–747. DOI: 10.1016/j.jpsychires.2008.09.012 PMID: 18996542

Koçak, Ç. V. (2018). How does regular exercise affect internet addiction level in university students? *Physical Education of Students*, *23*(4), 186–190. DOI: 10.15561/20755279.2019.0404

Koepp, M. J., Gunn, R. N., Lawrence, A. D., Cunningham, V. J., Dagher, A., Jones, T., Brooks, D. J., Bench, C. J., & Grasby, P. M. (1998). Evidence for striatal dopamine release during a video game. *Nature*, *393*(6682), 266–268. DOI: 10.1038/30498 PMID: 9607763

Koijam, A. S., Singh, K. D., Nameirakpam, B. S., Haobam, R., & Rajashekar, Y. (2024). Drug addiction and treatment: An epigenetic perspective. *Biomedicine and Pharmacotherapy*, *170*, 115951. DOI: 10.1016/j.biopha.2023.115951 PMID: 38043446

Kolaib, A. M. A., Al-Hazmi, A. H., & Kulaib, M. M. A. (2020). Prevalence of internet addiction and its associated factors among medical students at Taiba University, Saudi Arabia. *Journal of Family Medicine and Primary Care*, *9*(9), 4797. DOI: 10.4103/jfmpc.jfmpc_655_20 PMID: 33209802

Koob, G.F., Kandel, D.B., Baler, R.D., & Volkow, N.D. (2023). Neurobiology of addiction. *Tasman's Psychiatry,* 1-51. https://doi.org/DOI: 10.1007/978-3-030-42825-9_29-1

Koob, G. F., & Volkow, N. D. (2016). Neurobiology of addiction: A neurocircuitry analysis. *The Lancet. Psychiatry*, *3*(8), 760–773. DOI: 10.1016/S2215-0366(16)00104-8 PMID: 27475769

Koo, C., Wati, Y., Lee, C. C., & Oh, H. Y. (2011). Internet-addicted kids and South Korean government efforts: Boot-camp case. *Cyberpsychology, Behavior, and Social Networking*, *14*(6), 391–394. DOI: 10.1089/cyber.2009.0331 PMID: 21204693

Krahé, B., & Möller, I. (2004). Playing violent electronic games, hostile attributional style, and aggression-related norms in German adolescents. *Journal of Adolescence*, *27*(1), 53–69. DOI: 10.1016/j.adolescence.2003.10.006 PMID: 15013260

Kroemer, N. B., Lee, Y., Pooseh, S., Eppinger, B., Goschke, T., & Smolka, M. N. (2019). L-DOPA reduces model-free control of behavior by attenuating the transfer of value to action. *NeuroImage*, *186*, 113–125. DOI: 10.1016/j.neuroimage.2018.10.075 PMID: 30381245

Krych, R. (1989). Abnormal consumer behavior: A model of addictive behaviors. *Advances in Consumer Research. Association for Consumer Research (U. S.)*, *16*, 745–748.

Kühn, S., & Gallinat, J. (2014). Brain Structure and Functional Connectivity Associated With Pornography Consumption. *JAMA Psychiatry*, *71*(7), 827. DOI: 10.1001/jamapsychiatry.2014.93 PMID: 24871202

Kumar, M., & Jha, A. K. (2024). Adolescent Brain Development: Limbic System and Emotions. In *Encyclopedia of Religious Psychology and Behavior* (pp. 1–10). Springer Nature Switzerland. DOI: 10.1007/978-3-031-38971-9_10-1

Kumbhare, K. (2022). Effect Pornography has on an Individual's Personality. *International Journal of Indian Psychology*, *10*(3). Doi.org/10.25215/1003.156

Kuss, D. J., & Griffiths, M. D. (2011). Online Social Networking and Addiction—A Review of the Psychological Literature. *International Journal of Environmental Research and Public Health*, *8*(9), 3528–3552. DOI: 10.3390/ijerph8093528 PMID: 22016701

Kuss, D. J., & Griffiths, M. D. (2012). Online gaming addiction in children and adolescents: A review of empirical research. *Journal of Behavioral Addictions*, *1*(1), 3–22. DOI: 10.1556/JBA.1.2012.1.1 PMID: 26166826

Kuss, D. J., & Griffiths, M. D. (2017). Internet and gaming addiction: A systematic literature review of neuroimaging studies. *Brain Sciences*, *7*(5), 46. PMID: 28441336

Kuss, D. J., & Lopez-Fernandez, O. (2016). Internet addiction and problematic Internet use: A systematic review of clinical research. *World Journal of Psychiatry*, *6*(1), 143. DOI: 10.5498/wjp.v6.i1.143 PMID: 27014605

Laier, C., Pawlikowski, M., Pekal, J., Schulte, F. P., & Brand, M. (2013). Cybersex addiction: Experienced sexual arousal when watching pornography and not real-life sexual contacts makes the difference. *Journal of Behavioral Addictions*, *2*(2), 100–107. DOI: 10.1556/JBA.2.2013.002 PMID: 26165929

Laier, C., Wegmann, E., & Brand, M. (2018). Personality and cognition in gamers: Avoidance expectancies mediate the relationship between maladaptive personality traits and symptoms of Internet-gaming disorder. *Frontiers in Psychiatry*, *9*, 304. DOI: 10.3389/fpsyt.2018.00304 PMID: 30042702

Landolfi, E. (2013). Exercise addiction. *Sports Medicine (Auckland, N.Z.)*, *43*(2), 111–119. DOI: 10.1007/s40279-012-0013-x PMID: 23329605

Landripet, I., & Štulhofer, A. (2015). Is Pornography Use Associated with Sexual Difficulties and Dysfunctions among Younger Heterosexual Men? *Journal of Sexual Medicine*, *12*(5), 1136–1139. DOI: 10.1111/jsm.12853 PMID: 25816904

Laskowski, C. (2022). *Impacts of reward schedules and a dopamine agonist on dopamine receptor expression in an animal model of gambling addiction* (Doctoral dissertation, University of Lethbridge (Canada)).

Lebni, J. Y., Toghroli, R., & Abbas, J. (2020). A study of internet addiction and its effects on mental health: A study based on Iranian University Students. *Journal of Education and Health Promotion*, *9*(1), 205. DOI: 10.4103/jehp.jehp_148_20 PMID: 33062738

Lechan, R. M., & Toni, R. (2016). *Functional anatomy of the hypothalamus and pituitary*. Endotext. [Internet]

Lee, D., Lee, J., Lee, J. E., & Jung, Y. C. (2017). Altered functional connectivity in the default mode network in Internet gaming disorder: Influence of childhood ADHD. *Progress in Neuro-Psychopharmacology & Biological Psychiatry, 75*, 135–141. DOI: 10.1016/j.pnpbp.2017.02.005 PMID: 28174127

Lee, D., Namkoong, K., Lee, J., & Jung, Y. C. (2018). Abnormal gray matter volume and impulsivity in young adults with Internet gaming disorder. *Addiction Biology, 23*(5), 1160–1167. DOI: 10.1111/adb.12552 PMID: 28884950

Lee, J. H. (2023). Understanding Parkinson's Disorders: Classification and Evaluation Methods, Movement Disorders, and Treatment Methods. *International Journal of Advanced Culture Technology, 11*(3), 9–17.

Lee, J. H.. (2014). Neurobiological mechanisms of compulsive buying: A review of the literature. *Journal of Psychiatric Research, 57*, 79–86.

Lee, S., & Mysyk, A. (2004). The medicalization of compulsive buying. *Social Science & Medicine, 58*(9), 1709–1718. DOI: 10.1016/S0277-9536(03)00340-X PMID: 14990372

Leftwich, B. M. (2022). Compulsive buying behavior and its association with emotional distress, depression, and impulsivity in general population: An online survey. 1–15. https://doi.org/DOI: 10.1017/S1092852922001109

Leite, P. L., Pereira, V. M., Nardi, A. E., & Silva, A. C. (2014). Psychotherapy for compulsive buying disorder: A systematic review. *Psychiatry Research, 219*(3), 411–419. DOI: 10.1016/j.psychres.2014.05.037 PMID: 25023363

Lejoyeux, M., Avril, M., Richoux, C., Embouazza, H., & Nivoli, F. (2008). Prevalence of exercise dependence and other behavioral addictions among clients of a Parisian fitness room. *Comprehensive Psychiatry, 49*(4), 353–358. https://doi.org/ . 2007.12.005DOI: 10.1016/j.comppsych

Lejoyeux, M., & Ades, J. (1994). Les achats pathologiques: Une addiction comportementale. *Neuro-Psy, 9*(1), 25–32.

Lejoyeux, M., Andes, J., & Tassian, V.. (1996). Phenomenology and psychopathology of uncontrolled buying. *The American Journal of Psychiatry, 152*, 1524–1529. PMID: 8942446

Lejoyeux, M., & Weinstein, A. (2010). Compulsive Buying. *The American Journal of Drug and Alcohol Abuse, 36*(5), 248–253. DOI: 10.3109/00952990.2010.493590 PMID: 20560822

Leménager, T., Hoffmann, S., Dieter, J., Reinhard, I., Mann, K., & Kiefer, F. (2018). The links between healthy, problematic, and addicted internet use regarding comorbidities and self-concept-related characteristics. *Journal of Behavioral Addictions*, *7*(1), 31–43. DOI: 10.1556/2006.7.2018.13 PMID: 29444606

Lemmens, J. S., Valkenburg, P. M., & Peter, J. (2009). Development and validation of a game addiction scale for adolescents. *Media Psychology*, *12*(1), 77–95. DOI: 10.1080/15213260802669458

Lemmens, J. S., Valkenburg, P. M., & Peter, J. (2023). Psychosocial causes and consequences of pathological gaming. *Computers in Human Behavior*, *103*, 118–124.

Leonhardt, M., & Overå, S. (2021). Are there differences in video gaming and use of social media among boys and girls?—A mixed methods approach. *International Journal of Environmental Research and Public Health*, *18*(11), 6085. DOI: 10.3390/ijerph18116085 PMID: 34200039

Lerner, T. N., Holloway, A. L., & Seiler, J. L. (2021). Dopamine, updated: Reward prediction error and beyond. *Current Opinion in Neurobiology*, *67*, 123–130. DOI: 10.1016/j.conb.2020.10.012 PMID: 33197709

Lewis, R. G., Florio, E., Punzo, D., & Borrelli, E. (2021). The brain's reward system in health and disease. *Advances in Experimental Medicine and Biology*, *1344*, 57–69. DOI: 10.1007/978-3-030-81147-1_4 PMID: 34773226

Lew-Starowicz, M., & Coleman, E. (2022). Mental and sexual health perspectives of the international classification of diseases (icd-11) compulsive sexual behavior disorder •. *Journal of Behavioral Addictions*, *11*(2), 226–229. DOI: 10.1556/2006.2022.00032 PMID: 35895453

Ley, D., Prause, N., & Finn, P. (2014). The emperor has no clothes: A review of the 'pornography addiction' model. *Current Sexual Health Reports*, *6*(2), 94–105. DOI: 10.1007/s11930-014-0016-8

Lezhari, E. (2020). Addictions and tensions: the Psychomotor rehabilitation regarding the regulation of stress and anxiety among people suffering from addiction.

Li, B., Nguyen, T. P., Ma, C., & Dan, Y. (2020). Inhibition of impulsive action by projection-defined prefrontal pyramidal neurons. *Proceedings of the National Academy of Sciences of the United States of America*, *117*(29), 17278–17287. DOI: 10.1073/pnas.2000523117 PMID: 32631999

Lichtenstein, M. B. & Hinze, C. J. (2020). Exercise addiction. *Adolescent Addiction*, 265–288. DOI: 10.1016/B978-0-12-818626-8.00010-4

Lichtenstein, M. B., Christiansen, E., Elklit, A., Bilenberg, N., & Støving, R. K. (2014). Exercise addiction: A study of eating disorder symptoms, quality of life, personality traits and attachment styles. *Psychiatry Research*, *215*(2), 410–416. DOI: 10.1016/j.psychres.2013.11.010 PMID: 24342179

Lichtenstein, M. B., Hinze, C. J., Emborg, B., Thomsen, F., & Hemmingsen, S. D. (2017). Compulsive exercise: Links, risks and challenges faced. *Psychology Research and Behavior Management*, *10*, 85–95. DOI: 10.2147/PRBM.S113093 PMID: 28435339

Lichtenstein, M. B., Melin, A. K., Szabo, A., & Holm, L. (2021). The prevalence of exercise addiction symptoms in a sample of national level elite athletes. *Frontiers in Sports and Active Living*, *3*, 635418. Advance online publication. DOI: 10.3389/fspor.2021.635418 PMID: 34179773

Lim, M. A. (2021). Exercise addiction and COVID-19-associated restrictions. *Journal of Mental Health (Abingdon, England)*, *30*(2), 135–137. DOI: 10.1080/09638237.2020.1803234 PMID: 32755432

Lim, M. S., Carrotte, E. R., & Hellard, M. E. (2016). The impact of pornography on gender-based violence, sexual health and well-being: What do we know? *Journal of Epidemiology and Community Health*, *70*(1), 3–5. DOI: 10.1136/jech-2015-205453 PMID: 26022057

Lindenberg, K., Kindt, S., & Szász-Janocha, C. (2022). Effectiveness of cognitive behavioral therapy–based intervention in preventing gaming disorder and unspecified internet use disorder in adolescents: A cluster randomized clinical trial. *JAMA Network Open*, *5*(2), e2148995–e2148995. DOI: 10.1001/jamanetworkopen.2021.48995 PMID: 35179587

Lind, K., Marionneau, V., Järvinen-Tassopoulos, J., & Salonen, A. H. (2021). Sociodemographics, gambling participation, gambling settings, and addictive behaviors associated with gambling modes: A population-based study. *Journal of Gambling Studies*, *38*(4), 1–16. DOI: 10.1007/s10899-021-10074-7 PMID: 34623554

Li, S., Wu, Q., Tang, C., Chen, Z., & Liu, L. (2020). Exercise-Based Interventions for Internet Addiction: Neurobiological and Neuropsychological Evidence. *Frontiers in Psychology*, *11*, 1296. Advance online publication. DOI: 10.3389/fpsyg.2020.01296 PMID: 32670157

Lischer, S., Jeannot, E., Brülisauer, L., Weber, N., Khazaal, Y., Bendahan, S., & Simon, O. (2022). Response to the regulation of video games under the Youth Media Protection Act: A public health perspective. *International Journal of Environmental Research and Public Health*, *19*(15), 9320. DOI: 10.3390/ijerph19159320 PMID: 35954678

Liu, S., Xiao, T., Yang, L., & Loprinzi, P. D. (2019). Exercise as an alternative approach for treating smartphone addiction: A systematic review and meta-analysis of random controlled trials. *International Journal of Environmental Research and Public Health*, *16*(20), 3912. DOI: 10.3390/ijerph16203912 PMID: 31618879

Liu, S., Xu, B., Zhang, D., Tian, Y., & Wu, X. (2022). Core symptoms and symptom relationships of problematic internet use across early, middle, and late adolescence: A network analysis. *Computers in Human Behavior*, *128*, 107090. DOI: 10.1016/j.chb.2021.107090

Liu, X., Zheng, Y., Niculescu, M., Liang, Q., Yang, A., Dong, G., Gao, Z., Lin, P., Liu, Y., Chen, L., & Xu, D. (2023). The involvement of spontaneous brain activity in natural recovery from internet gaming disorder: A resting-state fMRI study. *Frontiers in Psychiatry*, *14*, 1093784. DOI: 10.3389/fpsyt.2023.1093784 PMID: 36896348

Liu, Y., Duan, L., Shen, Q., Xu, L., & Zhang, T. (2024). The relationship between childhood psychological abuse and depression in college students: Internet addiction as mediator, different dimensions of alexithymia as moderator. *BMC Public Health*, *24*(1), 2744. Advance online publication. DOI: 10.1186/s12889-024-20232-2 PMID: 39379902

Li, Z., Xia, X., Sun, Q., & Li, Y. (2023). Exercise intervention to reduce mobile phone addiction in adolescents: A systematic review and meta-analysis of randomized controlled trials. *Frontiers in Psychology*, *14*, 1294116. Advance online publication. DOI: 10.3389/fpsyg.2023.1294116 PMID: 38192396

Lo, C. K. M., Yu, L., Cho, Y. W., & Chan, K. L. (2020). A qualitative study of practitioners' views on family involvement in treatment process of adolescent internet addiction. *International Journal of Environmental Research and Public Health*, *18*(1), 86. DOI: 10.3390/ijerph18010086 PMID: 33374348

Long, J., Bhad, R., Potenza, M. N., Orsolini, L., Phan, V., Kanabar, M., & Achab, S. (2022). Public health approaches and policy changes after the inclusion of gaming disorder in ICD-11: Global needs. *BJPsych International*, *19*(3), 63–66. DOI: 10.1192/bji.2021.57 PMID: 36287819

Lough, E., & Fisher, M. H. (2016). Internet use and online safety in adults with Williams syndrome. *Journal of Intellectual Disability Research, 60*(10), 1020–1030. DOI: 10.1111/jir.12281 PMID: 27174494

Love, T., Laier, C., Brand, M., Hatch, L., & Hajela, R. (2015). Neuroscience of internet pornography addiction: A review and update. *Behavioral Sciences (Basel, Switzerland), 5*(3), 388–433. DOI: 10.3390/bs5030388 PMID: 26393658

Lozano-Blasco, R., Latorre-Martínez, M. P., & Cortes-Pascual, A. (2021). Analyzing adolescents: An analysis from the perspective of gamers on YouTube. *Sustainability (Basel), 13*(20), 11391. DOI: 10.3390/su132011391

Lukavská, K., Hrabec, O., Lukavský, J., Demetrovics, Z., & Király, O. (2022). The associations of adolescent problematic internet use with parenting: A meta-analysis. *Addictive Behaviors, 135*, 107423. DOI: 10.1016/j.addbeh.2022.107423 PMID: 35933287

Lu, R. (2023). Adolescents' internet addiction: Influence factors, risks, and neuroscience connectivity. *Journal of Education. Humanities and Social Sciences, 8*, 483–490. DOI: 10.54097/ehss.v8i.4293

Maan, J. S., Ershadi, M., Khan, I., & Saadabadi, A. (2023). Quetiapine. In *StatPearls*. StatPearls Publishing., https://www.ncbi.nlm.nih.gov/books/NBK459145

Maceri, R. M., Cherup, N. P., Buckworth, J., & Hanson, N. J. (2019). Exercise addiction in long distance runners. *International Journal of Mental Health and Addiction, 19*(1), 62–71. DOI: 10.1007/s11469-019-00122-0

Machado, B., de Faria, P. L., Araújo, I., & Caridade, S. (2024). Cyber interpersonal violence: Adolescent perspectives and digital practices. *International Journal of Environmental Research and Public Health, 21*(7), 832. DOI: 10.3390/ijerph21070832 PMID: 39063409

Magee, C. A., Buchman, I., & Barrie, L. (2016). Profiles of exercise dependence symptoms in ironman participants. *Psychology of Sport and Exercise, 24*, 48–55. DOI: 10.1016/j.psychsport.2016.01.005

Mahendra, Y., Jundi, R., Wulandari, G., & Munawar, A. (2024). The Urgency of Digital Literacy in Shaping Students' Civic Virtue: Challenges and Opportunities in the Technological Era. *ICoCSE Proceedings*, 1, 17-22.

Malak, M. Z. (2018). *Internet addiction and cognitive behavioral therapy*. Cognitive Behavioral Therapy and Clinical Applications., DOI: 10.5772/intechopen.71277

Manfredi, P. (2022). Benefits, risks and gender differences in sport, and exercise dependence: Key role of alexithymia. *International Journal of Environmental Research and Public Health, 19*(9), 5288. DOI: 10.3390/ijerph19095288 PMID: 35564683

Manning, J. C. (2006). The impact of internet pornography on marriage and the family: A review of the research. *Sexual Addiction & Compulsivity, 13*(2–3), 131–165. DOI: 10.1080/10720160600870711

Marcinko, D., & Karlovi, D. (2005). Oniomania—successful treatment with fluvoxamine and cognitive-behavioral psychotherapy. *Psychiatria Danubina, 17*, 97–100. PMID: 16395851

Marques, A., Peralta, M., Sarmento, H., Loureiro, V., Gouveia, É. R., & de Matos, M. G. (2019). Prevalence of risk for exercise dependence: A systematic review. *Sports Medicine (Auckland, N.Z.), 49*(2), 319–330. DOI: 10.1007/s40279-018-1011-4 PMID: 30374944

Martini, F., Fregna, L., Bosia, M., Perrozzi, G., & Cavallaro, R. (2022). Substance-related disorders. In *Fundamentals of Psychiatry for Health Care Professionals* (pp. 263–295). Springer International Publishing. DOI: 10.1007/978-3-031-07715-9_9

Masaeli, N., & Farhadi, H. (2021). Prevalence of internet-based addictive behaviors during COVID-19 pandemic: A systematic review. *Journal of Addictive Diseases, 39*(4), 1–27. DOI: 10.1080/10550887.2021.1895962 PMID: 33749537

Matar, R., & Abdelfattah, N. (2023). Neurobiological underpinnings of compulsive buying disorder: A multimodal imaging study. *Archives of Clinical Psychiatry, 50*(5).

Matheson, F. I., Hamilton-Wright, S., Hahmann, T., McLuhan, A., Tacchini, G., Wendaferew, A., & Dastoori, P. (2022). Filling the GAP: Integrating a gambling addiction program into a shelter setting for people experiencing poverty and homelessness. *PLoS One, 17*(3), e0264922. DOI: 10.1371/journal.pone.0264922 PMID: 35290379

Mattebo, M., Larsson, M., Tydén, T., & Häggström-Nordin, E. (2013). Professionals' perceptions of the effect of pornography on Swedish adolescents. *Public Health Nursing (Boston, Mass.), 31*(3), 196–205. DOI: 10.1111/phn.12058 PMID: 24720654

Mauer-Vakil, D., & Bahji, A. (2020). The addictive nature of compulsive sexual behaviours and problematic online pornography consumption: A review. *The Canadian Journal of Addiction, 11*(3), 42–51. DOI: 10.1097/CXA.0000000000000091

Mayo Foundation for Medical Education and Research. (2023, April 11). *Psychotherapy*. Mayo Clinic. https://www.mayoclinic.org/tests-procedures/psychotherapy/about/pac-20384616

Mc-Bride, J. F. (2019). Addiction and mindfulness; pornography addiction and mindfulness-based therapy act. *Sexual Addiction & Compulsivity*, *26*(1–2), 42–53. DOI: 10.1080/10720162.2019.1576560

McDaniel, C. C., Kavookjian, J., & Whitley, H. P. (2022). Telehealth delivery of motivational interviewing for diabetes management: A systematic review of randomized controlled trials. *Patient Education and Counseling*, *105*(4), 805–820. DOI: 10.1016/j.pec.2021.07.036 PMID: 34366228

McElroy, S., Keck, P. E.Jr, & Pope, H. G.Jr. (1994). Compulsive buying: A report of 20 cases. *The Journal of Clinical Psychiatry*, *55*, 242–248. PMID: 8071278

McHugh, B. C., Wisniewski, P., Rosson, M. B., & Carroll, J. M. (2018). When social media traumatizes teens: The roles of online risk exposure, coping, and post-traumatic stress. *Internet Research*, *28*(5), 1169–1188. DOI: 10.1108/IntR-02-2017-0077

Menon, V. A., Prasad, A., Puthur, L. A., K K, S., & Joseph, L. (2023). Social Media Dependency and Facebook Usage among the Older Adults of Kerala. *Studies in Media and Communication*, *11*(4), 202–208. DOI: 10.11114/smc.v11i4.6060

Mestre-Bach, G., Fernandez-Aranda, F., & Jiménez-Murcia, S. (2022). Exploring Internet gaming disorder: An updated perspective of empirical evidence (from 2016 to 2021). *Comprehensive Psychiatry*, *116*, 152319. DOI: 10.1016/j.comppsych.2022.152319 PMID: 35526417

Meyer, C., Taranis, L., Goodwin, H., & Haycraft, E. (2011). Compulsive exercise and eating disorders. *European Eating Disorders Review*, *19*(3), 174–189. DOI: 10.1002/erv.1122 PMID: 21584911

Meyer, M., Sattler, I., Schilling, H., Lang, U. E., Schmidt, A., Colledge, F., & Walter, M. (2021). Mental disorders in individuals with exercise addiction—A cross-sectional study. *Frontiers in Psychiatry*, *12*, 751550–751550. DOI: 10.3389/fpsyt.2021.751550 PMID: 34955915

Miller, K. J., & Mesagno, C. (2014). Personality traits and exercise dependence: Exploring the role of narcissism and perfectionism. *International Journal of Sport and Exercise Psychology*, *12*(4), 368–381. DOI: 10.1080/1612197X.2014.932821

Miller, W. R., & Rollnick, S. (2012). *Motivational interviewing: Helping people change*. Guilford Press.

Minarcik, J., Wetterneck, C. T., & Short, M. B. (2016). The effects of sexually explicit material use on romantic relationship dynamics. *Journal of Behavioral Addictions*, *5*(4), 700–707. DOI: 10.1556/2006.5.2016.078 PMID: 27784182

Minarini, A., Ferrari, S., Galletti, M., Giambalvo, N., Perrone, D., Rioli, G., & Galeazzi, G. M. (2017). N -acetylcysteine in the treatment of psychiatric disorders: Current status and future prospects. *Expert Opinion on Drug Metabolism & Toxicology*, *13*(3), 279–292. DOI: 10.1080/17425255.2017.1251580 PMID: 27766914

Minutillo, A., Di Trana, A., Aquilina, V., Ciancio, G. M., Berretta, P., & La Maida, N. (2024). Recent insights in the correlation between social media use, personality traits and exercise addiction: A literature review. *Frontiers in Psychiatry*, *15*, 1392317–1392317. DOI: 10.3389/fpsyt.2024.1392317 PMID: 38800058

Mitchell, J. E., Burgard, M., Faber, R., Crosby, R. D., & deZwaan, M. (2006). Cognitive behavioral therapy for compulsive buying disorder. *Behaviour Research and Therapy*, *44*(12), 1859–1865. DOI: 10.1016/j.brat.2005.12.009 PMID: 16460670

Modolo, V. B., Antunes, H. K. M., de Gimenez, P. R. B., De Mello Santiago, M. L., Tufik, S., & de Mello, M. T. (2011). Negative addiction to exercise: Are there differences between genders? *Clinics (São Paulo, Brazil)*, *66*(2), 255–260. https://doi.org/DOI: 10.1590/S1807-59322011000200013

Molla, M. D., Shirazi, M., & Nikmanesh, Z. (2018). The role of difficulties in emotion regulation and thought control strategies on pornography use. *Practice in Clinical Psychology*, *6*(2), 119–128. DOI: 10.29252/nirp.jpcp.6.2.119

Monaghan, S., & Blaszczynski, A. (2009). *Internet-based interventions for the treatment of problem gambling*. Centre for Addiction and Mental Health., https://www.academia.edu/download/30708795/InternetTreatmentforProblemGamblingCAMH2009_Final.pdf

Monahan, P., Black, D. W., & Gabel, J. (1996). Reliability and validity of a scale to measure change in persons with compulsive buying. *Psychiatry Research*, *64*(1), 59–67. DOI: 10.1016/0165-1781(96)02908-3 PMID: 8888365

Mooy, M. E., Natalia, M., & Taneo, J. (2023). The Effectiveness of Reality Group Counseling in Reducing Social Media Dependency. *Bulletin of Counseling and Psychotherapy*, *5*(3). Advance online publication. DOI: 10.51214/00202305459000

Moriarity, D. P., McArthur, B. A., Ellman, L. M., Coe, C. L., Abramson, L. Y., & Alloy, L. B. (2018). Immunocognitive model of depression secondary to anxiety in adolescents. *Journal of Youth and Adolescence*, *47*(12), 2625–2636. DOI: 10.1007/s10964-018-0905-7 PMID: 30088131

Mousa, S. E. A. (2023). The effectiveness of cognitive-behavioral therapy in alleviating social media addiction among university youth groups. *Egyptian Journal of Social Work*, *15*(1), 175–200. DOI: 10.21608/ejsw.2023.164679.1163

Mueller, A., Mitchell, J. E., Mertens, C., Mueller, U., Silbermann, A., Burgard, M., & deZwaan, M. (2007). Comparison of treatment seeking compulsive buyers in Germany and the United States. *Behaviour Research and Therapy*, *45*(7), 1629–1638. DOI: 10.1016/j.brat.2006.08.005 PMID: 17049486

Mueller, A., Mueller, U., Silbermann, A., Reinecker, H., Bleich, S., Mitchell, J. E., & deZwaan, M. (2008). A randomized, controlled trial of group cognitive-behavioral therapy for compulsive buying disorder: Posttreatment and 6-month follow-up results. *The Journal of Clinical Psychiatry*, *69*(7), 1131–1138. DOI: 10.4088/JCP.v69n0713 PMID: 18557665

Müller, A., Claes, L., Birlin, A., Georgiadou, E., Laskowski, N. M., Steins-Loeber, S., Brand, M., Brand, M., & de Zwaan, M. (2020). Associations of buying-shopping disorder symptoms with identity confusion, materialism, and socially undesirable personality features in a community sample. *European Addiction Research*, *27*(2), 142–150. DOI: 10.1159/000511078 PMID: 33120395

Müller, A., & de Zwaan, M. (2010). Pathological buying. A review of the current knowledge regarding this condition of behavioral excess. *Bundesgesundheitsblatt, Gesundheitsforschung, Gesundheitsschutz*, *53*(4), 289–294. PMID: 20182679

Müller, A., Laskowski, N. M., Trotzke, P., Ali, K., Fassnacht, D. B., de Zwaan, M., Brand, M., Häder, M., & Kyrios, M. (2021). Proposed diagnostic criteria for compulsive buying-shopping disorder: A Delphi expert consensus study. *Journal of Behavioral Addictions*, *10*(2), 208–222. DOI: 10.1556/2006.2021.00013 PMID: 33852420

Müller, A., Laskowski, N. M., Wegmann, E., Steins-Loeber, S., & Brand, M. (2021). Problematic Online Buying-Shopping: Is it Time to Consider the Concept of an Online Subtype of Compulsive Buying-Shopping Disorder or a Specific Internet-Use Disorder? *Current Addiction Reports*, *8*(4), 494–499. DOI: 10.1007/s40429-021-00395-3

Müller, A., Loeber, S., Söchtig, J., Te Wildt, B. T., & De Zwaan, M. (2015). Risk for exercise dependence, eating disorder pathology, alcohol use disorder and addictive behaviors among clients of fitness centers. *Journal of Behavioral Addictions*, *4*(4), 273–280. DOI: 10.1556/2006.4.2015.044 PMID: 26690622

Müller, A., & Mitchell, J. E. (2011). Overview of Treatment for Compulsive Buying. In *Compulsive Buying* (pp. 145–164). Routledge., https://www.taylorfrancis.com/chapters/edit/10.4324/9780203840962-18/overview-treatment-compulsive-buying DOI: 10.4324/9780203840962

Müller, A., Mitchell, J. E., & de Zwaan, M. (2015). Compulsive buying. *Journal of Behavioral Addictions*, *4*(3), 132–137. PMID: 26551898

My People Patterns. (2023, February 1). *Building rapport with teens so they talk in therapy*. Building Rapport With Teens So They Talk In Therapy. https://www.mypeoplepatterns.com/blog/rapport

Naassila, M. (2014). Chapitre 3. Neurobiologie de l'addiction. Dans Benyamina, A. (dir.), Addictions et comorbidités. (p. 25 -54). Dunod.

Nagata, J. M., Ganson, K. T., Iyer, P., Chu, J., Baker, F. C., Gabriel, K. P., & Bibbins-Domingo, K. (2022). Sociodemographic correlates of contemporary screen time use among 9- and 10-year-old children. *The Journal of Pediatrics*, *240*, 213–220. DOI: 10.1016/j.jpeds.2021.08.077 PMID: 34481807

Napier, T. C., Kirby, A., & Persons, A. L. (2020). The role of dopamine pharmacotherapy and addiction-like behaviors in Parkinson's disease. *Progress in Neuro-Psychopharmacology & Biological Psychiatry*, *102*, 109942. DOI: 10.1016/j.pnpbp.2020.109942 PMID: 32272129

Narayanan, A. H., Rajasekar, V. D., Danasekaran, R., Surya, B., Manoj, P., Kumar, S., Syed, R. N., & Ramesh, H. (2025). Compulsive buying disorder among medicine, dentistry, and nursing undergraduate students from Chengalpattu District, Tamil Nadu, India: A cross-sectional study. *Journal of Clinical and Diagnostic Research : JCDR*. Advance online publication. DOI: 10.7860/JCDR/2025/76372.20551

Nasser, A. S. (2021). Teenagers' Addiction to Pornography. *Psychology (Savannah, Ga.)*, *58*(2), 979–993. Doi.org/10.17762/pae.v58i1.847. DOI: 10.17762/pae.v58i1.847

National Eating Disorders Association. (2022). *National Eating Disorders Awareness Week: Expanding the scope*. https://www.nationaleatingdisorders.org

National Institutes of Health. (2022). *Video gaming may be associated with better cognitive performance in children*. National Institutes of Health.

Nazish, N. (2024, December 30). *Is the TikTok-viral 75 Hard Challenge right for you? Experts explain*. Verywell Mind. https://www.verywellmind.com/75-hard-challenge-8750715

Negash, S., Sheppard, N. V., Lambert, N. M., & Fincham, F. D. (2016). Trading later rewards for current pleasure: Pornography consumption and delay discounting. *Journal of Sex Research*, *53*(6), 689–700. DOI: 10.1080/00224499.2015.1025123 PMID: 26305628

Nesi, J., & Prinstein, M. J. (2015). Using social media for social comparison and feedback-seeking: Gender and popularity moderate associations with depressive symptoms. *Journal of Abnormal Child Psychology, 43*(8), 1427–1438. DOI: 10.1007/s10802-015-0020-0 PMID: 25899879

Nestler, E. J., & Lüscher, C. (2019). The molecular basis of drug addiction: Linking epigenetic to synaptic and circuit mechanisms. *Neuron, 102*(1), 48–59. DOI: 10.1016/j.neuron.2019.01.016 PMID: 30946825

New York Times. (2022, February 8). Parents and adolescentss: Finding balance when it comes to screen time. https://www.nytimes.com/guides/well/family/screen-time

Nguyen, H. V., Huang, H. C., Wong, M. K., Yang, Y. H., Huang, T. L., & Teng, C. I. (2018). Moderator roles of optimism and weight control on the impact of playing exergames on happiness: The perspective of social cognitive theory using a randomized controlled trial. *Games for Health Journal, 7*(4), 246–252. DOI: 10.1089/g4h.2017.0165 PMID: 29708775

Niemann, A., Hillerich, V., Wasem, J., Dieris-Hirche, J., Bottel, L., Pape, M., Herpertz, S., Timmesfeld, N., Basten, J., Theodor, B., Wölfling, K., Beckers, R., Henningsen, P., Neusser, S., & Neumann, A. (2023). Health Economic Evaluation of an online-based motivational program to reduce problematic media use and promote treatment motivation for internet use disorder—Results of the OMPRIS study. *International Journal of Environmental Research and Public Health, 20*(24), 7144. DOI: 10.3390/ijerph20247144 PMID: 38131696

Nwufo, J. I., Ike, O. O., Nwoke, M. B., Eze, J., Chukwuorji, J. C., & Kanu, G. C. (2022). Social anxiety and internet addiction among adolescent students in a sub-Saharan African country: Does family functioning make a difference? *South African Journal of Psychology. Suid-Afrikaanse Tydskrif vir Sielkunde, 53*(2), 275–285. DOI: 10.1177/00812463221140224

Oberoi, T. (2024). *Common Mechanisms of Change in Mindfulness-Based Cognitive Therapy (MBCT) and Traditional Cognitive Behavioral Therapy (CBT)*. Implications for Therapeutic Effectiveness.

Oberst, U., Wegmann, E., Stodt, B., Brand, M., & Chamarro, A. (2017). Negative consequences from heavy social networking in adolescents: The mediating role of fear of missing out. *Journal of Adolescence, 55*(1), 51–60. DOI: 10.1016/j.adolescence.2016.12.008 PMID: 28033503

Olave, L., Momeñe, J., Rodríguez Pérez, J. G., Estévez, A., & Iruarrizaga, I. (2019). ¿Existen diferencias en los esquemas cognitivos y en la autoestima entre las personas con adicción al ejercicio físico o con dismorfia muscular? [Are there differences in cognitive patterns and self-esteem among people with exercise addiction or muscle dysmorphia?]. *Revista Española de Drogodependencias*, *44*(2), 43–61. https://www.aesed.com/upload/files/v44n2_art2-dismorfia.pdf

Ong, R. H. S., Sim, H. S., Bergman, M. M., How, C. H., Png, C. A. L., Lim, C. S., Peh, L. H., & Oh, H. C. (2024). Prevalence and associations of problematic smartphone use with smartphone activities, psychological well-being, and sleep quality in a household survey of Singapore adults. *PLoS One*, *19*(12), e0315364. Advance online publication. DOI: 10.1371/journal.pone.0315364 PMID: 39693321

Onukwuli, V. O., Onyinye, E. N., Udigwe, I. B., Umeh, U. M., Enebe, J. T., & Umerah, A. T. (2023). Internet addiction during the COVID-19 pandemic among adolescents in southeast Nigeria and implications for adolescent care in the post-pandemic era: A cross-sectional study. *SAGE Open Medicine*, *11*, 205031212311527–205031212311527. DOI: 10.1177/20503121231152763 PMID: 36860685

Ordabayeva, N., Lisjak, M., & Jones, A. C. (2022). How social perceptions influence consumption for self, for others, and within the broader system. *Current Opinion in Psychology*, *43*, 30–35. DOI: 10.1016/j.copsyc.2021.06.009 PMID: 34274563

Orosz, G., Faragó, L., Paskuj, B., & Krekó, P. (2024). Strategies to combat misinformation: Enduring effects of a 15-minute online intervention on critical-thinking adolescents. *Computers in Human Behavior*, *159*, 108338. DOI: 10.1016/j.chb.2024.108338

Outar, L., Turner, M. J., Wood, A. G., & Lowry, R. (2018). "I need to go to the gym": Exploring the use of rational emotive behaviour therapy upon exercise addiction, irrational and rational beliefs. *Performance Enhancement & Health*, *6*(2), 82–93. DOI: 10.1016/j.peh.2018.05.001

Pálfi, V., Kovacsik, R., & Szabo, A. (2021). Symptoms of exercise addiction in aerobic and anaerobic exercises: Beyond the components model of addiction. *Psychology of Sport and Exercise*, *57*, 101952. DOI: 10.1016/j.psychsport.2021.101952 PMID: 34938830

Pallanti, S., Marras, A., & Makris, N. (2021). A research domain criteria approach to gambling disorder and behavioral addictions: Decision-making, response inhibition, and the role of cannabidiol. *Frontiers in Psychiatry*, *12*, 634418. DOI: 10.3389/fpsyt.2021.634418 PMID: 34603091

Pangarkar, T. (2025, January 13). *Fitness tracker statistics 2025 by health activities.* Market.us News. https://www.news.market.us/fitness-tracker-statistics/

Panksepp, J., & Wilson, C. G. (2016). Brain SEEKING circuitry in neuroeconomics: a unifying hypothesis for the role of dopamine-energized arousal of the medial forebrain bundle in enthusiasm-guiding decision-making. *Neuroeconomics*, 231-252.

Pan, Y.-C., Chiu, Y.-C., & Lin, Y.-H. (2020). Systematic Review and Meta-Analysis of Epidemiology of Internet Addiction. *Neuroscience and Biobehavioral Reviews, 118*(1), 612–622. Advance online publication. DOI: 10.1016/j.neubiorev.2020.08.013 PMID: 32853626

Paolucci, E. O., Genuis, M., & Violato, C. (1997). *A meta-analysis of the published research on the effects of pornography. The Changing Family and Child Development*. Ashgate Publishing Ltd.

Park, S. K., Kim, J. Y., & Cho, C. B. (2008). Prevalence of Internet addiction and correlations with family factors among South Korean adolescents. *Adolescence, 43*(172). PMID: 19149152

Pascoli, V., Terrier, J., & Lüscher, C. (2016). Addiction par stimulation des neurones dopaminergiques mésolimbiques. *médecine/sciences, 32*(8-9), 692-696.

Pathmendra, P., Raggatt, M., Lim, M. S., Marino, J. L., & Skinner, S. R. (2023). Exposure to pornography and adolescent sexual behavior: Systematic review. *Journal of Medical Internet Research, 25*, e43116. DOI: 10.2196/43116 PMID: 36853749

Peng, Z., Jia, Q., Mao, J., Luo, X., Huang, A., Zheng, H., Jiang, S., Ma, Q., Ma, C., & Yi, Q. (2025). Neurotransmitters crosstalk and regulation in the reward circuit of subjects with behavioral addiction. *Frontiers in Psychiatry, 15*, 1439727. DOI: 10.3389/fpsyt.2024.1439727 PMID: 39876994

Pessoa, L. (2017). A network model of the emotional brain. *Trends in Cognitive Sciences, 21*(5), 357–371. DOI: 10.1016/j.tics.2017.03.002 PMID: 28363681

Peter, J., & Valkenburg, P. M. (2008). Adolescents' exposure to sexually explicit internet material and sexual preoccupancy: A three-wave panel study. *Media Psychology, 11*(2), 207–234. DOI: 10.1080/15213260801994238

Peter, J., & Valkenburg, P. M. (2011). The influence of sexually explicit internet material on sexual risk behavior: A comparison of adolescents and adults. *Journal of Health Communication, 16*(7), 750–765. DOI: 10.1080/10810730.2011.551996 PMID: 21476164

Peter, J., & Valkenburg, P. M. (2016). Adolescents and pornography: A review of 20 years of research. *Journal of Sex Research*, *53*(4-5), 509–531. DOI: 10.1080/00224499.2016.1143441 PMID: 27105446

Petry, N. M., Ginley, M. K., & Rash, C. J. (2017). A systematic review of treatments for problem gambling. *Psychology of Addictive Behaviors*, *31*(8), 951–961. DOI: 10.1037/adb0000290 PMID: 28639817

Pettorruso, M., Valle, S., Cavic, E., Martinotti, G., & Grant, J. E. (2020). Problematic Internet use (PIU), personality profiles and emotion dysregulation in a cohort of young adults: Trajectories from risky behaviors to addiction. *Psychiatry Research*, *289*, 113036. DOI: 10.1016/j.psychres.2020.113036 PMID: 32450451

Pew Research Center. (2024, November 13). *Social Media Fact Sheet.*https://www.pewresearch.org/internet/fact-sheet/social-media/

Pierce, E. F., Daleng, M. L., & McGowan, R. W. (1993). Scores on exercise dependence among dancers. *Perceptual and Motor Skills*, *76*(2), 531–535. DOI: 10.2466/pms.1993.76.2.531 PMID: 8483663

Pinna, F. E. D. E. R. I. C. A., Dell'Osso, B., Di Nicola, M., Janiri, L., Altamura, A. C., Carpiniello, B. E. R. N. A. R. D. O., & Hollander, E. (2015). Behavioural addictions and the transition from DSM-IV-TR to DSM-5. *Journal of Psychopathology*, *21*(4), 380–389.

Planzer, S., Gray, H. M., & Shaffer, H. J. (2014). Associations between national gambling policies and disordered gambling prevalence rates within Europe. *International Journal of Law and Psychiatry*, *37*(2), 217–229. DOI: 10.1016/j.ijlp.2013.11.002 PMID: 24370209

Pluhar, E., Kavanaugh, J. R., Levinson, J. A., & Rich, M. (2019). Problematic interactive media use in teens: Comorbidities, assessment, and treatment. *Psychology Research and Behavior Management*, *12*, 447–455. DOI: 10.2147/PRBM.S208968 PMID: 31308769

Poll, M. (2020, January 20). Game on: Adolescentss and video games (Vol. 35, Issue 4). Mott Poll. https://mottpoll.org/reports/game-adolescentss-and-video-games

Pontes, H. M., & Griffiths, M. D. (2015). Measuring DSM-5 internet gaming disorder: Development and validation of a short psychometric scale. *Computers in Human Behavior*, *45*, 137–143. DOI: 10.1016/j.chb.2014.12.006

Pontes, H. M., & Griffiths, M. D. (2019). A new era for gaming disorder research: Time to shift from consensus to consistency. *Addictive Behaviors*. PMID: 31473045

Potenza, M. N. (2014). Non-substance addictive behaviors in the context of DSM-5. *Addictive Behaviors*, *39*(1), 1–2. DOI: 10.1016/j.addbeh.2013.09.004 PMID: 24119712

Potenza, M. N. (2017). Clinical neuropsychiatric considerations regarding nonsubstance or behavioral addictions. *Dialogues in Clinical Neuroscience*, *19*(3), 281–291. DOI: 10.31887/DCNS.2017.19.3/mpotenza PMID: 29302225

Pradana, P. H., Agustini, K., Dantes, G. R., & Sudatha, I. G. W. (2024). The urgency of digital literacy learning in educational units: Systematic literature review. *Child Education Journal*, *6*(1), 25–33. DOI: 10.33086/cej.v6i1.6100

Primack, B. A., Shensa, A., Sidani, J. E., Whaite, E. O., Lin, L., Rosen, D., Colditz, J. B., Radovic, A., & Miller, E. (2017). Social media use and perceived social isolation among young adults in the US. *American Journal of Preventive Medicine*, *53*(1), 1–8. DOI: 10.1016/j.amepre.2017.01.010 PMID: 28279545

Privara, M., & Bob, P. (2023). Pornography consumption and cognitive-affective distress. *The Journal of Nervous and Mental Disease*, *211*(8), 641–646. DOI: 10.1097/NMD.0000000000001669 PMID: 37505898

Priyono, D., & Fradianto, I. (2022). Coping strategies in adolescents with online games addiction. *International Journal of Progressive Sciences and Technologies*, *34*(1), 20. DOI: 10.52155/ijpsat.v34.1.4534

Prochaska, J. O., & DiClemente, C. C. (1983). Stages and processes of self-change of smoking: Toward an integrative model of change. *Journal of Consulting and Clinical Psychology*, *51*(3), 390–395. DOI: 10.1037/0022-006X.51.3.390 PMID: 6863699

Qi-Lytle, X., Sayers, S., & Wagner, E. J. (2023). Current Review of the Function and Regulation of Tuberoinfundibular Dopamine Neurons. *International Journal of Molecular Sciences*, *25*(1), 110. DOI: 10.3390/ijms25010110 PMID: 38203281

Quinones, M. P., & Kaddurah-Daouk, R. (2009). Metabolomics tools for identifying biomarkers for neuropsychiatric diseases. *Neurobiology of Disease*, *35*(2), 165–176. DOI: 10.1016/j.nbd.2009.02.019 PMID: 19303440

Qureshi, F. H., Sokić, K., & Khawaja, S. (2024). Impulsive buying tendencies and personality: Cognitive and affective aspects. https://doi.org/DOI: 10.20944/preprints202409.2097.v1

Raab, G., Elger, C. E., Neuner, M., & Weber, B. (2011). A neurological study of compulsive buying behaviour. *Journal of Consumer Policy*, *34*(4), 401–413. DOI: 10.1007/s10603-011-9168-3

Rachubińska, K., Cybulska, A. M., Szylińska, A., Kupcewicz, E., Ćwiek, D., Walaszek, I., & Grochans, E. (2024). Psychosocial functioning of individuals at risk of developing compulsive buying disorder. *Journal of Clinical Medicine, 13*(5), 1339. DOI: 10.3390/jcm13051339 PMID: 38592171

Raimo, S., Cropano, M., Trojano, L., & Santangelo, G. (2021). The neural basis of gambling disorder: An activation likelihood estimation meta-analysis. *Neuroscience and Biobehavioral Reviews, 120*, 279–302. DOI: 10.1016/j.neubiorev.2020.11.027 PMID: 33275954

Raising Children Network. (2024, February 8). Parents as role models for pre-adolescents and adolescents. Raising Children Network.

Rana, M., & Malik, P. (2023). Determinants of compulsive buying behavior: Psychosomatic- social analysis of maladaptive spending. *Journal of Positive School Psychology, 7*, 204–224.

Ratković, D., Knežević, V., Dickov, A., Fedrigolli, E., & Čomić, M. (2023, April). Comparison of binge-eating disorder and food addiction. *The Journal of International Medical Research, 51*(4), 3000605231171016. DOI: 10.1177/03000605231171016 PMID: 37115520

Raymer, D. L., Jr. (2021, September). Internet gaming disorder: A real mental health issue on the rise in adolescents and young adults. *Counseling Today*. https://www.counseling.org/publications/counseling-today-magazine/article-archive/article/legacy/internet-gaming-disorder--a-real-mental-health-issue-on-the-rise-in-adolescents-and-young-adults#:~:text=It%20is%20important%20to%20establish,time%20spent%20playing%20video%20games

Rehbein, F., Mößle, T., Rumpf, H. J., Bischof, G., & Bischof, A. (2015). Lebenszeit-und 12-Monatsprävalenz der Internet Gaming Disorder in der deutschen Erwachsenenbevölkerung: Wie sich das Spielverhalten Betroffener von unauffälligen Spielern unterscheidet. *Suchttherapie, 16*(S 01), S_07_02.

Remon, H. (2024). Online Addiction: A New Form of Mental Health Issue. *Science Insights, 44*(3), 1291–1300. DOI: 10.15354/si.24.re938

Renard, J., Rushlow, W. J., & Laviolette, S. R. (2018). Effects of adolescent THC exposure on the prefrontal GABAergic system: Implications for schizophrenia-related psychopathology. *Frontiers in Psychiatry, 9*, 281. DOI: 10.3389/fpsyt.2018.00281 PMID: 30013490

Reuter, M., & Montag, C. (2017). *Internet addiction neuroscientific approaches and therapeutical implications including smartphone addiction*. Springer International Publishing.

Ricciutti, N. M., & Zhang, S. (2024). A pilot study of the behavioral addictions knowledge survey: Ensuring students' knowledge about process/behavioral addictions. *Journal of Addictions & Offender Counseling*, *45*(2), 205–220. DOI: 10.1002/jaoc.12132

Rich, F. (2001). Naked capitalists. In Stombler, M., Burgess, E. O., Donnelly, D., & Simonds, W. (Eds.), *Sex matters: The sexuality and society reader* (pp. 462–466). Pearson Education Inc.

Ridgway, N. M., Kukar-Kinney, M., & Monroe, K. B. (2008). An expanded conceptualization and a new measure of compulsive buying. *The Journal of Consumer Research*, *35*(4), 622–639. DOI: 10.1086/591108

Roberts, A. G., & Lopez-Duran, N. L. (2019). Developmental influences on stress response systems: Implications for psychopathology vulnerability in adolescence. *Comprehensive Psychiatry*, *88*, 9–21. DOI: 10.1016/j.comppsych.2018.10.008 PMID: 30466015

Roberts, J. A., Manolis, C., & Tanner, J. F.Jr. (2003). Family structure, materialism, and compulsive buying: A reinquiry and extension. *Journal of Technological Advancements*, *31*(3), 300–311. DOI: 10.1177/0092070303031003007

Roberts, T. A., Daniels, E. A., Weaver, J. M., & Zanovitch, L. S. (2022). "Intermission!" A short-term social media fast reduces self-objectification among pre-teen and teen dancers. *Body Image*, *43*, 125–133. DOI: 10.1016/j.bodyim.2022.08.015 PMID: 36152479

Rolls, E. T. (2019). The cingulate cortex and limbic systems for emotion, action, and memory. *Brain Structure & Function*, *224*(9), 3001–3018. DOI: 10.1007/s00429-019-01945-2 PMID: 31451898

Rosenberg, K. P. (2014). *Behavioral addictions : Criteria, evidence, and treatment*. Academic Press.

Rosenthal, A., Levin, M. E., Garland, E. L., & Romanczuk-Seiferth, N. (2021). Mindfulness in treatment approaches for addiction—Underlying mechanisms and future directions. *Current Addiction Reports*, *8*(2), 282–297. DOI: 10.1007/s40429-021-00372-w

Rosenthal, S. R., Cha, Y., & Clark, M. A. (2018). The Internet Addiction Test in a Young Adult U.S. Population. *Cyberpsychology, Behavior, and Social Networking*, *21*(10), 661–666. DOI: 10.1089/cyber.2018.0143 PMID: 30334654

Ross, M. W., Månsson, S. A., & Daneback, K. (2012). Prevalence, severity, and correlates of problematic sexual internet use in swedish men and women. *Archives of Sexual Behavior*, *41*(2), 459–466. DOI: 10.1007/s10508-011-9762-0 PMID: 21562915

Royse, S. K., Lopresti, B. J., Mathis, C. A., Tollefson, S., & Narendran, R. (2023). Beyond monoamines: II. Novel applications for PET imaging in psychiatric disorders. *Journal of Neurochemistry*, *164*(3), 401–443. DOI: 10.1111/jnc.15657 PMID: 35716057

Rueda, C. (2020). Neuroeducation: Teaching with the brain. *Journal of Neuroeducation*, *1*(1), 108–113. DOI: 10.1344/joned.v1i1.31657

Sadagheyani, H. E., & Tatari, F. (2021). Investigating the role of social media on mental health. *Mental Health and Social Inclusion*, *25*(1), 41–51. DOI: 10.1108/MHSI-06-2020-0039

Sancho, M., De Gracia, M., Rodriguez, R. C., Mallorquí-Bagué, N., Sánchez-González, J., Trujols, J., Sánchez, I., Jiménez-Murcia, S., & Menchón, J. M. (2018). Mindfulness-based interventions for the treatment of substance and behavioral addictions: A systematic review. *Frontiers in Psychiatry*, *9*, 95. DOI: 10.3389/fpsyt.2018.00095 PMID: 29651257

Sandua, d. (2024). Overcoming addictions: strategies for breaking free from compulsive patterns.

Sathya, J., Babu, M., Gayathri, J., Indhumathi, G., Samad, Z. A., & Anandhi, E. (2023). Compulsive buying behavior and online shopping addiction of women. *Information Science Letters*, *12*(5), 1641–1650. DOI: 10.18576/isl/120512

Satici, S. A., Gocet Tekin, E., Deniz, M. E., & Satici, B. (2023). Doomscrolling scale: Its association with personality traits, psychological distress, social media use, and wellbeing. *Applied Research in Quality of Life*, *18*(2), 833–847. DOI: 10.1007/s11482-022-10110-7 PMID: 36275044

Sayin, H. U. (2019). Getting high on dopamine: Neuro scientific aspects of pleasure. *SexuS J*, *4*, 883–906.

Scerri, M., Anderson, A., Stavropoulos, V., & Hu, E. (2019). Need fulfilment and internet gaming disorder: A preliminary integrative model. *Addictive Behaviors Reports*, *9*, 100144. DOI: 10.1016/j.abrep.2018.100144 PMID: 31193898

Schneider, J. P. (2000). Effects of cybersex addiction on the family: Results of a survey. *Sexual Addiction & Compulsivity*, *7*(1), 31–58. DOI: 10.1080/10720160008400206

Schneider, L. A., King, D. L., & Delfabbro, P. H. (2017). Family factors in adolescent problematic Internet gaming: A systematic review. *Journal of Behavioral Addictions*, *6*(3), 321–333. DOI: 10.1556/2006.6.2017.035 PMID: 28762279

Schultz, W. (2015, July). Neuronal Reward and Decision Signals: From Theories to Data. *Physiological Reviews*, *95*(3), 853–951. DOI: 10.1152/physrev.00023.2014 PMID: 26109341

Schwebel, F. J., Korecki, J. R., & Witkiewitz, K. (2020). Addictive Behavior Change and Mindfulness-Based Interventions: Current Research and Future Directions. *Current Addiction Reports*, *7*(2), 117–124. DOI: 10.1007/s40429-020-00302-2 PMID: 33585158

Sears, S. M., & Hewett, S. J. (2021). Influence of glutamate and GABA transport on brain excitatory/inhibitory balance. *Experimental Biology and Medicine*, *246*(9), 1069–1083. DOI: 10.1177/1535370221989263 PMID: 33554649

Setyawati, R., Hartini, N., & Suryanto, S. (2020). The psychological impacts of internet pornography addiction on adolescents. *Humaniora*, *11*(3), 235–244. DOI: 10.21512/humaniora.v11i3.6682

Sharif, S. P., & Yeoh, K. K. (2018). Excessive Social Networking Sites Use and Online Compulsive Buying in Young Adults: The Mediating Role of Money Attitude. *Young Consumers*, *19*(3), 310–327. DOI: 10.1108/YC-10-2017-00743

Sharma, M. K., Bhargav, H., Kumar, A., Digambhar, V., & Mani, T. A. (2021). Mindfulness-based interventions: Potentials for management of internet gaming disorder. *International Journal of Yoga*, *14*(3), 244–247. DOI: 10.4103/ijoy.ijoy_46_21 PMID: 35017867

Sharma, M. K., & Palanichamy, T. S. (2018). Psychosocial interventions for technological addictions. *Indian Journal of Psychiatry*, *60*(8), 541. DOI: 10.4103/psychiatry.IndianJPsychiatry_40_18 PMID: 29540928

Shaw, P., Eckstrand, K., Sharp, W., Blumenthal, J., Lerch, J. P., Greenstein, D. E. E. A., Clasen, L., Evans, A., Giedd, J., & Rapoport, J. L. (2007). Attention-deficit/hyperactivity disorder is characterized by a delay in cortical maturation. *Proceedings of the National Academy of Sciences of the United States of America*, *104*(49), 19649–19654. DOI: 10.1073/pnas.0707741104 PMID: 18024590

Shaw, P., Malek, M., Watson, B., Sharp, W., Evans, A., & Greenstein, D. (2012). Development of cortical surface area and gyrification in attention-deficit/hyperactivity disorder. *Biological Psychiatry*, *72*(3), 191–197. DOI: 10.1016/j.biopsych.2012.01.031 PMID: 22418014

Shehzadi, K., Ahmad-ur-Rehman, M., Cheema, A. M., & Ahkam, A. (2016). Impact of personality traits on compulsive buying behavior: Mediating role of impulsive buying. *Journal of Service Science and Management*, *9*(5), 416–432. DOI: 10.4236/jssm.2016.95046

Shin, S. M., Ryu, S. J., Kim, B. J., Lee, D., & Chung, Y. (2015). The development and effectiveness of MI group counseling program for adolescents internet-addiction. *Sangdamhag Yeon'gu*, *16*(4), 89–109. DOI: 10.15703/kjc.16.4.201508.89

Sicilia, Á., Paterna, A., Alcaraz-Ibáñez, M., & Griffiths, M. D. (2021). Theoretical conceptualisations of problematic exercise in Psychometric Assessment Instruments: A systematic review. *Journal of Behavioral Addictions*, *10*(1), 4–20. DOI: 10.1556/2006.2021.00019 PMID: 33822749

Šimić, G., Tkalčić, M., Vukić, V., Mulc, D., Španić, E., & Šagud, M. & R. Hof, P. (. (2021). Understanding emotions: Origins and roles of the amygdala. *Biomolecules*, *11*(6), 823. DOI: 10.3390/biom11060823 PMID: 34072960

Singha, R. (2025). Neuroeconomic Insights on Addiction: Integrating the Multidimensional Addiction Behaviour Scale for Treatment, Prevention, and Holistic Well-Being. In Behavioral Economics and Neuroeconomics of Health and Healthcare (p. 181-212). IGI Global. https://www.igi-global.com/chapter/neuroeconomic-insights-on-addiction/356626

Singh, R., & Nayak, J. K. (2016). Effect of family environment on adolescent compulsive buying: Mediating role of self-esteem. *Asia Pacific Journal of Marketing and Logistics*, *28*(3), 396–419. DOI: 10.1108/APJML-05-2015-0082

Singh, S., Khanna, D., & Kalra, S. (2020). Role of neurochemicals in schizophrenia. *Current Psychopharmacology*, *9*(2), 144–161. DOI: 10.2174/2211556009666200401150756

Sinha, R. (2024). Stress and substance use disorders: Risk, relapse, and treatment outcomes. *The Journal of Clinical Investigation*, *134*(16), e172883. DOI: 10.1172/JCI172883 PMID: 39145454

Soriano-Molina, E., Limiñana-Gras, R. M., Patró-Hernández, R. M., & Rubio-Aparicio, M. (2024). The Impact of Internet Addiction on Adolescents Mental Health: A Meta-analytic Review.

Spicer, S. G., Nicklin, L. L., Uther, M., Lloyd, J., Lloyd, H., & Close, J. (2022). Loot boxes, problem gambling and problem video gaming: A systematic review and meta-synthesis. *New Media & Society*, *24*(4), 1001–1022. DOI: 10.1177/1461444821102717 5

Staff, N. A. (2024, June 19). Teens & Video Games: New Research on Teenage Video Game Addiction. https://www.newportacademy.com/resources/treatment/teenage-video-game- addiction/

Stein, D. J., Szatmari, P., Gaebel, W., Berk, M., Vieta, E., Maj, M., de Vries, Y. A., Roest, A. M., de Jonge, P., Maercker, A., Brewin, C. R., Pike, K. M., Grilo, C. M., Fineberg, N. A., Briken, P., Cohen-Kettenis, P. T., & Reed, G. M. (2020). Mental, behavioral and neurodevelopmental disorders in the ICD-11: An international perspective on key changes and controversies. *BMC Medicine*, *18*(1), 1–24. DOI: 10.1186/s12916-020-1495-2 PMID: 31983345

Stevens, M. W. R., King, D. L., Dorstyn, D., & Delfabbro, P. H. (2019). Cognitive–behavioral therapy for Internet gaming disorder: A systematic review and meta-analysis. *Clinical Psychology & Psychotherapy*, *26*(2), 191–203. DOI: 10.1002/cpp.2341 PMID: 30341981

Stevens, M. W., Dorstyn, D., Delfabbro, P. H., & King, D. L. (2021). Global prevalence of gaming disorder: A systematic review and meta-analysis. *The Australian and New Zealand Journal of Psychiatry*, *55*(6), 553–568. DOI: 10.1177/0004867420962851 PMID: 33028074

Stoliaroff, S. (2003). Know the signs of unhealthy exercise addiction. *Running Fit News*, *18*(6), 4–5.

Strizhak, A., & Mancheva, I. K. (2022). The impact of sociocultural factors on demonstrative consumption: A theoretical analysis. *Vestnik Tomskogo Gosudarstvennogo Universiteta.Ekonomika (Nis)*, *58*(58), 5–23. DOI: 10.17223/19988648/58/1

Štulhofer, A., Jurin, T., & Briken, P. (2016). Is high sexual desire a facet of male hypersexuality? Results from an online study. *Journal of Sex & Marital Therapy*, *42*(8), 665–680. DOI: 10.1080/0092623X.2015.1113585 PMID: 26569650

Subramanian, A., Chitlangia, S., & Baths, V. (2022). Reinforcement learning and its connections with neuroscience and psychology. *Neural Networks*, *145*, 271–287. DOI: 10.1016/j.neunet.2021.10.003 PMID: 34781215

Su, H., Ye, T., Cao, S., & Hu, C. (2024). Understanding the shift to compulsion in addiction: Insights from personality traits, social factors, and neurobiology. *Frontiers in Psychology*, *15*, 1416222. DOI: 10.3389/fpsyg.2024.1416222 PMID: 39315036

Sujarwoto, S., Saputri, R. A. M., & Yumarni, T. (2023). Social media addiction and mental health among university students during the COVID-19 pandemic in Indonesia. *International Journal of Mental Health and Addiction*, *21*(1), 96–110. DOI: 10.1007/s11469-021-00582-3 PMID: 34230820

Sun, C., Bridges, A., Johnason, J., & Ezzell, M. (2014). Pornography and the male sexual script: An analysis of consumption and sexual relations. *Archives of Sexual Behavior*, *45*(4), 983–994. Doi.org/10.1007/s10508-014-0391-2. DOI: 10.1007/s10508-014-0391-2 PMID: 25466233

Sussman, S., Lisha, N., & Griffiths, M. (2011). Prevalence of the addictions: A problem of the majority or the minority? *Evaluation & the Health Professions*, *34*(1), 3–56. DOI: 10.1177/0163278710380124 PMID: 20876085

Sweet, K. S., LeBlanc, J. K., Stough, L. M., & Sweany, N. W. (2020). Community building and knowledge sharing by individuals with disabilities using social media. *Journal of Computer Assisted Learning*, *36*(1), 1–11. DOI: 10.1111/jcal.12377

Szabo, A., Griffiths, M. D., Aarhus Høglid, R., & Demetrovics, Z. (2018). Drug, nicotine, and alcohol use among exercisers: Does substance addiction co-occur with exercise addiction? *Addictive Behaviors Reports, 7*, 26–31. https://doi.org/.2017.12.001DOI: 10.1016/j.abrep

Szabo, A. (1995). The impact of exercise deprivation on well-being of habitual exercises. *Australian Journal of Science and Medicine in Sport*, *27*, 68–75. PMID: 8599747

Szabo, A. (2010). *Addiction to exercise: A symptom or a disorder?* Nova Science Publishers, Incorporated.

Szabo, A., de la Vega, R., Kovácsik, R., Jiménez Almendros, L., Ruíz-Barquín, R., Demetrovics, Z., Boros, S., & Köteles, F. (2022). Dimensions of passion and their relationship to the risk of exercise addiction: Cultural and gender differences. *Addictive Behaviors Reports*, *16*, 100451–100451. DOI: 10.1016/j.abrep.2022.100451 PMID: 36092546

Szabo, A., & Demetrovics, Z. (2022). *Passion and addiction in sports and exercise*. Routledge. DOI: 10.4324/9781003173595

Szabo, A., & Kovacsik, R. (2019). When passion appears, exercise addiction disappears. *Swiss Journal of Psychology*, *78*(3–4), 137–142. DOI: 10.1024/1421-0185/a000228

Szabo, A., & Rendi, M. (2008). Exercise addiction. In Lane, A. (Ed.), *Sport and exercise psychology: Topics in applied psychology* (pp. 186–203). Hodder Education., https://perpus.univpancasila.ac.id/repository/EBUPT180160.pdf#page=186

Tadpatrikar, A., Sharma, S., Sharma, M. K., Bhargav, H., Anand, N., & Mishra, P. (2023). An integrated yoga and cognitive behavioral therapy intervention for managing excessive use of internet among the youth: A case series. *International Journal of Yoga*, *16*(1), 56–60. DOI: 10.4103/ijoy.ijoy_47_23 PMID: 37583538

Tambunan, H. R., Kumboyono, K., & Lestari, R. (2023). Cognitive Behaviour Therapy (CBT) lowers online game addiction rates in adolescents. *Jurnal Aisyah: Jurnal Ilmu Kesehatan*, *8*(S1), 361–368. DOI: 10.30604/jika.v8iS1.1665

Tamir, D. I., & Mitchell, J. P. (2012). Disclosing information about the self is intrinsically rewarding. *Proceedings of the National Academy of Sciences of the United States of America*, *109*(21), 8038–8043. DOI: 10.1073/pnas.1202129109 PMID: 22566617

Tandoc, E. C.Jr. (2020). Tools of disinformation: How fake news gets to deceive. In *Disinformation and fake news* (pp. 35–46). Springer Singapore.

Tang, C. S. K., & Koh, Y. Y. W. (2017). Online social networking addiction among college students in Singapore: Comorbidity with behavioral addiction and affective disorder. *Asian Journal of Psychiatry*, *25*, 175–178. DOI: 10.1016/j.ajp.2016.10.027 PMID: 28262144

Tang, C. S.-K., Koh, Y. W., & Gan, Y. (2017). Addiction to Internet Use, Online Gaming, and Online Social Networking Among Young Adults in China, Singapore, and the United States. *Asia-Pacific Journal of Public Health*, *29*(8), 673–682. DOI: 10.1177/1010539517739558 PMID: 29191049

Tang, H., Li, Y., Dong, W., Guo, X., Wu, S., Chen, C., & Lu, G. (2024). The relationship between childhood trauma and internet addiction in adolescents: A meta-analysis. *Journal of Behavioral Addictions*, *13*(1), 36–50. DOI: 10.1556/2006.2024.00001 PMID: 38340148

Tarka, P., & Harnish, R. J. (2023). Toward better understanding the materialism-hedonism and the Big Five personality-compulsive buying relationships: A new consumer cultural perspective. *Journal of Global Marketing*, *36*(3), 165–192. DOI: 10.1080/08911762.2023.2188509

Tateno, M., Teo, A. R., Ukai, W., Kanazawa, J., Katsuki, R., Kubo, H., & Kato, T. A. (2019). Internet addiction, smartphone addiction, and Hikikomori trait in Japanese young adult: Social isolation and social network. *Frontiers in Psychiatry*, *10*, 455. DOI: 10.3389/fpsyt.2019.00455 PMID: 31354537

Tavares, H., Sabbatini, D., Lobo, S., & Fuentes, D. (2008). Compras compulsivas: uma revisão e um relato de caso Compulsive buying disorder: a review and a Case Vignette. *Revista Brasileira de Psiquiatria : Orgão Oficial da Associação Brasileira de Psiquiatria, Asociación Psiqui´trica de la América Latina*, •••, 30.

Teicher, M. H., Samson, J. A., Anderson, C. M., & Ohashi, K. (2016). The effects of childhood maltreatment on brain structure, function and connectivity. *Nature Reviews. Neuroscience*, *17*(10), 652–666. DOI: 10.1038/nrn.2016.111 PMID: 27640984

Teng, Z., Pontes, H. M., Nie, Q., Griffiths, M. D., & Guo, C. (2021). Depression and anxiety symptoms associated with internet gaming disorder before and during the COVID-19 pandemic: A longitudinal study. *Journal of Behavioral Addictions*, *10*(1), 169–180. DOI: 10.1556/2006.2021.00016 PMID: 33704085

Throuvala, M. A., Griffiths, M. D., Rennoldson, M., & Kuss, D. J. (2019). School-based prevention for adolescent internet addiction: Prevention is the key. A systematic literature review. *Current Neuropharmacology*, *17*(6), 507–525. DOI: 10.2174/1570159X16666180813153806 PMID: 30101714

Tiggemann, M., & Zaccardo, M. (2015). "Exercise to be fit, not skinny": The effect of fitspiration imagery on women's body image. *Body Image*, *15*, 61–67. DOI: 10.1016/j.bodyim.2015.06.003 PMID: 26176993

Torres-Rodríguez, A., Griffiths, M. D., Carbonell, X., & Oberst, U. (2018). Internet gaming disorder in adolescence: Psychological characteristics of a clinical sample. *Journal of Behavioral Addictions*, *7*(3), 707–718. DOI: 10.1556/2006.7.2018.75 PMID: 30264606

Tracy, K., & Wallace, S. P. (2016). Benefits of peer support groups in the treatment of addiction. *Substance Abuse and Rehabilitation*, *7*, 143–154. DOI: 10.2147/SAR.S81535 PMID: 27729825

Tran, L. T., Wardle, H., Colledge-Frisby, S., Taylor, S., Lynch, M., Rehm, J., Volberg, R., Marionneau, V., Saxena, S., Bunn, C., Farrell, M., & Degenhardt, L. (2024). The prevalence of gambling and problematic gambling: A systematic review and meta-analysis. *The Lancet. Public Health*, *9*(8), e594–e613. DOI: 10.1016/S2468-2667(24)00126-9 PMID: 39025095

Trivedi, R. H., & Teichert, T. (2018). Attitudes, beliefs and impulsivity in online gambling addiction. *International Gambling Studies*, *18*(2), 327–342. DOI: 10.1080/14459795.2018.1466188

Trott, M., Jackson, S. E., Firth, J., Jacob, L., Grabovac, I., Mistry, A., Stubbs, B., & Smith, L. (2020). A comparative meta-analysis of the prevalence of exercise addiction in adults with and without indicated eating disorders. *Eating and Weight Disorders, 26*(1), 37–46. DOI: 10.1007/s40519-019-00842-1 PMID: 31894540

Trott, M., Johnstone, J., Pardhan, S., Barnett, Y., & Smith, L. (2021). Changes in body dysmorphic disorder, eating disorder, and exercise addiction symptomology during the COVID-19 pandemic: A longitudinal study of 319 health club users. *Psychiatry Research, 298*, 113831–113831. DOI: 10.1016/j.psychres.2021.113831 PMID: 33652248

Trotzke, P., Starcke, K., Pedersen, A., & Brand, M. (2021). Dorsal and ventral striatum activity in individuals with buying-shopping disorder during cue-exposure: A functional magnetic resonance imaging study. *Addiction Biology, 26*(6), e13073. DOI: 10.1111/adb.13073 PMID: 34156751

Turel, O., & Bechara, A. (2019). Little video-gaming in adolescents can be protective, but too much is associated with increased substance use. *Substance Use & Misuse, 54*(3), 384–395. DOI: 10.1080/10826084.2018.1496455 PMID: 30654698

Turner, M. J., Carrington, S., & Miller, A. (2019). Psychological distress across sport participation groups: The mediating effects of secondary irrational beliefs on the relationship between primary irrational beliefs and symptoms of anxiety, anger, and depression. *Journal of Clinical Sport Psychology, 13*(1), 17–40. DOI: 10.1123/jcsp.2017-0014

Twenge, J. M., Joiner, T. E., Rogers, M. L., & Martin, G. N. (2018). Increases in depressive symptoms, suicide-related outcomes, and suicide rates among US adolescents after 2010 and links to increased new media screen time. *Clinical Psychological Science, 6*(1), 3–17. DOI: 10.1177/2167702617723376

Twenge, J. M., Martin, G. N., & Spitzberg, B. H. (2019). Trends in US Adolescents' media use, 1976–2016: The rise of digital media, the decline of TV, and the (near) demise of print. *Psychology of Popular Media Culture, 8*(4), 329–345. DOI: 10.1037/ppm0000203

Uhl, G. R., Koob, G. F., & Cable, J. (2019). The neurobiology of addiction. *Annals of the New York Academy of Sciences, 1451*(1), 5–28. DOI: 10.1111/nyas.13989 PMID: 30644552

Ulfatari, N., Wibowo, M. E., & Japar, M. (2022). The effectiveness of reality group counseling with confrontation techniques to reduce smartphone addiction symptoms in college students. *Jurnal Bimbingan Konseling, 11*(1), 53–59.

Ünübol, B., Ünsalver, B. Ö., Ünübol, H., & Sayar, G. H. (2022, January 3). The prevalence and psychological relation of problem shopping: Data from a large-scale sample from Turkey. *BMC Psychology*, *10*(1), 1. DOI: 10.1186/s40359-021-00711-6 PMID: 34980253

Vadlin, S., Åslund, C., Hellström, C., & Nilsson, K. W. (2016). Associations between problematic gaming and psychiatric symptoms among adolescents in two samples. *Addictive Behaviors*, *61*, 8–15. DOI: 10.1016/j.addbeh.2016.05.001 PMID: 27203825

Valence, G., d'Astous, A., & Fortier, L. (1988). Compulsive buying: Concept and measurement. *Journal of Consumer Policy*, *11*(4), 419–433. DOI: 10.1007/BF00411854

Van Brunt, B. (2014). *Treating video game addiction: Three brief sessions*. American Counseling Association.

van der Schyff, E. L., Forsyth, R., Amon, K. L., Ridout, B., & Campbell, A. J. (2023). Increasing access to mental health services: Videogame players' perspectives. *International Journal of Environmental Research and Public Health*, *20*(6), 4772. DOI: 10.3390/ijerph20064772 PMID: 36981681

van Namen, D. M., Hilberink, S. R., de Vries, H., Nagelhout, G. E., & van Staa, A. (2024). "Please, see me"; Informal and professional support of students with relatives with addiction problems: A three-year longitudinal qualitative study. *BMC Public Health*, *24*(1), 3092. Advance online publication. DOI: 10.1186/s12889-024-20531-8 PMID: 39516781

Van Rooij, A. J., Ferguson, C. J., Colder Carras, M., Kardefelt-Winther, D., Shi, J., Aarseth, E., Bean, A. M., Bergmark, K. H., Brus, A., Coulson, M., Deleuze, J., Dullur, P., Dunkels, E., Edman, J., Elson, M., Etchells, P. J., Fiskaali, A., Granic, I., Jansz, J., & Przybylski, A. K. (2018). A weak scientific basis for gaming disorder: Let us err on the side of caution. *Journal of Behavioral Addictions*, *7*(1), 1–9. DOI: 10.1556/2006.7.2018.19 PMID: 29529886

van Timmeren, T., Jansen, J. M., Caan, M. W., Goudriaan, A. E., & van Holst, R. J. (2017). White matter integrity between left basal ganglia and left prefrontal cortex is compromised in gambling disorder. *Addiction Biology*, *22*(6), 1590–1600. DOI: 10.1111/adb.12447 PMID: 27612435

Vasile, D., & Vasiliu, O. (2021). Evidence-based pharmacological strategies for gambling disorder. Psihiatru. ro, 66(3).

Vasiliu, O., & Vasile, D. (2017). Compulsive buying disorder: A review of current data. *02*.https://www.iaras.org/iaras/home/caijems/compulsive-buying-disorder-a-review-of-current-data

Vasiliu, O. (2022). Therapeutic management of buying/shopping disorder: A systematic literature review and evidence-based recommendations. *Frontiers in Psychiatry*, *13*, 1047280. DOI: 10.3389/fpsyt.2022.1047280 PMID: 36405896

Veale, D. M. (1987). Exercise dependence. *British Journal of Addiction*, *82*(7), 735–740. DOI: 10.1111/j.1360-0443.1987.tb01539.x PMID: 3311101

Veale, D. M. (1995). Does primary exercise dependence really exist? In Annett, J., Cripps, B., & Steinberg, H. (Eds.), *Exercise addiction: Motivation for participation in sport and exercise: Proceedings of British Psychology, Sport and Exercise Psychology Section* (pp. 71–75). British Psychological Society.

Vecchio, L. M. (2016). *Investigating Monoamine Regulation: The Transport Of The Dopamine Transporter To Striatal Terminals And The Effects Of Tyrosine Hydroxylase Overexpression On Dopaminergic and Noradrenergic-Related Phenotypes*. University of Toronto.

Veit, R., Schag, K., Schopf, E., Borutta, M., Kreutzer, J., Ehlis, A. C., Zipfel, S., Giel, K. E., Preissl, H., & Kullmann, S. (2021). Diminished prefrontal cortex activation in patients with binge eating disorder associates with trait impulsivity and improves after impulsivity-focused treatment based on a randomized controlled IMPULS trial. *NeuroImage. Clinical*, *30*, 102679. DOI: 10.1016/j.nicl.2021.102679 PMID: 34215149

Verma, T.el. (2019). Managing online video gaming-related addictive behaviors through motivational interviewing. *Indian Journal of Social Psychiatry*, *35*(3), 217–219. DOI: 10.4103/ijsp.ijsp_113_18

Villella, C., Martinotti, G., Di Nicola, M., Cassano, M., La Torre, G., Gliubizzi, M. D., Messeri, I., Petruccelli, F., Bria, P., Janiri, L., & Conte, G. (2011). Behavioural addictions in adolescents and young adults: Results from a prevalence study. *Journal of Gambling Studies*, *27*(2), 203–214. DOI: 10.1007/s10899-010-9206-0 PMID: 20559694

Vinberg, M., Wetterborg, D., & Enebrink, P. (2021). Gambling at work: A qualitative study of Swedish elite athletes, coaches, and managers. *Journal of Gambling Studies*, *37*(4), 1197–1217. DOI: 10.1007/s10899-021-10007-4 PMID: 33527302

Volkow, N. D., Michaelides, M., & Baler, R. (2019). The neuroscience of drug reward and addiction. *Physiological Reviews*, *99*(4), 2115–2140. DOI: 10.1152/physrev.00014.2018 PMID: 31507244

Volkow, N. D., Wang, G. J., Fowler, J. S., Tomasi, D., Telang, F., & Baler, R. (2010, September). Addiction: Decreased reward sensitivity and increased expectation sensitivity conspire to overwhelm the brain's control circuit. *BioEssays*, *32*(9), 748–755. DOI: 10.1002/bies.201000042 PMID: 20730946

Volkow, N. D., Wise, R. A., & Baler, R. (2017). The dopamine motive system: Implications for drug and food addiction. *Nature Reviews. Neuroscience*, *18*(12), 741–752. DOI: 10.1038/nrn.2017.130 PMID: 29142296

Von Deneen, K. M., Hussain, H., Waheed, J., Xinwen, W., Yu, D., & Yuan, K. (2022). Comparison of frontostriatal circuits in adolescent nicotine addiction and internet gaming disorder. *Journal of Behavioral Addictions*, *11*(1), 26–39. DOI: 10.1556/2006.2021.00086 PMID: 35049521

Von der Heiden, J. M., Braun, B., Müller, K. W., & Egloff, B. (2019). The association between video gaming and psychological functioning. *Frontiers in Psychology*, *10*, 1731. DOI: 10.3389/fpsyg.2019.01731 PMID: 31402891

Vosoughi, S., Roy, D., & Aral, S. (2018). The spread of true and false news online. *science*, 359(6380), 1146-1151.

Wacks, Y., & Weinstein, A. M. (2021). Excessive smartphone use is associated with health problems in adolescents and young adults. *Frontiers in Psychiatry*, *12*, 669042. DOI: 10.3389/fpsyt.2021.669042 PMID: 34140904

Wakefield, J. C. (2013). DSM-5: An overview of changes and controversies. *Clinical Social Work Journal*, *41*(2), 139–154. DOI: 10.1007/s10615-013-0445-2

Wang, H., La Russa, M., & Qi, L. S. (2016). CRISPR/Cas9 in genome editing and beyond. *Annual Review of Biochemistry*, *85*(1), 227–264. DOI: 10.1146/annurev-biochem-060815-014607 PMID: 27145843

Wang, H., Li, X., Lok, G. K. I., Meng, C., Tan, Y., Lee, U. M., & Chan, N. (2024). Family-based therapy for internet addiction among adolescents and young adults: A meta-analysis. *Journal of Behavioral Addictions*, *13*(2), 295–312.

Wang, Y., Qin, Y., Li, H., Yao, D., Sun, B., Gong, J., Dai, Y., Wen, C., Zhang, L., Zhang, C., Luo, C., & Zhu, T. (2023). Acupuncture modulates the functional connectivity among the subcortical nucleus and fronto-parietal network in adolescents with internet addiction. *Brain and Behavior*, *13*(11), e3241. Advance online publication. DOI: 10.1002/brb3.3241 PMID: 37721727

Wang, Z., Potenza, M. N., Song, K., Dong, G., Fang, X., & Zhang, J. (2022). Subgroups of internet gaming disorder based on addiction-related resting-state functional connectivity. *Addiction (Abingdon, England), 118*(2), 327–339. DOI: 10.1111/add.16047 PMID: 36089824

Watkins, M. (Ed.). (2024, November 29). Video game addiction symptoms and treatment. American Addiction Centers. https://americanaddictioncenters.org/behavioral-addictions/video-gaming-addiction

Weinstein, A. & Szabo, A. (2023). Exercise addiction: A narrative overview of research issues. *Dialogues in Clinical Neuroscience, 25*(1), 1–13. https://doi.org/.2023.2164841DOI: 10.1080/19585969

Weinstein, A., & Lejoyeux, M. (2020). Neurobiological mechanisms underlying internet gaming disorder. *Dialogues in Clinical Neuroscience, 22*(2), 113–126. DOI: 10.31887/DCNS.2020.22.2/aweinstein PMID: 32699511

Weinstein, A., Maraz, A., Griffiths, M. D., Lejoyeux, M., & Demetrovics, Z. (2016). Compulsive buying—features and characteristics of addiction. In *Neuropathology of drug addictions and substance misuse* (pp. 993–1007). Academic Press. DOI: 10.1016/B978-0-12-800634-4.00098-6

Weinstein, A., & Weinstein, Y. (2013). Exercise addiction- diagnosis, bio-psychological mechanisms and treatment issues. *Current Pharmaceutical Design, 20*(25), 4062–4069. DOI: 10.2174/13816128113199990614 PMID: 24001300

Weinstein, A., Weinstein, Y., & Maayan, G. (2015). A study on the relationship between compulsive exercise, depression and anxiety. *Journal of Behavioral Addictions, 4*(4), 315–318. DOI: 10.1556/2006.4.2015.034 PMID: 26690627

Wei, Z., Hassan, N. C., Hassan, S. A., Ismail, N., Gu, X., & Dong, J. (2025). Psychometric validation of Young's Internet Addiction Test among Chinese undergraduate students. *PLoS One, 20*(4), e0320641. Advance online publication. DOI: 10.1371/journal.pone.0320641 PMID: 40273278

Wendt, L. M., Austermann, M. I., Rumpf, H. J., Thomasius, R., & Paschke, K. (2021). Requirements of a group intervention for adolescents with internet gaming disorder in a clinical setting: A qualitative interview study. *International Journal of Environmental Research and Public Health, 18*(15), 7813. DOI: 10.3390/ijerph18157813 PMID: 34360106

Wijman, T. (2021, December 22). *The games market and beyond in 2021: The Year in numbers | newzoo*. The Games Market and Beyond in 2021: The Year in Numbers. https://newzoo.com/resources/blog/the-games-market-in-2021-the-year -in-numbers- esports-cloud-gaming

Williams, W. A., Grant, J. E., Winstanley, C. A., & Potenza, M. N. (2008). Current concepts in the classification, treatment, and modeling of pathological gambling and other impulse control disorders. Animal and translational models for CNS drug discovery, 317-357.

Workman, L., & Paper, D. (2010). Compulsive Buying: A Theoretical Framework. *Journal of Business Inquiry*, •••, 9.

World Health Organization. (2020, October 22). Addictive behaviours: Gaming disorder. https://www.who.int/news-room/questions-and-answers/item/addictive -behaviours-gaming-disorder

World Health Organization. (2024). *Clinical descriptions and diagnostic requirements for ICD-11 mental, behavioural and neurodevelopmental disorders*. World Health Organization.

Xiao, L. Y. (2021). People's Republic of China legal update: The notice on further strictly regulating and effectively preventing online video gaming addiction in minors (published August 30, 2021, effective september 1, 2021). *Gaming Law Review, 25*(9), 379–382. DOI: 10.1089/glr2.2021.0026

Xie, L., Zhao, J., Li, Y., & Bai, J. (2024). PET brain imaging in neurological disorders. *Physics of Life Reviews*. PMID: 38574584

Xin, M., Xing, J., Pengfei, W., Houru, L., Mengcheng, W., & Hong, Z. (2018). Online activities, prevalence of internet addiction and risk factors related to family and school among adolescents in China. *Addictive Behaviors Reports, 7*, 14–18. DOI: 10.1016/j.abrep.2017.10.003 PMID: 29450251

Xu, L., Wu, L., Geng, X., Wang, Z., Guo, X., Song, K., Liu, G., Deng, L., Zhang, J., & Potenza, M. N. (2021). A review of psychological interventions for internet addiction. *Psychiatry Research, 302*, 114016. DOI: 10.1016/j.psychres.2021.114016 PMID: 34087672

Yar, A., Gündoğdu, Ö. Y., Tural, Ü., & Memik, N. Ç. (2019). Prevalance of internet addiction among adolescents with psychiatric disorders. *Archives of Neuropsychiatry*. DOI: 10.29399/npa.23045

Yaunin, Y., Darwin, E., Yanwirasti, Y., Nurdin, A., Yetti, H., & Liza, R. (2019). The difference of dopamine transporter and serotonin transporter level between addicted and non-addicted internet user experiencing stress in senior high school students in Padang, Indonesia. *Proceedings of the Proceedings of the 1st EAI International Conference on Medical and Health Research, ICoMHER November 13-14th.* DOI: 10.4108/eai.13-11-2018.2283690

Yau, Y. H., Crowley, M. J., Mayes, L. C., & Potenza, M. N. (2012). Are Internet use and video- game-playing addictive behaviors? Biological, clinical and public health implications for youths and adults. *Minerva Psichiatrica*, *53*(3), 153. PMID: 24288435

Yen, J. Y., Yeh, Y. C., Wang, P. W., Liu, T. L., Chen, Y. Y., & Ko, C. H. (2018). Emotional regulation in young adults with internet gaming disorder. *International Journal of Environmental Research and Public Health*, *15*(1), 30. DOI: 10.3390/ijerph15010030 PMID: 29295597

Yen, J.-Y., Lin, P.-C., Wu, H.-C., & Ko, C.-H. (2022). The withdrawal-related affective, gaming urge, and anhedonia symptoms of internet gaming disorder during abstinence. *Journal of Behavioral Addictions*. Advance online publication. DOI: 10.1556/2006.2022.00008 PMID: 35338772

Ye, X. L., Zhang, W., & Zhao, F. F. (2023). Depression and internet addiction among adolescents: A meta-analysis. *Psychiatry Research*, *326*, 115311. DOI: 10.1016/j.psychres.2023.115311 PMID: 37348449

Yılmazer, E. (2024). Hormonal Underpinnings of Emotional Regulation: Bridging Endocrinology and Psychology. *The Journal of Neurobehavioral Sciences*, *11*(2), 60–75.

Yip, S. W., Worhunsky, P. D., Xu, J., Morie, K. P., Constable, R. T., Malison, R. T., Carroll, K. M., & Potenza, M. N. (2018). Gray-matter relationships to diagnostic and transdiagnostic features of drug and behavioral addictions. *Addiction Biology*, *23*(1), 394–402. DOI: 10.1111/adb.12492 PMID: 28150390

Young, K. S. (2009). Internet addiction test. Center for on-line addictions.

Young, K. S. (2010). When gaming becomes an obsession: Help for parents and their children to treat online gaming addiction. *Retrieved October, 17*, 2013.

Young, P. A. (2023). *Investigating the Role of the Lateral Nigrostriatal Pathway in Modulating Voluntary Movement* (Doctoral dissertation).

Young, K. (2009). Understanding online gaming addiction and treatment issues for adolescents. *The American Journal of Family Therapy*, *37*(5), 355–372. DOI: 10.1080/01926180902942191

Young, K. S. (2004). Internet addiction: A new clinical phenomenon and its consequences. *The American Behavioral Scientist*, *48*(4), 402–415. DOI: 10.1177/0002764204270278

Young, K. S. (2007). Cognitive behavior therapy with Internet addicts: Treatment outcomes and implications. *Cyberpsychology & Behavior*, *10*(5), 671–679. DOI: 10.1089/cpb.2007.9971 PMID: 17927535

Youngman, J., & Simpson, D. (2014). Risk for exercise addiction: A comparison of triathletes training for sprint-, olympic-, half-ironman-, and ironman-distance triathlons. *Journal of Clinical Sport Psychology*, *8*(1), 19–37. DOI: 10.1123/jcsp.2014-0010

Yue, Y., Jun, Z., Yao, N., Yanwen, F., Yiting, Z., & Yiting, F. (2024). The influence of adolescents' internet adaptation on internet addiction: The mediating role of internet cultural adaptation. *Frontiers in Psychiatry*, *14*, 1338343. Advance online publication. DOI: 10.3389/fpsyt.2023.1338343 PMID: 38260791

Zack, M., George, R. S., & Clark, L. (2020). Dopaminergic signaling of uncertainty and the aetiology of gambling addiction. *Progress in Neuro-Psychopharmacology & Biological Psychiatry*, *99*, 109853. DOI: 10.1016/j.pnpbp.2019.109853 PMID: 31870708

Zeidi, I. M., Divsalar, S., Morshedi, H., & Alizadeh, H. (2020). The effectiveness of group cognitive-behavioral therapy on general self-efficacy, self-control, and internet addiction prevalence among medical university students. *Social Health and Behavior*, *3*(3), 93–102. DOI: 10.4103/SHB.SHB_20_20

Zeng, X., Sun, Y. H., Gao, F., Hua, L., Xu, S., & Yuan, Z. (2024). Concurrent behavioral modeling and multimodal neuroimaging reveals how feedback affects the performance of decision making in internet gaming disorder. *NeuroImage*, *297*, 120726. DOI: 10.1016/j.neuroimage.2024.120726 PMID: 38986794

Zhang, F., Xie, H., Wang, S., Li, F., Gong, Q., & Jia, Z. (2023). The role of the orbitofrontal cortex in exercise addiction and exercise motivation: A brain imaging study based on multimodal magnetic resonance imaging. *Journal of Affective Disorders*, *325*, 240–247. DOI: 10.1016/j.jad.2023.01.030 PMID: 36638963

Zhang, J., Wang, E., Zhang, L., & Chi, X. (2024). Internet addiction and depressive symptoms in adolescents: Joint trajectories and predictors. *Frontiers in Public Health*, *12*, 1374762. DOI: 10.3389/fpubh.2024.1374762 PMID: 38894983

Zhao, S., Grasmuck, S., & Martin, J. (2008). Identity construction on Facebook: Digital empowerment in anchored relationships. *Computers in Human Behavior*, *24*(5), 1816–1836. DOI: 10.1016/j.chb.2008.02.012

Zhou, N., Cao, H., Li, X., Zhang, J., Yao, Y., Geng, X., Lin, X., Hou, S., Liu, F., Chen, X., & Fang, X. (2018). Internet addiction, problematic internet use, nonproblematic internet use among Chinese adolescents: Individual, parental, peer, and sociodemographic correlates. *Psychology of Addictive Behaviors*, *32*(3), 365–372. DOI: 10.1037/adb0000358 PMID: 29771562

Zhou, X., Rau, P. L. P., Yang, C. L., & Zhou, X. (2021). Cognitive behavioral therapy-based short-term abstinence intervention for problematic social media use: Improved well-being and underlying mechanisms. *The Psychiatric Quarterly*, *92*(2), 761–779. DOI: 10.1007/s11126-020-09852-0 PMID: 32989636

Zhu, Y., Chen, H., Li, J., Mei, X., & Wang, W. (2023). Effects of different interventions on internet addiction: A systematic review and network meta-analysis. *BMC Psychiatry*, *23*(1), 921. Advance online publication. DOI: 10.1186/s12888-023-05400-9 PMID: 38066462

About The Contributors

Rommel Johnson, PhD, NCC, LPC, CAADC, CRC, is an Assistant Professor at the University of Texas, Rio Grande Valley, in the School of Rehabilitation Services and Counseling, where he teaches graduate and undergraduate courses on addiction and rehabilitation. He is a dedicated researcher, clinician, and educator with extensive experience in the field of addiction, particularly in the area of behavioral addictions. Dr. Johnson earned his Ph.D. in Counselor Education and Supervision from Western Michigan University and holds a Graduate Certificate in Alcohol and Drug Abuse Counseling. He is also a Board Certified Advanced Alcohol and Drug Addiction Counselor. Dr. Johnson's work emphasizes the psychological, social, and neurobiological factors that contribute to addictive patterns. Dr. Johnson is committed to bridging empirical evidence with practical insights to equip behavioral health professionals with the knowledge and skills to support individuals affected by behavioral addictions. He also maintains a clinical practice, providing counseling and addiction recovery services.

Reuben Mwangi is an Assistant Professor in the Department of Counseling, Educational Leadership & Higher Education at Central Michigan University. He earned his doctorate in Counselor Education and Supervision from Western Michigan University, and his scholarship is backed by extensive experience as a Licensed Professional Counselor. Dr. Mwangi holds certifications as a Certified Advanced Alcohol and Drug Counselor (CAADC) and through the International Certificate & Reciprocity Consortium (IC&RC) via the Michigan Certification Board for Addiction Professionals (MCBAP), demonstrating his commitment to expertise in addiction counseling. Grounded in person-centered and motivational interviewing techniques, Dr. Mwangi's counseling approach is further informed by cognitive behavioral therapy. He is dedicated to establishing a supportive therapeutic environment that empowers clients to confront mental health challenges and enhance their well-being. His dedication to theoretical integration and metatheory ensures that his practice and scholarship are continuously evolving. As an active member of the American Counseling Association (ACA) and other professional organizations, Dr. Mwangi is committed to maintaining the highest ethical and professional standards in counseling. His teaching interests cover a range of core counseling topics, including Professional Orientation and Ethics, Personal and Professional Development Across the Lifespan, Counseling Techniques, and specialized courses such as Introduction to Counseling Addiction and Etiology of Addiction. Dr. Mwangi's research examines help-seeking attitudes, multicultural counseling competencies, immigration and acculturation, substance abuse, and the intersection of mental health and spirituality. He shares his research findings through presentations at regional, national, and international conferences, contributing to the scholarly understanding of human growth and development.

***

Lakshmi Balakrishnan, Enthusiastic and passionate learner with 6+ years of experience providing learning support and instructions to students of all levels. Passionate learner who always listens to the needs of students and provides them with the tools they need to succeed academically, developing a passion for learning and working together as a team. Excellent communication and problem solving skills. Currently working as an Assistant Professor at St Francis de Sales College (Autonomous), Bangalore and serving as the program coordinator of the departmrnt.

Joselyn Barnhart is a student in the Master of Clinical Rehabilitation Counseling program at the University of Texas Rio Grande Valley. She holds a Bachelor's in Psychology with a minor in Addiction Studies. Joselyn is passionate about empowering individuals with disabilities so they may achieve their desired goals both personal and professional. She has a strong interest in mental health awareness, advocating for disability rights, and the impact of substance use disorders on individuals with disabilities. Currently, Joselyn is involved in a graduate research assistantship under the Rehabilitation Services and Counseling Department at the University of Texas Rio Grande Valley. She is also active in community involvement focused on the importance of mental health advocacy and inclusion for all. Upon graduation, Joselyn aims to pursue licensure as a professional counselor. She plans to work in a clinical setting to help support individuals with disabilities and substance use disorders.

Ayush Dwivedi is currently pursuing a Bachelor of Arts in Psychology at Graphic Era (Deemed to be University). As an undergraduate student, he started to do research in pursuit of knowledge and more understanding of the psychological field. he aims that one day he would be able to contribute his perspectives to this field.

Bilal El-Mansoury is a postdoctoral researcher specializing in Neuroscience and Neurology. His previous research focused on the role of glial cell dysfunction in the pathophysiology of hepatic encephalopathy and neurodegenerative disorders, investigating mechanisms such as neuroinflammation, oxidative stress, and neuronal dysfunction. Currently, Dr. El-Mansoury's work is centered on the regulatory roles of microRNAs and their implications in CDKL5 deficiency disorder, aiming to uncover novel therapeutic strategies for this rare neurodevelopmental condition.

Tiffany Lee is a Professor and Director of Western Michigan University's Addiction Studies Program (SPADA). She has experience as a counselor, circuit court advocate, and child protective investigator. Dr. Lee is also a trainer with the American Society of Addiction Medicine (ASAM). Her grant projects and research primarily focus on addiction training for mental health and medical professionals, and she is the author of the book, Embracing Diversity: Treatment and Care in Addiction Counseling (2nd ed.). From 2016 to 2022, Dr. Lee served on the Health Professional Recovery Committee (HPRC) for the Michigan Department of Licensing and Regulatory Affairs (LARA). She was appointed Vice-Chair of the HPRC (2018-2020) and Chair of Clinical and Policy Subcommittee (2017-2022), which worked with the Attorney General's office to update the policy manual during that time.

Lyndsay Nuyen, LMSW, CAADC, CCS IS a part-time instructor for the Addiction Studies program as well as the School of Social Work. She has been teaching at Western Michigan University (WMU) since 2016. She supervises a co-occurring substance use and mental health program at Integrated Services of Kalamazoo. She has worked in the field of addiction for the last 10 years and specializes in providing Integrated Dual Disorder Treatment (IDDT). Within IDDT, she is a practicing Dialectical Behavior Therapy (DBT) therapist and has been part of a comprehensive DBT team since 2014. Lyndsay is currently pursuing a PhD in Interdisciplinary Health Studies at WMU. Lyndsay received her B.A. in English with an Emphasis in Writing and Psychology from Kalamazoo College and her Masters in Social Work from WMU. She enjoys spending time with her family, pets, and playing pickleball.

Cameron Ortega is an Assistant Professor in the School of Rehabilitation Services and Counseling. She holds a Ph.D. in Rehabilitation Counseling (2022) and a Master's in Rehabilitation Counseling (2009) from the University of Texas Rio Grande Valley, as well as a Bachelor's in Fine Arts (2006) from the University of

Texas Pan American. With over 15 years of experience in mental health and substance use treatment, Dr. Ortega has worked with diverse populations in various settings, including inpatient, outpatient, and private practice. She currently serves as Secretary on the Board of Directors for the Texas Rehabilitation Association and is a Board Director for the Palmer Drug Abuse Program in McAllen. Dr. Ortega's research focuses on the intersection of substance use, disability, and psychiatric disorders, with a strong commitment to social justice, particularly within the LGBTQIA+ community. She utilizes a harm reduction framework to explore ways to mitigate risks and improve the quality of life for individuals experiencing substance use disorders. Her work examines the impact of systemic inequities on access to care and advocates for inclusive, person-centered approaches that prioritize safety, dignity, and empowerment. Through her research and advocacy, Dr. Ortega seeks to bridge gaps in service delivery and promote evidence-based strategies that support long-term recovery and well-being.

Leslie Reyes is a student in the Master of Science in Clinical Rehabilitation Counseling program at The University of Texas Rio Grande Valley. She has a strong interest in social justice, mental health accessibility, and supporting individuals with disabilities. Her desire is to understand the systemic inequities that impact marginalized communities. She is particularly passionate about advocating for minority groups, including individuals with disabilities and members of the LGBTQIA+ community, to ensure they receive impartial support and services. Currently, Leslie is involved in research under the mentorship of Dr. Ortega, contributing to projects that examine substance use and the barriers to mental health care for underserved populations. She is also active in community service, leadership roles, and volunteer initiatives, including her previous work at hospitals, schools, and university organizations. Leslie aims to become a licensed professional counselor (LPC) with a focus on rehabilitation counseling. She hopes to work in settings that address the mental health needs of diverse and underserved populations, advocating for systemic change and promoting inclusive, evidence-based interventions.

Papia Saraf, I am an educator and researcher in Psychology with 14 years of academic experience. Additionally, I have held corporate Human Resources roles for 11 years. My passion lies in guiding students through the intricate and fascinating world of Psychology, fostering their understanding and appreciation of the vast potential of the human psyche. As a researcher, I am committed to the systematic exploration of psychological concepts across diverse settings and sample populations, contributing to the advancement of knowledge and a deeper comprehension of the discipline.

Ravindra Singh has completed his Ph.D. from Banaras Hindu University (Institute of Eminence). Currently, he is working as an Assistant Professor of Psychology at Magadh University, Bodh Gaya, Bihar. Earlier he was Indian Youth Ambassador at BRICS. Beijing China 2017 during Indian delegation. Dr. Singh has also worked as a Junior Project Fellow, a funded project, in New Delhi in 2018. He worked as a Former Teaching Assistant at IIT, BHU. Recently he was the Youth Member at G20 Youth for India's G-20 Presidency. He served as an Independent Reviewer in Frontiers in Psychology Journal and a Member of APA, International Affiliate, Washington DC, and a member of the prestigious National Academy of Psychology, (NAOP) India. He has 7 Years of teaching experience and supervising 3 PhD candidates along with many posts' graduate thesis supervision.

Aditya Ratna Tripathi is currently pursuing a Bachelor of Arts in Psychology at Graphic Era (Deemed to be University). As an undergraduate student, Aditya has started to participate in the pursuit of knowledge to understand psychological science in depth. His core research interest belongs to exploring various psychological phenomena and backgrounds of cognition and health.

Blaire Zielke, LMSW, CAADC is the Executive and Clinical Director of Enlightened Recovery in Kalamazoo, Michigan, where she leads the strategic and clinical operations of a substance use disorder treatment facility grounded in a holistic and integrative approach to care. With over a decade of experience in behavioral health, she has worked across inpatient psychiatry, emergency services, and youth-focused programming, bringing a trauma-informed and equity-driven lens to her leadership. Blaire is currently pursuing a PhD in Interdisciplinary Health Sciences at Western Michigan University. Her research focuses on disparities in behavioral health access, system-level outcomes, and evidence-based program development. In addition to her clinical and academic roles, Blaire has served as a consultant in youth professional development and anti-human trafficking initiatives, supporting policy advancement and organizational training. She also teaches social work courses, with a deep commitment to interdisciplinary education and cultivatin

Index

A

B

C

D

E

F

G

I

www.ingramcontent.com/pod-product-compliance
Lightning Source LLC
LaVergne TN
LVHW082051011026
849162LV00019B/465